Case Studies in Thyroid and Parathyroid Tumors

Amit Agarwal • Ranil Fernando •
Rajeev Parameswaran • Anand Mishra •
Roma Pradhan

Case Studies in Thyroid and Parathyroid Tumors

Springer

Amit Agarwal
Department of Endocrine and
Breast Surgery
Medanta Hospital
Lucknow, Uttar Pradesh, India

Rajeev Parameswaran
Department of Surgery
Yong Loo Lin School of Medicine
National University of Singapore
Singapore, Singapore

Roma Pradhan
Department of Endocrine and
Breast Surgery
Medanta Hospital
Lucknow, India

Ranil Fernando
Faculty of Medicine
University of Moratuwa
Moratuwa, Sri Lanka

Anand Mishra
Department of Endocrine Surgery
King George's Medical University
Lucknow, Uttar Pradesh, India

ISBN 978-981-99-0937-7 ISBN 978-981-99-0938-4 (eBook)
https://doi.org/10.1007/978-981-99-0938-4

This Springer imprint is published by the registered company Springer Nature Singapore Pte Ltd.
The registered company address is: 152 Beach Road, #21-01/04 Gateway East, Singapore 189721, Singapore

Acknowledgments

Although our names appear as authors, this book has been a result of the work of a large team who contributed towards making these cases. Their contribution to individual cases ranges from giving ideas and concepts for the cases, preparing the case summaries, citing, and preparing the relevant literature, including the pictures and discussion. We are naming them in alphabetical order along with their affiliation:

1. Ganesh Bhatt, MCh Fellow, Department of Endocrine Surgery, King George's Medical University, Lucknow, India
2. Kulranjan Singh, Mch, Associate Professor, Department of Endocrine Surgery, King George's Medical University, Lucknow, India
3. Mechteld C de Jong, Consultant Surgeon, Department of Endocrine Surgery, St. James's University Hospital, Leeds, United Kingdom
4. Nancy Raja, MCh Fellow, Department of Endocrine Surgery, King George's Medical University, Lucknow, India
5. Pooja Ramakant, Additional Professor, Department of Endocrine Surgery, King George's Medical University, Lucknow, India
6. Sheeja Sainulabdeen, MD, Division of Pathology, Medical College Kottayam, Kerala, India
7. Sushil K Gupta, Professor, Department of Endocrine Surgery, SGPGIMS, Lucknow, India
8. Upander Kumar, MCh Fellow, Department of Endocrine Surgery, King George's Medical University, Lucknow, India

Without them we would not have been able to complete this large book and we are deeply grateful for all the help they have given us.

Amit Agarwal, Rajeev Parmeshwaram, Ranil Fernando, Anand Mishra, Roma Pradhan

Contents

About the Authors

Amit Agarwal is presently Director and Head, Department of Endocrine and Breast Surgery at Medanta Hospital, Lucknow. He was previously Professor and Head, at the Department of Endocrine Surgery, Sanjay Gandhi Postgraduate Institute of Medical Sciences (SGPGIMS), Lucknow, India. He has formally trained more than 55 endocrine surgeons. He has been an immediate past president of the Indian Thyroid Society, past president of the Indian Association of Endocrine Surgeons, past president of the International Society of Oncoplastic Endocrine Surgeons (ISOPES), council coordinator of International Association of Endocrine Surgeons, and council member of Asian Association of Endocrine Surgeons. He is on the editorial advisory board of *Thyroid Research and Practice*. Dr. Agarwal has published more than 200 peer-reviewed articles in national and international journals and has written numerous book chapters. He has authored four books: *Evidence-Based Endocrine Surgery*, *Endocrine Surgery Made Easy*, *IAES Textbook of Endocrine Surgery*, and *Atlas of Thyroid Surgery*. He is the founding Editor-in-Chief of the *World Journal of Endocrine Surgery*, the official journal of the Asian Association of Endocrine Surgeons. His clinical interests include robotic and endoscopic thyroid and parathyroid surgery. His research interests include the study of the molecular biology of thyroid and parathyroid tumors and minimally invasive endocrine surgery. He is an invited faculty to deliver prestigious orations and has given more than 200 lectures, including Harvard University and Mayo Clinic, USA.

Ranil Fernando, MS, FRCS, FCPS, FAIS, PhD is the former senior professor and head, Department of Surgery, Faculty of Medicine, University of Moratuwa, Moratuwa, Sri Lanka. He retired from Kelaniya University on 30th Sept 2022. He is the founder dean of the Faculty of Medicine University of Moratuwa where he is currently working.He has delivered several orations and memorial lectures and invited lectures nationally and internationally. Prof. Fernando has published many articles in national and international journals, books, and book chapters. He is a member of the editorial board of various journals and a recipient of many national and international awards and medals. His main research interests are the diseases of the thyroid and parathyroid.

Rajeev Parameswaran is a senior consultant and head at the general surgery division (thyroid and endocrine surgery) at the National University Hospital, Singapore, specializing in thyroid and endocrine surgical disorders. He also serves at Alexandra Hospital, National Cancer Institute of Singapore, and is a faculty at the Yong Loo Lin School of Medicine, Singapore. Dr. Rajeev completed his specialist endocrine surgical training and fellowship in endocrine surgery from Oxford. He was later employed as a consultant in endocrine and general surgery in the UK. Dr. Rajeev was awarded an M Phil from Oxford for his research on aberrant glycoproteins in thyroid tumors. Dr. Rajeev has a particular interest in managing endocrine cancers (cancers of the thyroid, parathyroid, and adrenal glands), minimally invasive surgery of the adrenal and parathyroid glands, and re-operative endocrine surgery. His main research area is the aberrant expression of glycoproteins in endocrine cancers. He has published many peer-reviewed articles and textbook chapters.

Anand Mishra is professor and head, Department of Endocrine Surgery at King George's Medical University, Lucknow, India. He completed MCh from Sanjay Gandhi Postgraduate Institute of Medical Sciences, Lucknow, and is the first MCh in this specialty in the country. Dr. Mishra established the Department of Endocrine Surgery at King George's Medical University. He is the governing council member of Uttar Pradesh Association of Surgeons of India, vice president of Indian Association of Surgeons of India, member and adviser to Asian Association of Endocrine Surgeons, and director of education, north zone, Association of Breast Surgeons of India. He has received International guest scholarship 2015 by American College of Surgeons, ICMR travel grant for St Gallen Breast cancer conference, Vienna, Austria 2015, developing nations fellowship for ninth European Breast Cancer conference Glasgow, Scotland, March 2014, IDEA (International Development and Education Award) from American Society of Clinical Oncology 2011, Young Surgeon Travel grant by Japan Surgical Society, Japan, in 2009, 2008, 2005, 2003, 1999, Betadine young surgeon award 2005 by Association of Surgeons of India in 2005, Dr. Ramesh Nigam Memorial oration 2013 by Association of Surgeons of India 2013, and many invited lectures at various national conferences in India. Dr. Mishra has edited books, published book chapters, and indexed publications.

Roma Pradhan, MS, MCh Endocrine surgery is a dedicated endocrine and breast surgeon and has established the Department of Endocrine and Breast Surgery, Medanta Hospital, Lucknow, India and currently heading it. She is the council member of the Indian Association of Endocrine Surgeons. She has published many peer-reviewed articles in national and international journals and has written numerous book chapters. She is on the editorial board of the *World Journal of Endocrine Surgery*, the official journal of the Asian Association of Endocrine Surgeons. Dr. Pradhan was the first to use continuous neuromonitoring in entire north India in thyroid surgery. Her clinical interests include thyroid, minimally invasive parathyroid surgery, and oncoplastic breast surgery. She is an invited faculty to deliver lectures in many national and international meetings.

Part I

Primary Hyperparathyroidism (PHPT): Unusual Clinical Presentation

PHPT Presenting as Osteitis Fibrosa Cystica

Case

A 15-year-old girl presented to the dental OPD with maxillary swelling (Fig. 1). A biopsy was done from the maxillary swelling was suggestive of brown tumor. Hence the patient was referred to the Endocrine surgery department. Biochemical evaluation showed raised serum calcium, low phosphorus, and high intact parathyroid hormone. A review of plain radiographs revealed multiple fractures with diffuse osteopenia. Brown tumors were also observed at multiple sites (shaft of the left femur, and the shaft of the left tibia). These findings were consistent with osteitis fibrosa cystica. Localizing investigation pointed to right superior enlarged

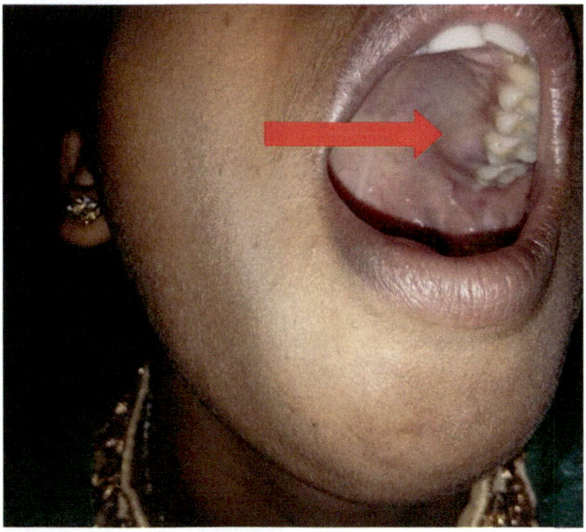

Fig. 1 Red arrow pointing to maxillary swelling

Roma Pradhan is the lead author of this chapter.

A. Agarwal et al., *Case Studies in Thyroid and Parathyroid Tumors*,
https://doi.org/10.1007/978-981-99-0938-4_1

parathyroid gland. Focused parathyroidectomy was done with 50% drop in iPTH level at 10 min (Miami's criteria). Postoperatively patient was started on prophylactic calcium infusion and was continued for 5 days along with oral calcium and active vitamin D (Figs. 2 and 3).

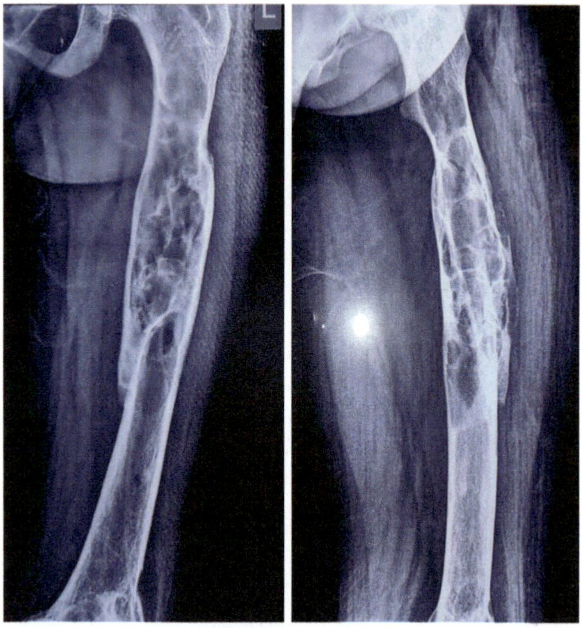

Fig. 2 Brown tumor in femur

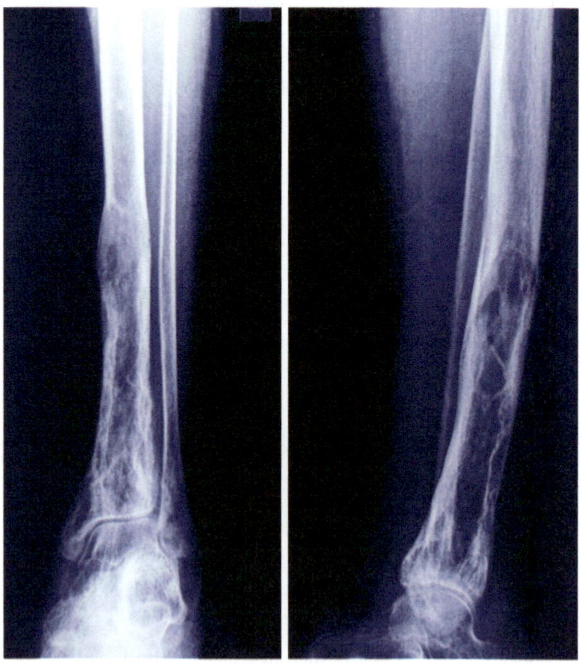

Fig. 3 Brown tumors at lower end of tibia

Discussion

Bone disease in severe primary hyperparathyroidism is described classically as osteitis fibrosa cystica or Von Recklinghausen's bone disease and is a classical manifestation of this disease. OFC happens due to prolonged exposure of bone to high PTH levels. This manifestation is not seen in the western world because of early detection of PHPT. However in this part of the world, it's still quite commonly seen in patients of PHPT. Osteitis fibrosa cystica is characterized clinically by presence of bone pain and radiologically by pathological fractures of the long bones [1], a demineralized skeleton, a salt-and-pepper appearance of the skull, subperiosteal resorption of the phalanges, multi-lobular bone cysts, and brown tumors. A collage of osteitis fibrosa cystica from different patients showing various X-ray findings is shown in Figs. 4a–f and 5. Brown tumors are non-neoplastic lesions. Their histopathology is characterized by multinucleated giant cells (osteoclasts), repetitive granulation tissue, vascular and proliferating fibrous tissue, and a brown hemosiderin deposition that imparts the brown color after which the lesions are named as brown tumors [2]. There are some features to differentiate brown tumors from other conditions which may mimic them. The intensity of the bone pain arising from a brown tumor is milder than that from malignant bone lesions. Although symptoms of benign bone lesions (e.g., an aneurysmal bone cyst, simple bone cyst, or fibrous dysplasia) can mimic those of brown tumors, certain signs are only found with brown tumors, specifically, subperiosteal bone resorption on the skull, or a salt-and-pepper appearance and osteosclerosis of the upper and lower end plates of vertebrae (the rugger-jersey spine) [3]. If treated properly, PHPT is reversible. Remineralization

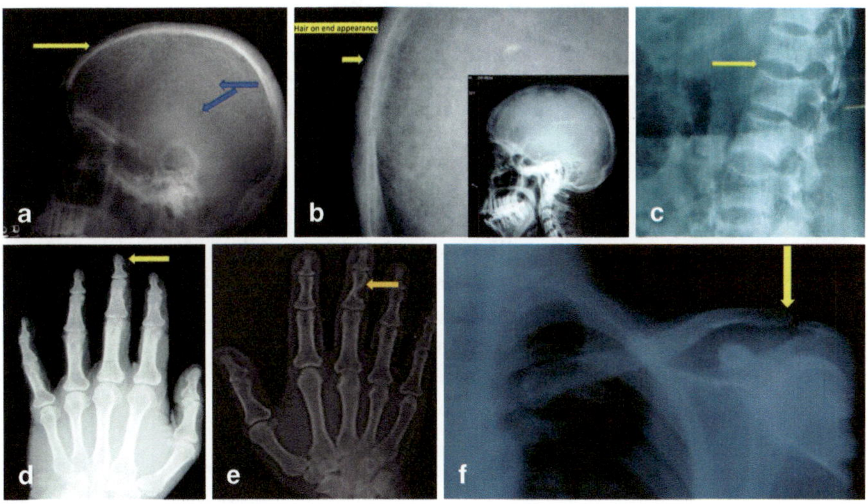

Fig. 4 (**a**) Yellow arrow: loss of outer table, blue arrow: spotty loss of bone density of skull vault, (**b**) hair on end appearance, (**c**) fish mouth appearance of lumbar vertebra, (**d**) resorption of tip of distal phalanx, (**e**) gross subperiosteal bone resorption, (**f**) erosion of outer end of clavicle

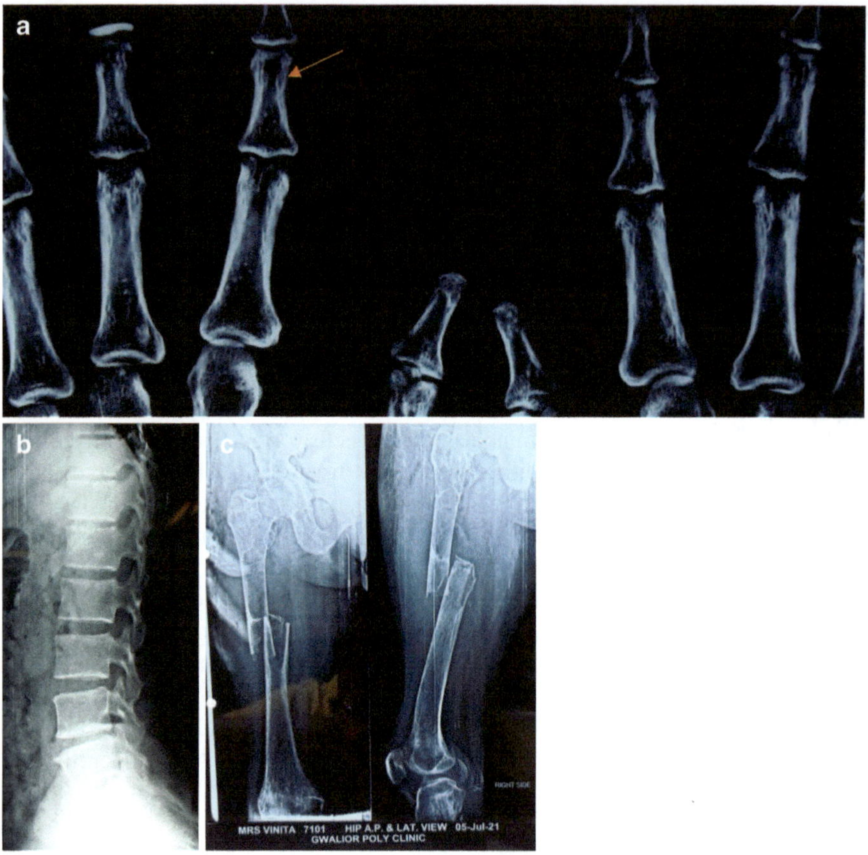

Fig. 5 (**a**) Lucent striations within the cortex of the long axis of the phalanges (also known as cortical tunneling). (**b**) A plain radiograph of the spine showing prominent density of the subchondral endplate at multiple lumbar spines. Rugger-jersey appearance. (**c**) Pathological fracture through the brown tumor in femur

starts as early as 1 week after the procedures. In the case of the pelvis and spine, an improvement in osteopenia is usually observed within 3 weeks to 3 months, whereas recovery of the subperiosteal and cortical resorption of the skull and hands takes 6–9 months. Although this condition has evolved to an asymptomatic disease for the majority of patients, its classic skeletal involvement should not be overlooked, particularly in young patients who present with multiple pathological fractures.

References

1. Panagopoulos A, Tatani I, Kourea HP, Kokkalis ZT, Panagopoulos K, Megas P. Osteolytic lesions (brown tumors) of primary hyperparathyroidism misdiagnosed as multifocal giant cell tumor of the distal ulna and radius: a case report. J Med Case Rep. 2018;12(1):176.
2. Rodríguez-Gutiérrez R, Hinojosa-Amaya JM. Brown tumors: severe osteitis fibrosa cystica. Mayo Clin Proc. 2015;90(5):699–700.
3. Nikodimopoulou M, Liakos S. Secondary hyperparathyroidism and target organs in chronic kidney disease. Hippokratia. 2011;15(Suppl 1):33–8.

Truncal Calciphylaxis in Primary Hyperparathyroidism Without Renal Failure

Case

A 38-year-old lady with a history of on and off abdominal pain and progressive limb weakness presented to the emergency department for acute abdomen. The patient was diagnosed to have pancreatitis and was managed conservatively. On evaluation she was found to have renal calculi and referred to urology. She was evaluated in the urology department and found to have high serum calcium and intact PTH levels and referred to the endocrine surgery department. The patient was well nourished and bed bound presented with painful, tender violaceous plaque-like cutaneous lesions with patchy skin necrosis along with hard tender nodules under these lesions on lower abdomen extending to upper thighs (Fig. 1). Her lower limb power was 3/5 in bilateral limbs. With high serum calcium of 16 mg/dL (8.6–10.6) and intact PTH of 1438 ($N = 10–65$) a diagnosis of primary hyperparathyroidism was made with normal vitamin D and creatinine levels. Localizing studies identified the

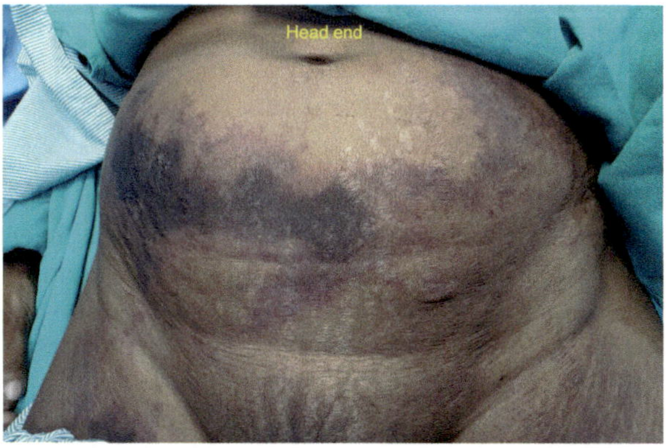

Fig. 1 Tender violaceous plaque-like cutaneous lesions

Roma Pradhan is the lead author of this chapter.

A. Agarwal et al., *Case Studies in Thyroid and Parathyroid Tumors*,
https://doi.org/10.1007/978-981-99-0938-4_2

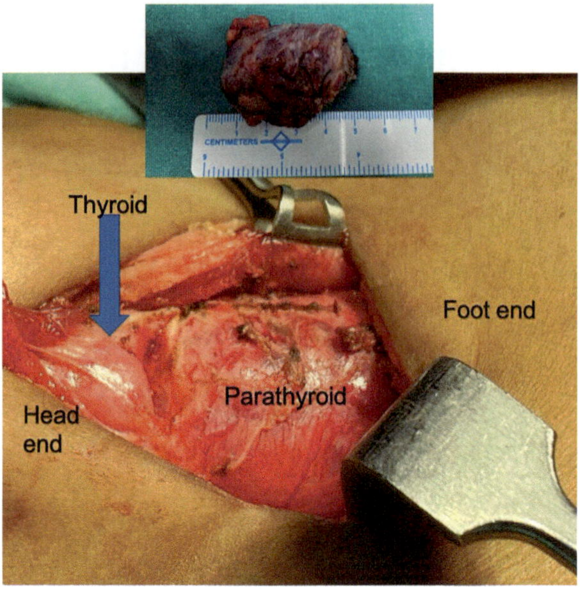

Fig. 2 Intraoperative picture

enlarged lesion as right inferior parathyroid gland. Due to poor general condition of the patient, right inferior parathyroidectomy was done under regional block. A 4.5 cm enlarged right inferior parathyroid gland was removed (Fig. 2) with fall in IOPTH to more than 50% (Miami's criteria). Postoperatively patient improved and was able to stand with support; however the trunk lesions became more painful and began to ulcerate. This was managed with daily dressing and debridement. The patient's general condition improved but unfortunately, we lost the patient due to severe blood transfusion reaction on 20th POD.

Discussion

Calciphylaxis is usually seen in patients of secondary or tertiary hyperparathyroidism and in patients dependent on dialysis or those requiring renal transplant. Nonetheless, calciphylaxis can be also seen in patients of primary hyperparathyroidism in the absence of renal failure when the serum calcium and phosphate levels exceed their solubility levels in the blood [1]. This, in turn, leads to calcium phosphate deposits in small- and medium-sized arteries that compromise the vascular supply. Ischemia of the skin and soft tissue leads to necrosis though it typically spares the muscle. The ischemic changes result in violaceous, livedo reticularis, plaque-like lesions that progress to painful, subcutaneous nodules like the ones in our case. These nodules can then become nonhealing, leathery, eschar-like lesions with a predilection for becoming infected. Calciphylaxis of the buttocks and lower extremities is more prevalent and has an overall better prognosis than involvement of the trunk or upper extremities [2].

The diagnosis of calciphylaxis is based on examination, laboratory investigations, and histopathologic findings. Calciphylaxis should be part of the differential diagnosis if a patient presents with painful subcutaneous nodules as described above. These lesions, along with elevated serum calcium on admission laboratory assessment, are the hallmarks of calciphylaxis. Patients with primary hyperparathyroidism have an elevated serum parathyroid hormone level in conjunction with an elevated calcium level. However there are no definite laboratory investigations which can diagnose calciphylaxis certainly. A skin biopsy may aid in diagnosis; however it is generally avoided to prevent further infection of the wound. If necessary it can be performed to rule out other connective tissue disorders. Once calciphylaxis due to primary hyperparathyroidism is diagnosed, the management is much clearer than in cases due to secondary or tertiary hyperparathyroidism. However, early diagnosis and aggressive wound management with antibiotic therapy are two of the most important keys in managing this condition. Lastly, and most importantly, there is the role of surgery. Patients who undergo parathyroidectomy have a marked clinical improvement in calciphylaxis, when compared with those who do not. However, surgery is of the most benefit to patients if done before the skin lesions develop [1] Preoperative cinacalcet, 30 mg daily, can be started and be taken until the day of surgery. Although parathyroidectomy does not necessarily lead to complete regression of disease in all patients, it is often the recommended therapy [3, 4].

In our case calciphylaxis was seen in the patient of primary hyperparathyroidism without renal failure over abdomen or truncal calciphylaxis which is rare. Semi-emergency parathyroidectomy should be undertaken in order to avoid mortality which is very high due to sepsis.

References

1. Joukhadar R, Bright T. Calciphylaxis in primary hyperparathyroidism: a case report and brief review. South Med J. 2009;102:318–21.
2. Mirza I, Chaubay D, Gunderia H, Shih W, El-Fanek H. An unusual presentation of calciphylaxis due to primary hyperparathyroidism. Arch Pathol Lab Med. 2001;125:1351–3.
3. Duffy A, Schurr M, Warner T, Chen H. Long-term outcomes in patients with calciphylaxis from hyperparathyroidism. Ann Surg Oncol. 2006;13:96–102.
4. Roy R, Lee JA. Calciphylaxis due to hyperparathyroidism. Endocr Pract. 2011;17(Suppl 1):54–6.

Hypercalcemic Crisis Resulting in Acute Kidney Failure

Case
A 56-year-old woman presented with excessive vomiting and weakness and developed ARF. She had to be hemodialyzed and was also given steroids. She was then detected to have elevated calcium (17.2 mg/dL) and was diagnosed to be having hypercalcemic crisis. Subsequently she was found to have elevated PTH as well (1341 pg/mL) and low vitamin D (19.7 ng/mL). So, a diagnosis of PHPT-induced hypercalcemic crisis was made. USG and CECT (Fig. 1) suggested a left inferior adenoma while MIBI was reported as double adenoma. Prior to surgery, her serum calcium was 10.5 mg/dL. In view of discordant imaging she underwent bilateral exploration. At operation, left inferior adenoma was found while the other 3 glands were normal. The adenoma was inseparable from the thyroid (Fig. 2) so an en bloc excision with hemithyroidectomy was done. The hemithyroidectomy-adenoma specimen weighed 13.4 gm. The HPE was benign parathyroid adenoma.

Amit Agarwal is the lead author of this chapter.

A. Agarwal et al., *Case Studies in Thyroid and Parathyroid Tumors*,
https://doi.org/10.1007/978-981-99-0938-4_3

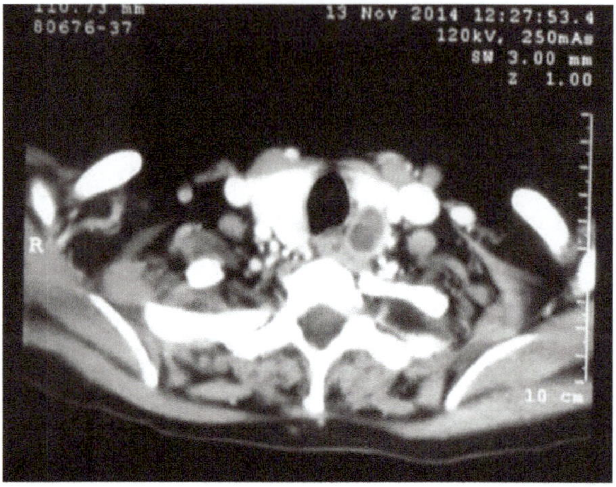

Fig. 1 CECT neck showing hypodense left inferior parathyroid adenoma posterior to left lobe of thyroid

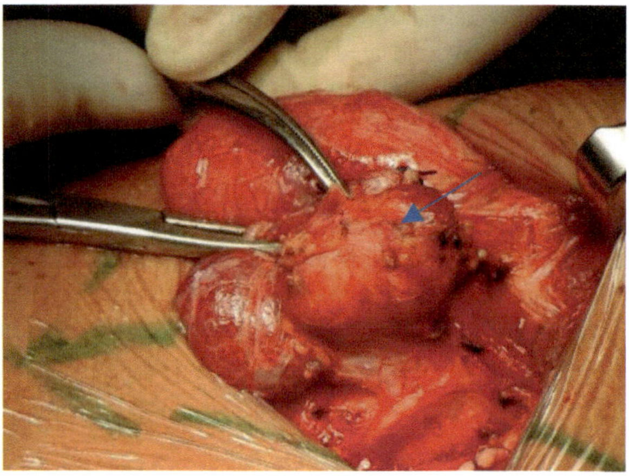

Fig. 2 Intraoperative picture showing adenoma (arrow) densely adhered to thyroid

Discussion

Hypercalcemic crisis is a rare, severe life-threatening complication of PHPT defined as serum calcium greater than 15 mg/dL (≥3.75 mmol/L) with signs and symptoms of acute calcium intoxication [1]. Patients usually present with end organ damage mostly affecting central nervous system, cardiac, gastrointestinal, and renal functions. Hypercalcemic crisis is seen in advanced PHPT occurring in 1–2% of patients. There are concerns about life-threatening cardiac arrhythmias when severe hyperparathyroid-induced hypercalcemic crisis (HIHC) is not treated promptly. Prompt recognition and aggressive measures to reduce serum calcium levels are responsible for dramatic reduction in morbidity and mortality seen in recent series. Management of patients in parathyroid crisis consists of emergency measures to acutely decrease serum calcium. First-line therapy consists of volume expansion with isotonic saline at an initial rate of 200–300 mL/h which is later adjusted to maintain a urine output of 100–150 mL/h. Other measures include use of bisphosphonates. Pamidronate may be given in 60–90 mg doses IV infusion with maximal response at 90 mg over 2–4 h. It causes decrease in calcium levels within 24 h. Zoledronic acid is the newer bisphosphonate agent which is more potent and can be administered in smaller doses of 4 mg over 15 min infusion. However, bisphosphonates take 2–4 days for maximum effect and the effect of bisphosphonates lasts for several weeks which can lead to postoperative hypocalcemia. Calcitonin at a dose of 6–8 IU/kg every 6 h acts rapidly and lowers serum calcium by 1–2 mg/dL. Calcitonin has a rapid onset but short duration of effect, and patients develop tolerance to the calcium-lowering effect. In hypercalcemia mediated by vitamin D and in hematologic malignancies (e.g., myeloma, lymphoma), glucocorticoids are the first line of therapy after fluids. Thus, when serum calcium fails to decrease with the standard treatments or if there is cardiac/neurological impairment, hemodialysis is effective as a last resort to rapidly lower serum calcium. The use of low calcium dialysate of 1.25 mmol/L is found to be more effective than standard calcium dialysate of 1.5 mmol/L. Calcium-free hemodialysis decreases the serum calcium levels more markedly and rapidly compared with hydration or the use of furosemide, bisphosphonates, glucocorticoids, calcitonin, and mithramycin [2]. Moreover, renal function impairment is very common in patients with hypercalcemia which also complicates the hydration procedure. Therefore, CFHD is beneficial for the treatment of hypercalcemia in the event of severe hypercalcemic symptoms, congestive heart failure, renal failure, or other conditions that contraindicate adequate hydration. Some institutions perform calcium-free hemodialysis in acute hypercalcemic crisis. However, some argue against use of calcium-free hemodialysis as hemodynamic instability and hypotension may occur due to suppression of myocardial contractility. However, hypotensive episodes occur in only one third of hemodialysis sessions. And these hypotensive episodes are usually transient and can be corrected by moderate fluid loading. Thus, CFHD facilitates the treatment of hypercalcemia and also serves as a safeguard against development of pulmonary edema during vigorous hydration in patients with renal failure or heart failure [3].

References

1. Singh DN, Gupta SK, Kumari N, Krishnani N, Chand G, Mishra A, Agarwal G, Verma AK, Mishra SK, Agarwal A. Primary hyperparathyroidism presenting as hypercalcemic crisis: Twenty-year experience. Indian J Endocrinol Metab. 2015;19(1):100–5.
2. Wang CC, Chen YC, Shiang JC, et al. Hypercalcemic crisis successfully treated with prompt calcium-free hemodialysis. Am J Emerg Med. 2009;27:1174.e1–3.
3. Sethi J, Kumar V, Rathi M, Gupta KL. Acute kidney injury associated with hypercalcaemic crisis in a patient with primary hyperparathyroidism. BMJ Case Rep. 2018;2018:bcr2018225235.

The teaching point of the case is that the patient survived such extreme hypercalcemia and had complete recovery of renal functions after parathyroidectomy.

Familial Isolated Hyperparathyroidism (FIHP)

Case

Sixteen affected members over 4 generations. First generation—65/F who died due to Upper GI Bleed and suffered from Gastritis for 20 years prior to death. Second generation—4 out of 5 siblings affected. The healthy sibling did not have any children and remains asymptomatic to date. The oldest sibling died of complications of PHPT–Acute on CKD. All affected individuals have symptoms of PHPT only. Third generation—8 out of 12 are affected: three exhibit isolated PHPT. Fourth generation—3 out of 11 affected. Flowchart of family tree of the four generations of one family in shown in (Fig. 1). While one has been operated for PHPT, 1 has asymptomatic hypercalcemia

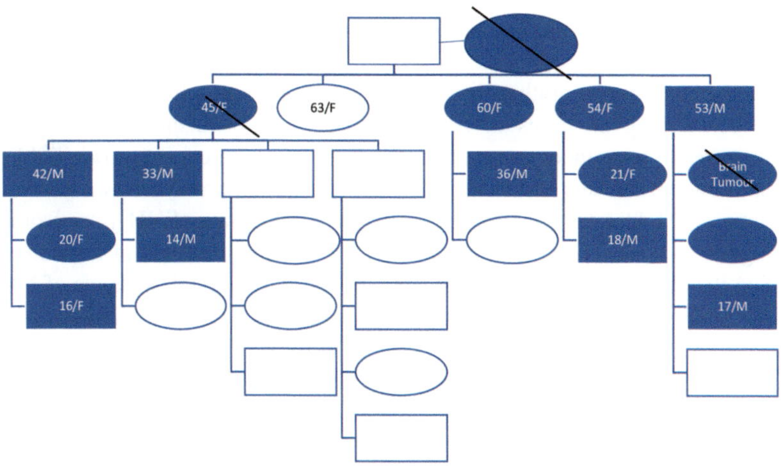

Fig. 1 Flowchart of family tree of the four generations of one family

---

Amit Agarwal is the lead author of this chapter.

A. Agarwal et al., *Case Studies in Thyroid and Parathyroid Tumors*,
https://doi.org/10.1007/978-981-99-0938-4_4

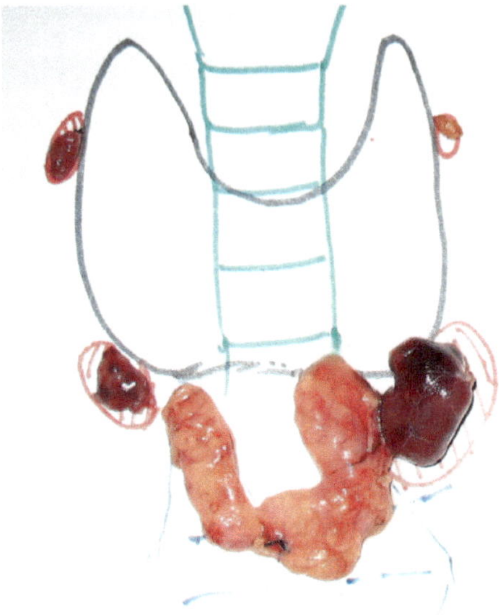

Fig. 2 Specimen picture of subtotal parathyroidectomy with cervical thymectomy in one family member

detected on screening and 1 has a collagenoma. Thus, 9 out of 16 affected have been operated for PHPT; five underwent 3.5 gland parathyroidectomy, two underwent excision of double adenoma, and two underwent single gland excision (Fig. 2).

Discussion

Familial isolated hyperparathyroidism (FIHP) occurs with a frequency of approximately 1% among all cases of primary hyperparathyroidism (PHPT). FIHP is thought to result from incomplete expression of a syndromic form of familial PHPT [multiple endocrine neoplasia type 1 (MEN 1), hyperparathyroidism–jaw tumor syndrome (HPT-JT), familial hypocalciuric hypercalcemia (FHH)], or from still unrecognized causes. The diagnosis of FIHP is essentially made in kindreds with PHPT in the absence of clinical, biochemical, and radiological evidence of MEN1, HPT-JT syndrome, or FHH [1–3]. FIHP is a genetically heterogeneous disease because mutations in MEN1, HRPT2, and CASR genes have all been reported. However, the majority of FIHP cases have still unrecognized causes and therefore novel genes related to FIHP. Studies have shown that a substantial proportion of kindreds clinically diagnosed as FIHP carry MEN1 gene mutations, suggesting that they are indeed an occult form of the MEN 1 syndrome [4]. It is recommended that MEN1 genotyping may be done in these FIHP families, as the finding of mutation(s) may predict multiglandular involvement and therefore would prompt the surgeon to carry out a bilateral exploration rather than a focused parathyroidectomy which may result in incomplete treatment [5]. Indeed, the detection of a MEN1 mutation should prompt further investigation in the family, with the possibility of identifying new cases.

References

1. Simonds WF, James-Newton LA, Agarwal SK, Yang B, Skarulis MC, Hendy GN, Marx SJ. Familial isolated hyperparathyroidism: clinical and genetic characteristics of 36 kindreds. Medicine (Baltimore). 2002;81(1):1–26.
2. Warner J, Epstein M, Sweet A, Singh D, Burgess J, Stranks S, Hill P, Perry-Keene D, Learoyd D, Robinson B, Birdsey P, Mackenzie E, Teh BT, Prins JB, Cardinal J. Genetic testing in familial isolated hyperparathyroidism: unexpected results and their implications. J Med Genet. 2004;41(3):155–60.
3. Mizusawa N, Uchino S, Iwata T, Tsuyuguchi M, Suzuki Y, Mizukoshi T, Yamashita Y, Sakurai A, Suzuki S, Beniko M, Tahara H, Fujisawa M, Kamata N, Fujisawa K, Yashiro T, Nagao D, Golam HM, Sano T, Noguchi S, Yoshimoto K. Genetic analyses in patients with familial isolated hyperparathyroidism and hyperparathyroidism-jaw tumour syndrome. Clin Endocrinol. 2006;65(1):9–16.
4. Marx SJ. New concepts about familial isolated hyperparathyroidism. J Clin Endocrinol Metab. 2019;104:4058–66.
5. Cetani F, Pardi E, Ambrogini E, Lemmi M, Borsari S, Cianferotti L, Vignali E, Viacava P, Berti P, Mariotti S, Pinchera A, Marcocci C. Genetic analyses in familial isolated hyperparathyroidism: implication for clinical assessment and surgical management. Clin Endocrinol. 2006;64:146–52.

PHPT Presenting as Pulmonary Thromboembolism

Case

A 28-year-old man presented to the Emergency Department with acute-onset, right-side chest pain, accompanied by dyspnea. His medical history was unremarkable except for history of previous surgery for renal stones 10 years back. He denied smoking, frequent alcohol intake, or therapy with any medication. Physical examination on presentation did not reveal any abnormal findings. His blood pressure was 110/70 mmHg, with pulse rate of 110/min, the respiratory rate 28/min. The oxygen saturation was 83–84% and the ECG demonstrated sinus tachycardia with normal axis, ST-caving, and delayed R-wave transition. Echocardiography revealed dilated RA/RV, mild TR, RSVP-40, PAT-60 mm, D-shaped LV cavity, No VSD/PDA, no pericardial effusion; Mc Connell's sign was positive. Laboratory evaluation revealed strongly positive d-dimer and serum calcium levels (14.4 mg/dL, 8.8–10.5, iCa = 2.1). The Wells score was 6. The aforementioned combination of clinical symptoms and laboratory findings raised the suspicion of Pulmonary Embolism (PE) and an urgent spiral CT angiography and Doppler study of lower limbs was ordered. Pulmonary CT angiogram revealed filling defect in right and left pulmonary artery and extending into descending pulmonary artery branches. Doppler study did not reveal DVT in bilateral lower limbs.

Low molecular weight heparin (LMWH, dalteparin, 5000 units, sc, twice a day) was administered for the treatment of PE, as well as intravenous hydration and denosumab for the management of hypercalcemia.

More laboratory tests were ordered in order to identify the cause of hypercalcemia. PTH was found to be significantly elevated (106.5 pmol/L, 1.6–6.9), along with elevated 24-h urinary calcium (516 mg/24 h, 100–250), reduced phosphorus—2.7 (1.5 mg/dL, 2.7–4.5), and deficient 25(OH)D3 (5.1).

Amit Agarwal is the lead author of this chapter.

A. Agarwal et al., *Case Studies in Thyroid and Parathyroid Tumors*,
https://doi.org/10.1007/978-981-99-0938-4_5

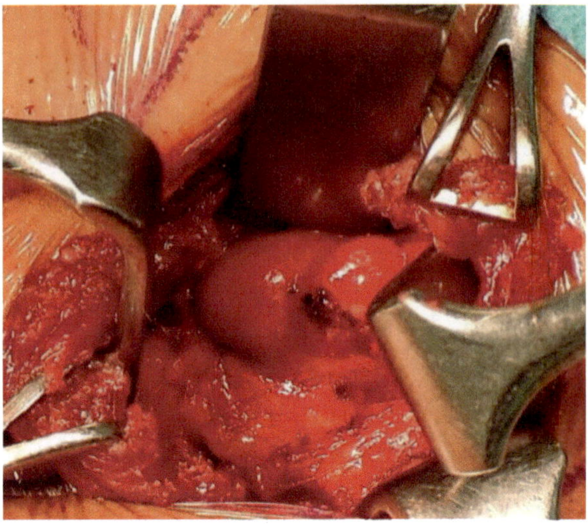

Fig. 1 Intraoperative picture showing the adenoma

Ultrasonography was suggestive of left inferior adenoma measuring 1.7 × 1.8 cm. This finding was also confirmed by Tc99m Sestamibi imaging. X-ray KUB revealed bilateral renal medullary nephrocalcinosis. Skeletal radiograph illustrated subperiosteal resorption of the phalanges. Bone densitometry (DXA scan) was indicative of osteoporosis (L1-L4 lumbar vertebras T-score—3.6, left neck femur T-score—2.8, right neck femur—3.8).

The assessment for blood coagulation abnormalities revealed high homocysteine levels (>50 μmol/lt, normal <15). However, lupus anticoagulant was negative and no mutation was found in factor V Leiden.

After recovering from PTE, the patient was referred for parathyroidectomy. In view of concordant findings of USG and MIBI scan, a focused parathyroidectomy was done under bilateral cervical block after withholding the injection Dalteparin for 24 h which was restarted 24 h after surgery and then switched to rivaroxaban 20 mg od. A 3.5 gm adenoma measuring 3.5 × 2.5 × 0.5 cm was removed (Fig. 1) and there was curative fall in IOPTH and histological examination of the lesion was compatible with parathyroid adenoma. Following surgery, PTH and calcium levels returned to normal and the patient remained in good physical condition during his follow-up over a period of 12 months.

Discussion

The association of PHPT and thrombotic events, which has been previously reported in the literature, still little is known in terms of the pathophysiological mechanisms that are responsible for hypercoagulable state in hypercalcemia [1]. It still remains uncertain whether the pathophysiological background of thrombosis in PHPT is related to prothrombotic factors acting indirectly (e.g., increased prevalence of risk factors for CVD), directly (causing disturbances of the hemostatic system), or even a combination of both. We describe a patient who presented with thrombotic event (pulmonary embolism) and after thorough investigation the diagnosis of PHPT—due to a parathyroid adenoma—was established. Several potential mechanisms have been proposed. It is suggested that calcium-triggered vasoconstriction activates several factors of the clotting system and also boosts platelet aggregation [2]. Additionally, renal mechanisms for the reabsorption of sodium and water are disturbed by the hypercalcemic state, and non-compensated polyuria due to nausea and anorexia can lead to dehydration and hypercoagulable state. Furthermore, elevated calcium concentrations can be potentially responsible for cytotoxic effects that stimulate cell death and result in thrombosis. It has been shown that increased platelet count, F VII and FX activities, and D-Dimer levels in patients with PHPT represent a potential hypercoagulable state, which might augment the risk for atherosclerotic and atherothrombotic complications [3].

References

1. Walker MD, Rubin M, Silverberg SJ. Nontraditional manifestations of primary hyperparathyroidism. J Clin Densitom. 2013;16(1):40–7.
2. Erem C, Kocak M, Hacihasanoglu A, et al. Blood coagulation, fibrinolysis and lipid profile in patients with primary hyperparathyroidism: increased plasma factor VII and X activities and D-dimer levels. Exp Clin Endocrinol Diabetes. 2008;116(10):619–24.
3. Koufakis T, Antonopoulou V, Grammatiki M, Karras SN, Ajjan R, Zebekakis P, Kotsa K. The relationship between primary hyperparathyroidism and thrombotic events: report of three cases and a review of potential mechanisms. Int J Hematol Oncol Stem Cell Res. 2018;12(3):175–80.

Juvenile PHPT

Case

A 14-year-old girl presented with a fracture of the left humerus sustained 25 days back following trivial trauma. The patient was managed conservatively with POP cast application, but the fracture showed no signs of healing. The patient was then referred to us with a possibility of hypercalcemia for further management. On questioning only positive history was that of recent irritability, depression and mood swings, and history of developing a limp. On examination, she had a waddling gait and her left arm was in POP cast. There were no features suggestive of Rickets and there were neurocutaneous markers and no bony swellings over the body. She also had widening of the left third metacarpal and proximal phalanx of the index finger and tenderness over the right lower tibiofibular joint. X-ray of forearm showing brown tumor of the distal end of left ulna (Fig. 1). On examination of the neck, there was no neck swelling. Her evaluation revealed hypercalcemia (11.9 mg% and 12.0 mg% on two occasions), elevated ALP (4722.4 IU/L), low phosphorous (1.38 mg%), elevated PTH (170.3 pmol/L, normal range 1.06–5.83 pmol/L), normal 24-h urinary calcium (271 mg/24 h), and insufficient Vitamin D (37.9 nmol/L, normal range: 50–250). With a biochemical diagnosis of hyperparathyroidism, localization was done with USG (29 × 11 mm hypoechoic, heterogenous lesion posterior to the left lobe of the thyroid, lower 1/3rd posteriorly) and MIBI scan (S/O Left inferior parathyroid) adenoma. Her BMD revealed severe osteoporosis with a *Z* score of −4.2 at the Lumbar vertebrae, −8.3 arc radius, and −4.1 at the femur. She underwent a focused parathyroidectomy with surgeon performed ultrasound (Fig. 2) and 2.5 cm parathyroid adenoma (Fig. 3) was removed with curative fall in IOPTH using Miami criteria. Histopathology was suggestive of a 1.8 g parathyroid adenoma. She developed severe hungry bone syndrome and was managed with intravenous calcium infusion followed by oral calcium and active vitamin D supplements. At subsequent visits, her fracture healed and she regained normal shoulder and arm movements.

Amit Agarwal is the lead author of this chapter.

A. Agarwal et al., *Case Studies in Thyroid and Parathyroid Tumors*,
https://doi.org/10.1007/978-981-99-0938-4_6

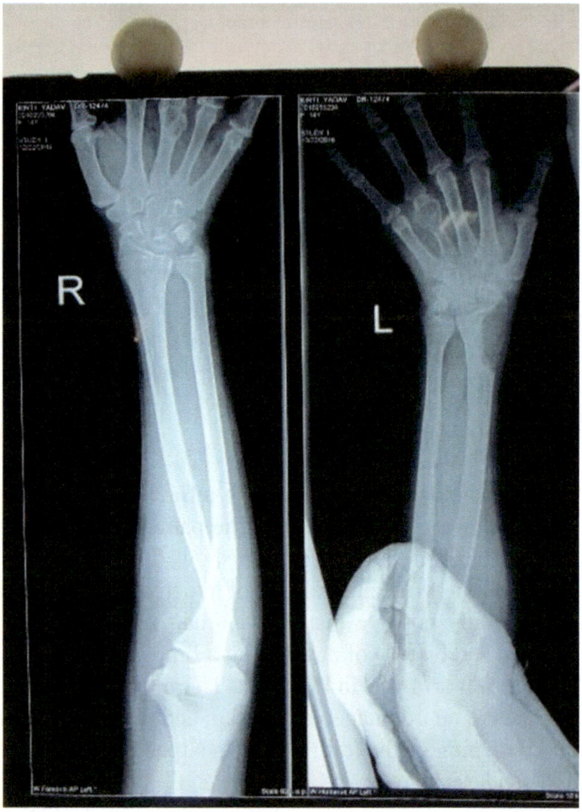

Fig. 1 X-ray of forearm showing brown tumor of the distal end of left ulna

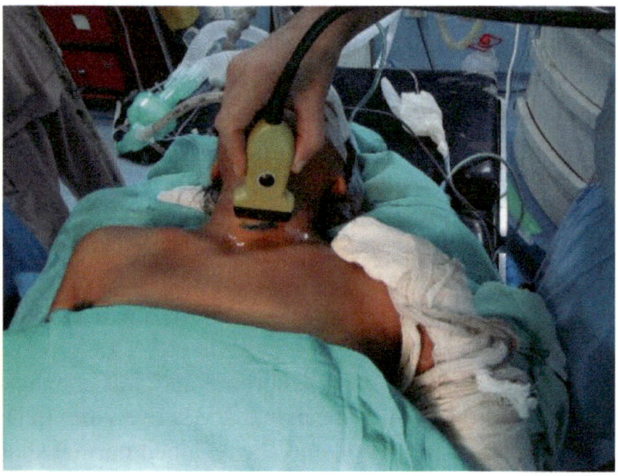

Fig. 2 The young PHPT patient undergoing surgeon-performed USG. Note the plaster in the left arm

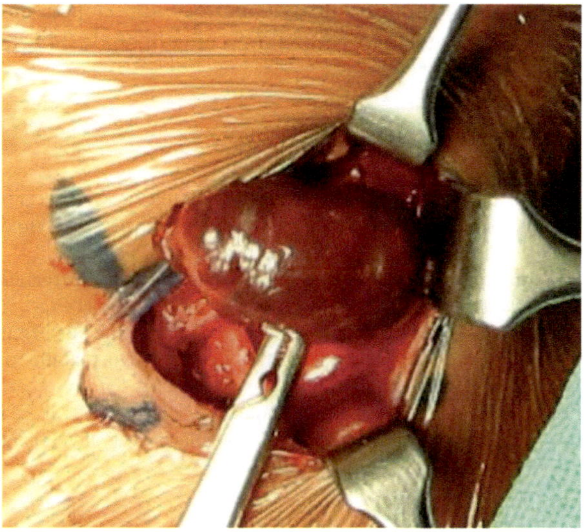

Fig. 3 Intraoperative picture showing the adenoma

Discussion

Primary hyperparathyroidism (PHPT) is a rare disease in juvenile patients. There are subtle differences in adult and juvenile PHPT than in adult patients. Females and males are equally affected in juvenile PHPT patients, contrary to the predomination of females in adult PHPT. Contrary to PHPT in adults, PHPT in children and young adults usually have more symptoms and the disease is more severe. Also, the diagnosis of PHPT is often delayed in children, which might lead to serious end-organ damages and finally familial forms of PHPT, like MEN 1 and MEN 2A syndromes, hyperparathyroid-jaw tumor syndrome and familial isolated primary hyperparathyroidism, which are more common in juvenile patients than in adults. Besides the difference in clinical presentation, the biochemistry is also different with juvenile PHPT children showing higher preoperative levels of serum calcium, urinary calcium, PTH, and lower levels of serum phosphorous. The reason for this biochemical difference is that the sensitivity of bones to the PTH effects is more increased in children than in adults. Young bones, during the growing process in juvenile PHPT patients, are responsible for the greater hypercalcemia in response to the same level of PTH as seen in adults. However, young PHPT patients had higher vitamin D level compared to adults. This might be due to the fact that renal production of vitamin D, which depends on PTH, is lowered with an increasing age. Also, as against the widely held belief, the rates of multiglandular disease are not higher in children with PHPT. A focused parathyroidectomy avoids the risk of postoperative hypoparathyroidism in juvenile PHPT. However, a world of caution. When a young patient presents with mild hypercalcemia the differential diagnosis should be made between J-PHPT and familial hypocalciuric hypercalcemic (FHH), a benign condition not requiring operation, due to inactivating mutations of the calcium-sensing receptor. Hence, unlike adult PHPT, the evaluation of hypercalcemia in children must include 24 urinary calcium estimations.

Further Reading

Jovanovic M, Paunovic I, Zdravkovic V, Djordjevic M, Rovcanin B, Tausanovic K, Slijepcevic N, Zivaljevic V. Case-control study of primary hyperparathyroidism in juvenile vs. adult patients. Int J Pediatr Otorhinolaryngol. 2020;131:109895.

Mukherjee S, Bhadada SK, Arya AK, et al. Primary hyperparathyroidism in the young: comparison with adult primary hyperparathyroidism. Endocr Pract. 2018;24:1051–6.

Roizen J, Levine MA. A meta-analysis comparing the biochemistry of primary hyperparathyroidism in youths to the biochemistry of primary hyperparathyroidism in adults. J Clin Endocrinol Metab. 2014;99:4555–64.

Saponaro F, Marcocci C, Cacciatore F, Miccoli M, Pardi E, Borsari S, Materazzi G, Miccoli P, Cetani F. Clinical profile of juvenile primary hyperparathyroidism: a prospective study. Endocrine. 2018;59(2):344–52.

Loss of Height in PHPT

Case

A 57-year-old woman presented with complaints of loss of height, approximately 2 in. in the past 5–6 years and back pain and bilateral lower leg pain since 6–7 years. She also had difficulty in climbing stairs. She was found to be having low serum phosphorus: 1.6, 1.8 (on 2 occasion); normal total calcium: 10.0, 10.2 (on 2 occasion) but elevated ionized calcium: 7.5, 7 (on 2 occasion); elevated serum alkaline phosphatase: 1416, elevated PTH: 743.8. Skeletal survey revealed diffuse osteopenia with brown tumors. Lateral spine radiograph demonstrated diffuse osteopenia with cortical thinning (Fig. 1), decreased height (Fig. 2), and biconcavity of lumbar vertebrae suggesting bone softening. BMD showed severe osteoporosis. USG and MIBI were concordant for left inferior adenoma and she underwent focused parathyroidectomy and 10.0 g adenoma was removed (Fig. 3).

Amit Agarwal is the lead author of this chapter.

A. Agarwal et al., *Case Studies in Thyroid and Parathyroid Tumors*,
https://doi.org/10.1007/978-981-99-0938-4_7

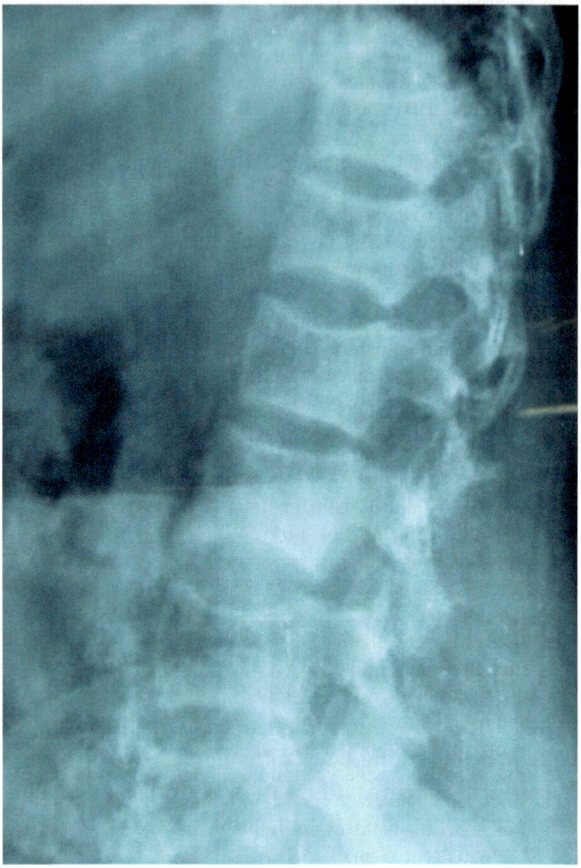

Fig. 1 Plain X-ray film of spine lateral spine radiograph demonstrates diffuse osteopenia with cortical thinning, decreased height, and biconcavity of lumbar vertebrae suggesting bone softening

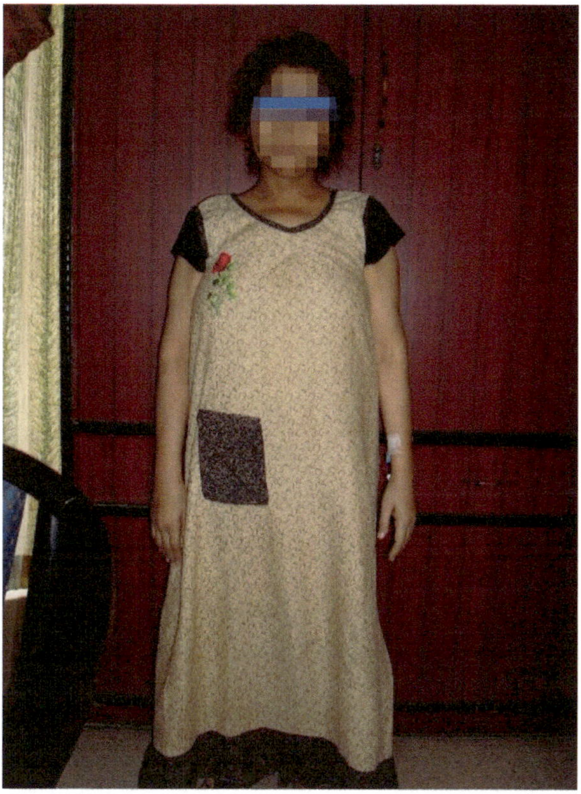

Fig. 2 Clinical photograph of patient showing loss of height

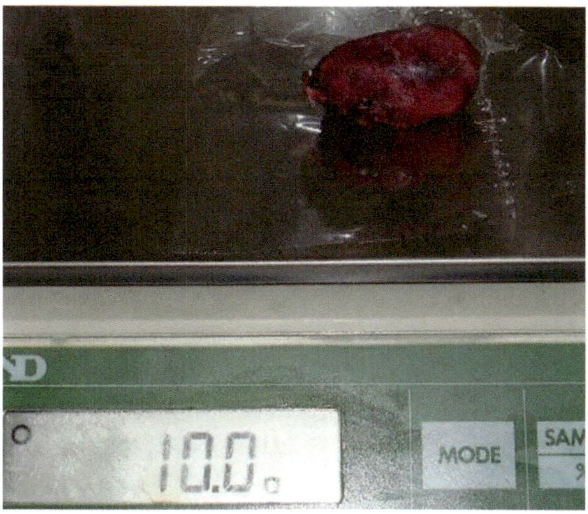

Fig. 3 Specimen of parathyroid adenoma

Discussion

Although PHPT occurs at all ages, the majority of patients are postmenopausal women [1]. A variable degree of bone loss is commonly found, with greater involvement of cortical sites, such as the forearm, than at trabecular sites, such as the lumbar spine. Despite the preferential involvement of cortical bone in PHPT, an increased rate of vertebral fractures has been reported in most studies, and two-thirds of vertebral fractures are clinically silent [2]. Vertebral X-ray examination is the gold standard by which vertebral fractures are detected. Findings on X-ray include [3]: Thinning of cortices and prominent vertical trabeculae, vertebral compression fracture and vertebra plana, decreased height of the vertebrae with biconcave endplates, and Rugger-Jersey spine (alternating bands of sclerosis along the endplates and areas of central lucency). Because of the vertebral fractures and loss of height of the thoracolumbar vertebrae, patients may experience a significant loss of height.

References

1. Silverberg SJ, Shane E, de la Cruz L, Dempster DW, Feldman F, Seldin D, Jacobs TP, Siris ES, Cafferty M, Parisien MV, Lindsay R, Clements TL, Bilezikian JP. Skeletal disease in primary hyperparathyroidism. J Bone Miner Res. 1989;4:283–91.
2. De Geronimo S, Romagnoli E, Diacinti D, D'Erasmo E, Minisola S. The risk of fractures in postmenopausal women with primary hyperparathyroidism. Eur J Endocrinol. 2006;155:415–20.
3. Panwar J, Kandagaddala M, Bhat TA, Hsu CC-T, Mitra P. The forgotten art of plain radiography in the evaluation of metabolic bone disease. IJMSR. 2019;2(1):319.

Maternal PHPT

Case 1

Gestational bilateral pelvic fractures: A 37-year-old woman presented with complaints of pain in both lower limbs for 3 years and difficulty in walking for 3 years. She had become pregnant 3 years back but became bedbound at 6 months gestation due to severe pain and was found to be having spontaneous fractures of ischiopubic rami on both sides (Fig. 1). She was given traction and bed rest for 1 month. Milk intake was adequate but exercise was nil and she was not on anti-convulsants or steroids. No history of neck swelling. No abdominal pain. No history of renal stones. She gave birth to a healthy child who now is 2/12 years old. The patient was evaluated for metabolic bone disease in view of the past history of pelvic fractures. She was given analgesics. Investigations were suggestive of primary hyperparathyroidism. Serum calcium (11.2 mg/dL) and serum PTH (402 pg/mL) were elevated, and 25 OH Vitamin D was extremely low (13.06 ng/mL). Both USG and MIBI scans were concordant for a left inferior adenoma. She underwent focused parathyroidectomy and a 2.6 g adenoma was removed.

Case 2 Neonatal Hypocalcemia and Seizure

A 24-year-old woman presented with a history of pain in her right leg on walking and a history of multiple fractures (forearm and pelvic). She sustained the pelvic fracture while she was 8 months pregnant. She delivered a baby by LSCS 1 month later but the baby expired at 1 month of age due to seizures. Subsequently, investigations revealed that she had Sr calcium total: 12.0, 14.5. Ionized calcium: 5.8, PTH; 492 pg/mL, SAP; 1539, 1497, Urine exam: Phosphate crystals+. She was diagnosed as suffering from PHPT and was taken up for a focused parathyroidectomy 2 months after LSCS. Superior parathyroid was found to be enlarged 2.4 × 1.5 × 1 cm, weighing 15 g. She became eucalcemic and subsequently she conceived and now has two healthy children.

Amit Agarwal is the lead author of this chapter.

A. Agarwal et al., *Case Studies in Thyroid and Parathyroid Tumors*,
https://doi.org/10.1007/978-981-99-0938-4_8

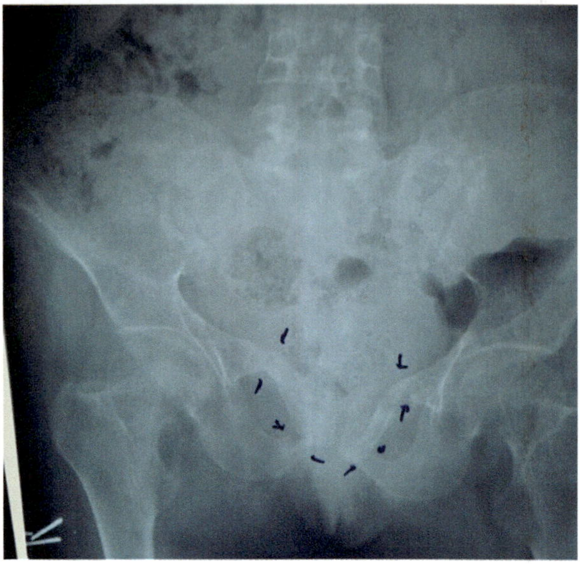

Fig. 1 Plain x-ray showing bilateral ischio-pubic rami fractures

Discussion

PHPT during pregnancy will have both maternal and fetal complications. *Maternal complications* include: Symptoms of primary hyperparathyroidism are reported in up to 67% of affected women, which are mainly nonspecific and overlap with the common complaints during pregnancy, of fatigue, nausea, vomiting, constipation, and difficulty in concentrating. Severe complications of hypercalcemia include nephrolithiasis (24–36%), bone disease (13–19%), pancreatitis (7–13%), and hypercalcemic crisis [1]. Hypercalcemic crisis can result, as the maternal efflux of calcium to the fetus is suddenly discontinued. Also, complications such as hyperemesis gravidarum and pre-eclampsia have been reported. The physiological changes in phosphor calcium homeostasis and calciotropic hormones during pregnancy may mask gestational PHPT or complicate its recognition. The total calcium level falls in pregnant women, due to gestational hypoalbuminemia, yet the level of ionized calcium (the physiologically active fraction) remains unchanged. Increased glomerular filtration results in maternal hypercalciuria. A total of 25–30 g of calcium is actively transported from the mother to the fetus through the placenta, to support fetal development and bone formation. Approximately 80% of this calcium accumulates during the third trimester. Active calcium transport through the placenta is independent of maternal PTH levels but is mediated by fetal and placental secretion of PTH-related protein (PTHrp). Most calcium demands are met by enhanced maternal intestinal calcium absorption, mediated by an increase in 1,25-dihydroxy vitamin D levels. 1-hydroxylase is regulated mainly by PTHrP levels during pregnancy. The above-mentioned physiological changes that occur during pregnancy, including hypoalbuminemia, increased glomerular filtration rate and transplacental transfer of calcium, contributing to lowering of serum calcium levels, which may mask gestational PHPT that remains undiagnosed in up to 80% of cases [2, 3].

- **Fetal complications of maternal PHPT:** neonatal hypocalcemia (with or without seizures), stillbirth, miscarriage. In the literature a three- to fivefold increase in the miscarriage rate in classical PHPT during pregnancy has been reported. Premature birth, intrauterine growth retardation, and low birth weight may also occur. However, recent cohort studies show that mild hypercalcemia in gestational PHPT is generally not associated with an increased risk of abortion rates and obstetrical complications. This reassuring data should be confirmed by prospective studies.
- *Neonatal Tetany*: Large quantities of calcium (20–30 g) are actively transported across the placenta from the mother to the fetus to facilitate normal bone mineralization. Most (80%) are transferred in the third trimester. Parathyroid hormone and calcitonin do not cross the placenta. Fetal 1,25-dihydroxyvitamin D, synthesized in both fetal kidney and placenta, acts as the major stimulus and regulator of calcium transfer across the placenta. In the fetus, maternal primary hyperparathyroidism results in high concentrations of serum calcium that act to suppress the parathyroid glands, resulting in a low fetal parathyroid hormone concentration. Fetal calcitonin concentrations are high to encourage bone mineralization. At birth, the neonate is suddenly deprived of this rich source of calcium. It is incapable of mobilizing calcium from bone owing to the low concentrations of parathyroid hormone and high concentrations of calcitonin. After delivery, the most dangerous complication is neonatal hypocalcemia [4]. Neonatal hypocalcemia occurs in more than 50% of cases and is usually transient, but in some cases, it can be permanent. Neonatal tetany occurs in 25% of cases. Neonatal hypocalcemia is secondary to elevated maternal calcium levels that suppress the fetal parathyroid glands. Neonatal hypocalcemia due to maternal hyperparathyroidism is classified into early onset (<48 h of life) and late onset (first week of life). Since maternal hypercalcemia due to hyperparathyroidism suppresses the fetal parathyroid glands leading to late-onset neonatal hypocalcemia, the neonate may present with seizures, poor feeding, apnea, and cyanosis. If the infant is breast fed, tetany can be delayed by 1 month or more.
- *Management:* In asymptomatic patients with mild hypercalcemia (<2.75 mmol/L), conservative treatment with oral hydration and low-calcium diet, with or without forced diuresis with a low dose of loop diuretic can produce good outcomes for both mother and child. Effectiveness and safety of treatment options for primary hyperparathyroidism in pregnancy remain unknown, but when calcium levels rise above 2.75 mmol/L, parathyroidectomy is increasingly recommended. The early diagnosis of primary hyperparathyroidism followed by appropriate management reduces these complications significantly. However, the optimal management of primary hyperparathyroidism during pregnancy needs to be individualized and should be based on the clinical course, gestational age, the severity of hypercalcemia, and the risk to benefit assessment for each treatment option for the mother and a child. Most clinical studies and guidelines recom-

mend parathyroidectomy as the treatment of choice for primary hyperparathyroidism occurring in pregnancy [5]. The efficacy and safety of medical treatment for primary hyperparathyroidism in pregnancy remain unknown. Conservative treatment might be used but only in primary hyperparathyroidism with mildly elevated calcium levels (<11 mg/dL). Intravenous or oral rehydration, with or without forced diuresis with a loop diuretic, is the first-line treatment, that has limited efficacy. Few drugs are available for the management of primary hyperparathyroidism during pregnancy. In particular, the use of subcutaneous calcitonin has a pregnancy category C rating (fetal risk not ruled out due to fetal abnormalities in animal studies alone) and calcitonin does not cross the placenta but has limited efficacy due to tachyphylaxis. The calcimimetic drug, cinacalcet, has also been used in combination with calcitonin and has demonstrated an effective reduction in PTH levels, but also has a category C rating and crosses the placenta. Bisphosphonates cross the placenta and are toxic to the fetus at high doses, and although they have been used during pregnancy in several cases, they are not recommended.

References

1. Schnatz PF, Curry SL. Primary hyperparathyroidism in pregnancy: evidence-based management. Obstet Gynecol Surv. 2002;57:365–76.
2. Hirsch D, Kopel V, Nadler V, Levy S, Toledano Y, Tsvetov G. Pregnancy outcomes in women with primary hyperparathyroidism. J Clin Endocrinol Metab. 2015;100:2115–22.
3. Abood A, Vestergaard P. Pregnancy outcomes in women with primary hyperparathyroidism. Eur J Endocrinol. 2014;171:69–76.
4. Beattie GC, Ravi NR, Lewis M, Williams H, Blair AW, Campbell W, Browning GGP. Rare presentation of maternal primary hyperparathyroidism. Br Med J. 2000;321:223–4.
5. McMullen TPW, Learoyd DL, Williams DC, Sywak MS, Sidhu SB, Delbridge LW. Hyperparathyroidism in pregnancy: options for localization and surgical therapy. World J Surg. 2010;34:1811–6.

PHPT Presenting with Psychiatric Symptoms

Case

A 35-year-old male presented with a complaint of altered behavior for 6 months with a history of delusion of prosecution and depressive episodes. He also had a fall from a moving train leading to a spine fracture which was fixed by screws (Fig. 1) but had temporary paraplegia. On examination, he had a brown tumor of the right clavicle and a 2 × 1 cm swelling noted in front of the neck. His medications included Tab Sertraline, 25 mg twice daily, and Clonotril (0.5 mg) once daily. BMD showed severe osteoporosis with a *T*-score of −5.5 at the distal ulna. USG Neck showed a 3.4 × 3 × 2.5 cm well-defined lesion in relation to the right inferior pole region posterior to the thyroid gland likely to be a parathyroid adenoma. He had elevated PTH (parathyroid hormone) >3000 pg/mL (12–88) and elevated calcium: 15.4 mg/dL. MIB showed a concordant right inferior parathyroid adenoma. He underwent focused parathyroidectomy with curative fall in IOPTH and 11.4 g adenoma was excised (Fig. 2). The patient had an uneventful perioperative course and remained free of any complications of anesthesia and surgery. His neuropsychiatric symptoms were recovering well with no need of any antipsychotic drugs.

Amit Agarwal is the lead author of this chapter.

A. Agarwal et al., *Case Studies in Thyroid and Parathyroid Tumors*,
https://doi.org/10.1007/978-981-99-0938-4_9

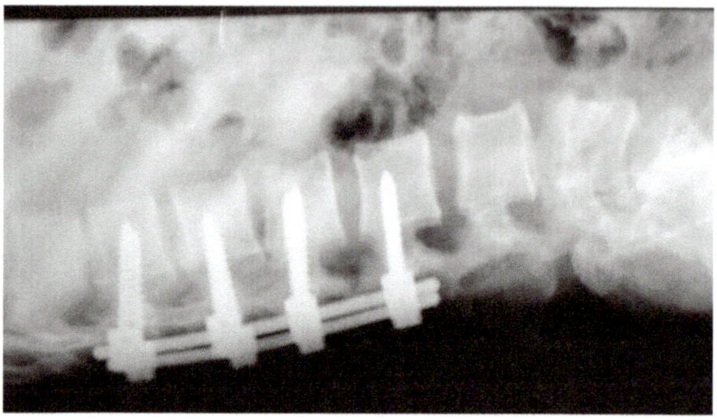

Fig. 1 X-ray of spine showing L5-S1 fracture with s/p fixation

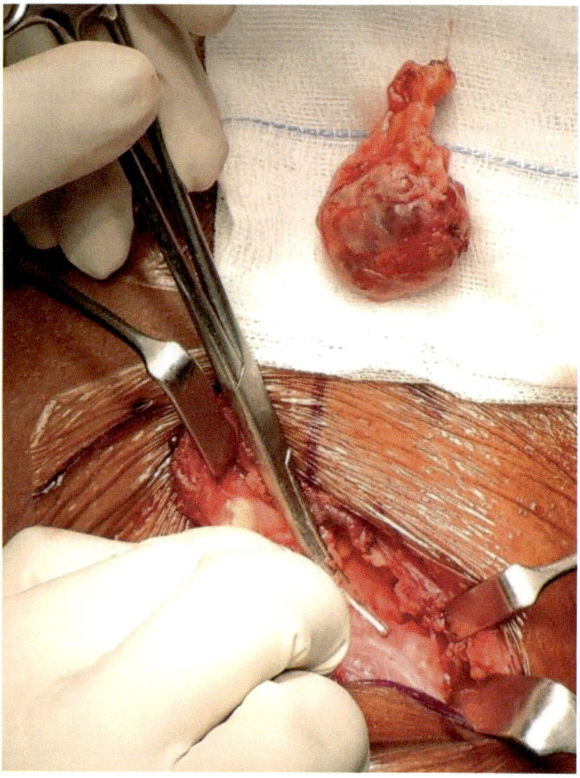

Fig. 2 Operative specimen of inferior parathyroid adenoma with part of thymus

Discussion

Hypercalcemia associated with PHPT has been linked to anxiety, personality changes, and depression. Several studies have focused on the evaluation of psychiatric disease and cognitive changes in patients with PHPT. Using rigorous neurocognitive and psychiatric testing, Roman et al. [1] prospectively evaluated 28 patients with PHPT undergoing parathyroidectomy and 27 control patients with benign euthyroid thyroid disease undergoing thyroidectomy The researchers found that patients with pHPT had more comorbidities than the age and sex-matched controls, were significantly more depressed preoperatively than the controls, and had significantly lower scores on the GMLT. Postoperatively, both groups improved significantly in depression scores. Assessing depression specifically, Wilhelm et al. [2] retrospectively analyzed 360 patients who underwent parathyroidectomy between 1994 and 2002 for PHPT. Thirty-five of these patients met the Diagnostic and Statistical Manual IV-Revised (DSM IV-R) criteria for major depression; after surgery, 90% of patients felt that depression no longer impacted their work, 52% had improved QOL, 27% discontinued their antidepressant medications, and 27% reduced their antidepressant medicine dose. Similarly, Liu et al. [3] showed that patients undergoing parathyroidectomy showed significant improvement in neuropsychiatric symptoms after surgery. Neuropsychiatric symptoms are more prevalent in patients with primary hyperparathyroidism. Neuropsychiatric symptoms should be assessed in all patients with primary hyperparathyroidism and should be considered a relative indication for parathyroidectomy.

References

1. Roman SA, Sosa JA, Mayes L, et al. Parathyroidectomy improves neurocognitive deficits in patients with primary hyperparathyroidism. Surgery. 2005;138:1121–9.
2. Wilhelm SM, Lee J, Prinz RA. Major depression due to primary hyperparathyroidism: a frequent and correctable disorder. Am Surg. 2004;70:175–18.
3. Liu JY, Peine BS, Mlaver E, et al. Neuropsychologic changes in primary hyperparathyroidism after parathyroidectomy from a dual-institution prospective study. Surgery. 2021;169(1):114–9.

PHPT Presenting with Severe Proximal Muscle Weakness

Case

A 61-year-old man presented with complaints of generalized bony pains for 2 years with extreme difficulty in getting up from a sitting position and difficulty in climbing stairs. The severity of his complaints are increasing so much so that he was bedridden for the past 2 weeks. There was no history of fracture. The patient was heavily built (Fig. 1), 110 kg, history of renal calculi, which resolved spontaneously after some medical treatment. He was a known diabetic for 7 years which was well controlled. Minimal sun exposure with more in-door work and a sedentary lifestyle. A neurological examination showed weakness of his grip strength (right hand: 15 kg, left hand: 110 kg), and a decreasing grade of muscle power in the iliopsoas (4+ grade), and gluteus (3+ grade). However, there was no muscle atrophy. Both Gowers' sign and Trendelenburg's sign were positive. He could not walk for more than 10 m because of fatigue. There were no extrapyramidal symptoms, and coordination disorders were not detected. Serum Intact PTH 466.7 pg/mL, 25-OHD: <1.6 pg/mL (19.6–54.3). Both USG neck and MIBI were concordant for left inferior parathyroid adenoma. He underwent focused parathyroidectomy and a 9.1 g adenoma (Fig. 2) was removed. He was put on prophylactic calcium infusion for 2 days and discharged on day 4 with calcium and Vitamin D supplements. One week after the operation, he was able to stand up from a chair without support. His grip strength and fatigability also improved. Three months later, he was able to walk without a cane and do squats and climb down the stairs without holding the handrail. Six months later, his fatiguability had disappeared, and he stopped taking calcium and vitamin D supplements and has fully and satisfactorily returned to work.

Amit Agarwal is the lead author of this chapter.

A. Agarwal et al., *Case Studies in Thyroid and Parathyroid Tumors*,
https://doi.org/10.1007/978-981-99-0938-4_10

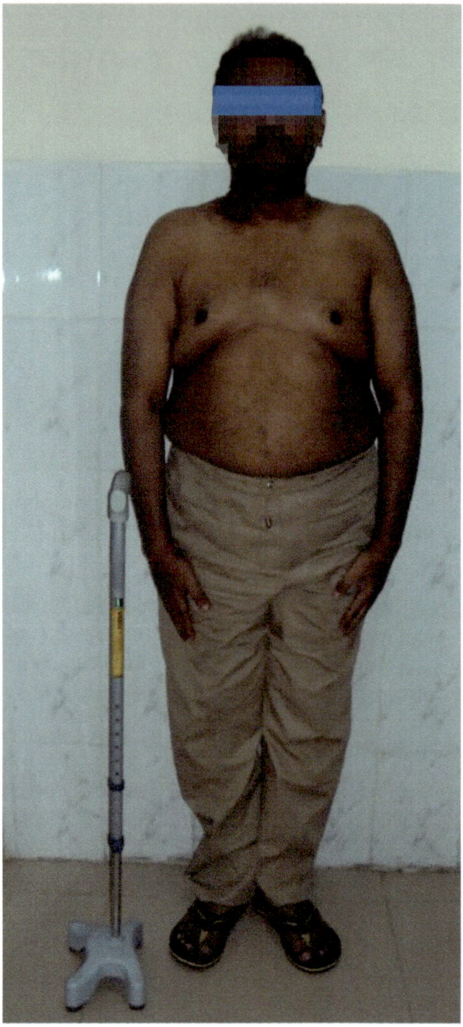

Fig. 1 Patient with his walker

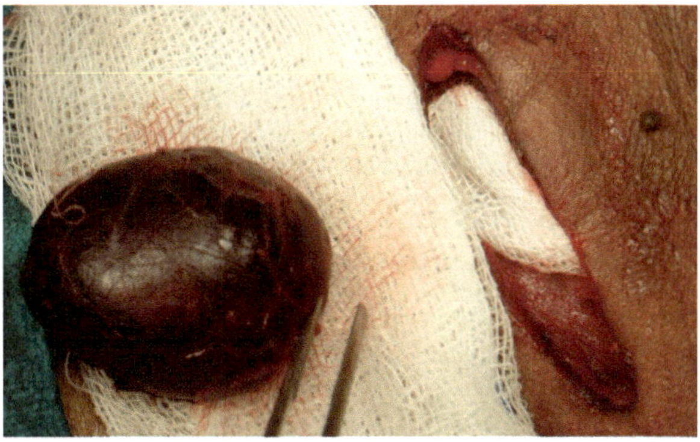

Fig. 2 Specimen and the small incision of focused parathyroidectomy

Discussion

PHPT patients are often diagnosed because of complaints of muscular weakness, easy muscle fatigability, and tiredness. Thus, it disguises itself like a myopathy-like disorder. Hyperparathyroidism has been reported to affect predominantly the proximal lower extremity muscles, e.g., the quadriceps muscle. Excessive levels of PTH rather than high calcium levels play a primary role in neuromuscular symptoms in PHPT. There are two main mechanisms underlying muscle weakness and fatigability due to PHPT [1]: The first mechanism is the reduced energy production (PTH interferes with the oxidation of long-chain fatty acid by blocking the transformation of free carnitine to acylcarnitine through the inhibition of carnitine palmitoyl transferase activity-carnitine cycle dysfunction). The second mechanism, involving the promotion of catabolism by PTH, is related to the inhibition of the synthesis of proteins, amino acids, and nucleic acids, which eventually leads to muscle atrophy. Various studies have shown improvement in muscle strength after parathyroidectomy. In the study by Deutch et al. [2], the authors concluded that women with PHPT increase knee extension force after parathyroidectomy as a result of increased force generation capacity of the muscle predominantly due to improvement in the strength of the quadriceps muscle. In the study by Quiros et al. [3] muscle strength was assessed using the ability to climb flights of stairs. In their study, the surveys from both postoperative 1 and 2 reflected a significant change in the patient's ability to climb stairs with most changes being obvious within the first 14 days after surgery.

References

1. Mihashi I, Ishii K, Ogawa Y, Uchida A, Hara H, Tamaoka A. Normocalcemic primary hyperparathyroidism presenting with muscle weakness and body pain. Intern Med. 2021;60:953–6.
2. Deutch S, Jensen MB, Christiansen PM, Hessov I. Muscular performance and fatigue in primary hyperparathyroidism. World J Surg. 2000;24:102–7.
3. Quiros RM, Alef MJ, Wilhelm SM, Djuricin G, Loviscek K, Prinz RA. Health-related quality of life in hyperparathyroidism measurably improves after parathyroidectomy. Surgery. 2003;134:675–80.

PHPT with CKD

Case

A 48-year-old lady presented with a history of pain in right lower limb for 3 years, pain radiating from lower back to right lower limb, severe pain with sleeplessness at night impairing ambulation. She also complained of facial puffiness on and off for 2 years and episodic nausea and vomiting episodes for 2 and ½ years with a history of loss of weight and loss of appetite. She also had generalized hyperpigmentation for 2 years. Symptoms aggravated over the past 6 months with fever, low grade with cough and minimal sputum from 15 days, and generalized fatiguability and history of constipation from 3 months. She also gave a history of hypertension for 10 years which was uncontrolled despite 3 anti-hypertensive drugs with peaks of 240 mmHg and had three episodes of accelerated hypertension and hospitalization. On examination of musculoskeletal system, she had antalgic gait with restriction of movements at the right hip joint with pain. Power was 4/5 B/L, UL, and LL. On evaluation for accelerated hypertension, she was found to have raised serum calcium levels and elevated PTH. Her serum creatinine was found to be 3.38 mg and her eGFR was 18 mL/min/1.73 m^2. Her 25-OH vit D was 71.6 nmol/L, serum phosphorous was consistently low: 3.32, 1.55, 1.71, 1.69, 2.0, 1.85, and serum ALP was 3616 IU/L.

	2017	2018	2019
Sr. Ca^{2+} (mg/dL)	9.9	13.2	12.0
PTH		1182 pg/mL	3045 pg/mL
Vit D		16.3 ng/mL	28.4 ng/mL

Her USG Neck and MIBI were concordant for right inferior parathyroid adenoma. She underwent focused parathyroidectomy (Fig. 1) with curative fall in

Amit Agarwal is the lead author of this chapter.

A. Agarwal et al., *Case Studies in Thyroid and Parathyroid Tumors*,
https://doi.org/10.1007/978-981-99-0938-4_11

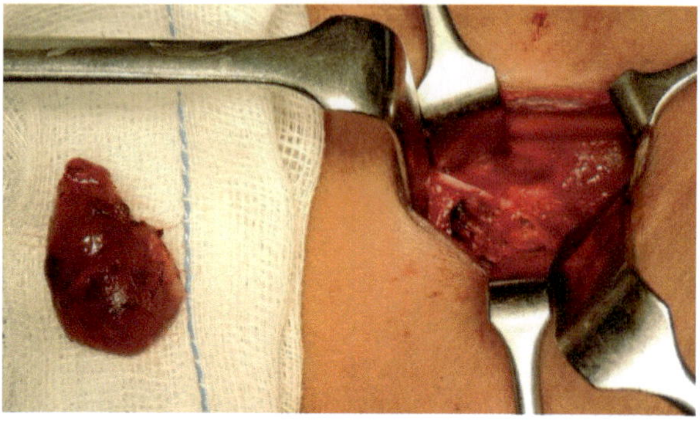

Fig. 1 Intraoperative view of the surgical field and the excised parathyroid adenoma

IOPTH (Miami criteria). She remained eucalcemic for 6 months. However, subsequently, she developed recurrent hypercalcemia with elevated PTH.

Discussion

Prolonged hypercalcemia impairs renal function, and a reduced GFR is common in advanced PHPT [1, 2]. In such cases, the differential diagnoses are: PHPT with co-existing CKD, SHPT, THPT, FHH, or ectopic PTH secretion. In PHPT with co-existing CKD there will be hypercalcemia and hypophosphatemia. While in SHPT there will be hypocalcemia, decreased vit D synthesis and increased phosphate levels. In tertiary HPT, there will be a history of prolonged SPHT (i.e., normo- or hypocalcemia with increased PTH), serum phosphorous will be increased or normal and it occurs usually following renal transplant after prolonged SHPT. Renal insufficiency in PHPT results from hypercalciuria which in turn causes damage to tubular cells in loop of Henle, Collecting duct, distal tubule, down-regulates aquaporin expression which reduces the urinary concentrating ability and reduces glomerular blood flow and glomerular filtration. Several clinicopathological features of PHPT are modified by renal insufficiency. Hypertension has been reported to be more prevalent in PHPT patients than in matched control subjects [3]. The high frequency of hypertension in PHPT patients together with peripheral insulin insensitivity may contribute to the increased risk of cardiovascular disease in these patients. PTH increases production of 1,25(OH)2D from 25OHD by stimulating renal 1-a-hydroxylase activity. An important point to remember is that progression of PHPT can be caused by loss of renal mass and resistance to PTH in patients with renal dysfunction. Serum 1,25(OH)2D concentrations start to decline early in the course of renal failure. Because 1,25(OH)2D is required to correct skeletal resistance to the calcemic action of PTH and it inhibits synthesis and secretion of PTH in vitro and in vivo, and reduced 1,25(OH)2D promotes proliferation of the parathyroid glands, resulting in a vicious cycle of HPT. This also explains the increased frequency of multiglandular disease in the renal insufficiency group [4]. A study by Tassone et al. [5] addresses renal function in primary hyperparathyroidism for the first time employing KDIGO GFR categories and GFR estimation using the CKD-EPI formula. In their series of PHPT patients, PTH levels did not rise as a result of renal impairment until GFR was below 45 mL/min/1.73 m^2. Their results support the hypothesis that the impact of moderate to severe renal insufficiency on the clinical expression of PHTP might be mediated by further PTH hypersecretion. Since multiglandular disease is more likely in such cases, bilateral exploration should be preferred. Further, in patients with primary hyperparathyroidism and concurrent stage III chronic kidney disease, a stricter criterion of a >50% intraoperative parathormone decrease to a normal range should be used for successful parathyroidectomy [6].

References

1. Jones DB, Jones JH, Lloyd HJ, Lucas PA, Wilkins WE, Walker DA. Changes in blood pressure and renal function after parathyroidectomy in primary hyperparathyroidism. Postgrad Med J. 1983;59:350–3.
2. Kristoffersson A, Backman C, Granqvist K, Jarhult J. Pre- and postoperative evaluation of renal function with five different tests in patients with primary hyperparathyroidism. J Intern Med. 1990;227:317–24.
3. Nainby-Luxmoore JC, Langford HG, Nelson NC, Watson RL, Barnes TY. A case-comparison study of hypertension and hyperparathyroidism. J Clin Endocrinol Metab. 1982;55:303–6.
4. Yamashita H, Noguchi S, Uchino S, Watanabe S, Murakami T, Ogawa T, Masatsugu T, Takamatsu Y. Eiji Miyatake and Hiroto Yamashita Influence of renal function on clinico-pathological features of primary hyperparathyroidism. Eur J Endocrinol. 2003;148:597–602.
5. Tassone F, Gianotti L, Emmolo I, Ghio M, Borretta G. Glomerular filtration rate and parathyroid hormone secretion in primary hyperparathyroidism. J Clin Endocrinol Metab. 2009;94:4458–61.
6. Liu SN, Yusufali AH, Mao ML, Khan ZF, Farrá JC, Lew JI. Stricter ioPTH criterion for successful parathyroidectomy in stage III CKD patients with primary hyperparathyroidism. Surgery. 2018;164(6):1306–10.

PHPT Presenting with Poor Mentation

Case
Relatives of a 72-year-old man presented with complaints of increased somnolescence and a history of recurrent episodes of altered sensorium and slurring of speech for 3 months and also gave a history that he was having pain in lower limbs for 1 year and generalized weakness, loss of appetite, and dysphagia for 3 months. He also had a history of abdominal pain on and off which was diagnosed as that of gallstones. There was no history of proximal muscle weakness, bony pains, recurrent fractures, renal stones, graveluria or hematuria, or mood swings. He was having NIDDM for 12 years and was also hypertensive. On examination he was conscious but was having impaired orientation. Evaluation revealed elevated Calcium: 12.3, 11.7 mmol/L (8.5–10.5) (on two occasions) low serum Phosphorous: 1.3 mg/dL (2.5–4.5), elevated serum PTH: 207, 145.6 pg/mL (9–55) (on two occasion), ALP: 74 IU/dL (55–150) and low 25 hydroxy vitamin D: 14.3 ng/mL (9–47). BMD revealed osteoporosis at forearm 3.2. Ultrasound neck showed 2.1 × 0.9 cm hypoechoic lesion with increased vascularity in left upper thyroid lobe—likely left superior parathyroid lesion and MIBI SPECT scan showed MIBI avid tumor (persistent focal uptake on delayed images) (Fig. 1) in relation to upper pole of left thyroid lobe. CT brain showed cerebral ischemic changes. He underwent focused parathyroidectomy with IOPTH monitoring and a 2 g adenoma (Fig. 2) was removed with more than 50% fall in IOPTH. Postoperatively there was subjective improvement in mentation.

Amit Agarwal is the lead author of this chapter.

A. Agarwal et al., *Case Studies in Thyroid and Parathyroid Tumors*,
https://doi.org/10.1007/978-981-99-0938-4_12

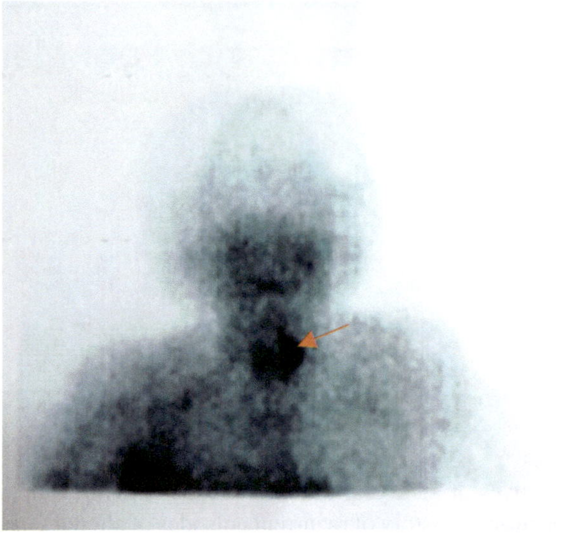

Fig. 1 MIBI scan showing left superior MIBI avid lesion (arrow)

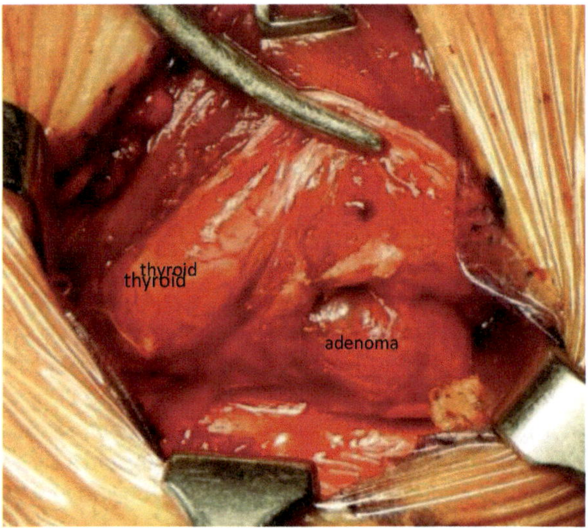

Fig. 2 Intraoperative view showing left superior adenoma

Discussion

Many studies suggest PHPT is associated with impaired quality of life (QOL) and depression [1, 2]. While less well studied, some have demonstrated reduced memory or impairment in other cognitive domains [3, 4]. More controversial is whether neuropsychological symptoms are specifically attributable to PHPT and reversible with surgical correction of the disorder. PTH-induced vascular dysfunction within the intracerebral circulation might compromise cerebral vascular function or blood flow regulation and thereby account for the observed cognitive changes in PHPT. Liu et al. [5] showed that although higher PTH was associated with worse intracerebral autoregulation, cerebrovascular function, cognition, and mood were normal in mild PHPT. PTX did not improve vascular or cognitive function. The observed improvement in mood cannot be clearly attributed to PTX.

References

1. Iacovelli E, Gilio F, Mascia ML, Scillitani A, Romagnoli E, Pichiorri F, Fucile S, Minisola S, Inghilleri M. Acute and chronic effects of hypercalcaemia on cortical excitability as studied by 5 Hz repetitive transcranial magnetic stimulation. J Physiol. 2011;589:1619–26.
2. Coker LH, Rorie K, Cantley L, Kirkland K, Stump D, Burbank N, Tembreull T, Williamson J, Perrier N. Primary hyperparathyroidism, cognition, and health-related quality of life. Ann Surg. 2005;242:642.
3. Chiang CY, Andrewes DG, Anderson D, Devere M, Schweitzer I, Zajac JD. A controlled, prospective study of neuropsychological outcomes post parathyroidectomy in primary hyperparathyroid patients. Clin Endocrinol. 2005;62:99.
4. Kastrup O, Maschke M, Wanke I, Diener HC. Posterior reversible encephalopathy syndrome due to severe hypercalcemia. J Neurol. 2002;249:1563–6.
5. Liu M, Sum M, Cong E, Colon I, Bucovsky M, Williams J, Kepley A, Kuo J, Lee JA, Lazar RM, Marshall R, Silverberg S, Walker MD. Cognition and cerebrovascular function in primary hyperparathyroidism before and after parathyroidectomy. J Endocrinol Investig. 2020;43(3):369–79.

PHPT Presenting as a Jaw Tumor

Case

A 35-year-old lady presented with a history of having undergone segmental resection of the mandible with plate reconstruction (Fig. 1) for a progressively increasing painless swelling of the lower jaw which was thought to be a giant cell tumor of the mandible. The HPE showed multinucleated giant cells with trabeculae and new bone formation. Orthopantogram and X-ray of the mandible showed a lytic, multifocal lesion without a sclerotic margin (Figs. 2, 3). HPE of resected jaw tumor (Fig. 4) was reported as brown tumor and hence the patient was referred for further management. On examination, she was found to be having an anterior neck swelling, 2 × 2 cm moving with deglutition. She was evaluated further and was found to be having elevated serum ionized calcium, 1.57 mmol/L (1.15–1.33 mmol/L), elevated PTH, 27.34 pmol/L (1.6–6.9 pool/L), low phosphorous, 2.38 mg/dL (2.3–4.7), elevated ALP, 1036 IU/L (60.0–270.0), extremely low Vitamin D levels, 18.79 nmol/L (50–250). Skeletal survey revealed brown tumors of skull and BMD showed osteoporosis with a *T*-score of −3.1 at fore arm, −3.2 at Hip, and −2.1 at spine. Hence a clinical diagnosis of primary hyperparathyroidism was made. Both USG (Fig. 5) and MIBI were concordant for an inferior parathyroid adenoma, 2.4 × 2.7 × 1.4 cm. She was taken up for parathyroidectomy and in view of intraoperative adhesions to thyroid, en-block hemithyroidectomy with excision of inferior parathyroid adenoma (Fig. 6) was done. IOPTH showed curative fall according to Miami criteria (pre-excision value of 28.78 pmol/L and 10 min value of 15.66 pmol/L). This case highlights the unnecessary and mutilating surgery performed for a curable systemic disease.

Amit Agarwal is the lead author of this chapter.

A. Agarwal et al., *Case Studies in Thyroid and Parathyroid Tumors*,
https://doi.org/10.1007/978-981-99-0938-4_13

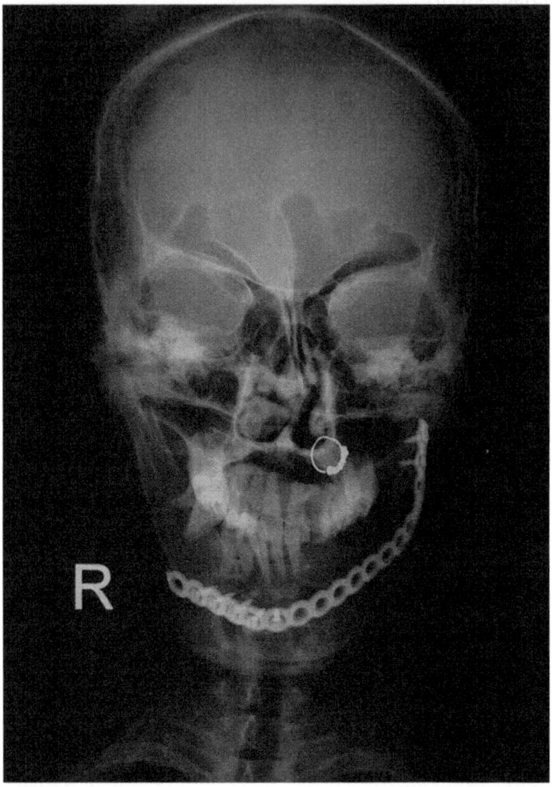

Fig. 1 Plain X-ray showing plate reconstruction after hemi-mandibulectomy

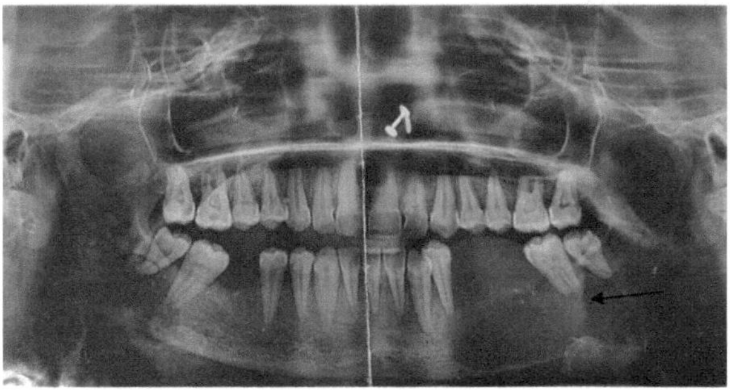

Fig. 2 An orthopantomogram of the patient that demonstrates a multifocal brown tumor of the left and right body of the mandible showing ground-glass attenuation with thin cortex and sharp margins

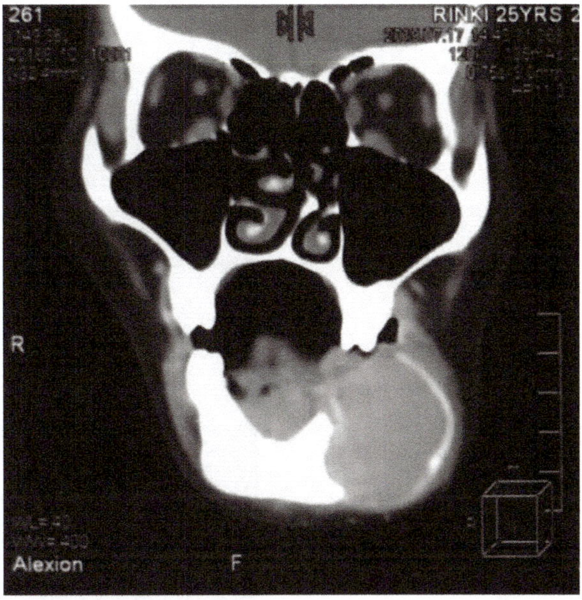

Fig. 3 Axial CT images showing brown tumor of left mandible

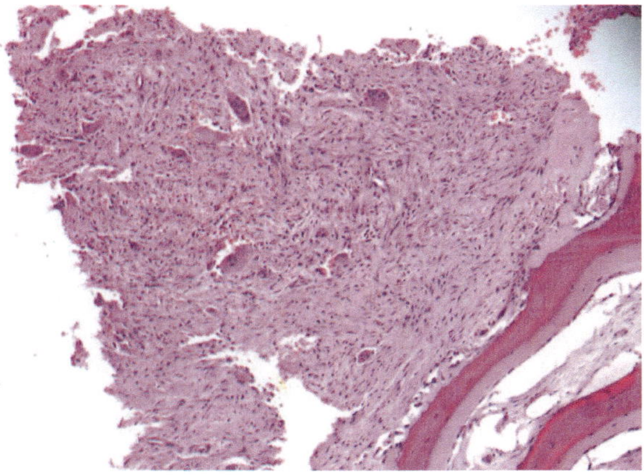

Fig. 4 HPE of the resected mandibular tumor showing: the image shows a zone of bone resorption in the center. The resulting defect has been filled with fibroblastic tissue. Around the periphery are osteoid-producing cells

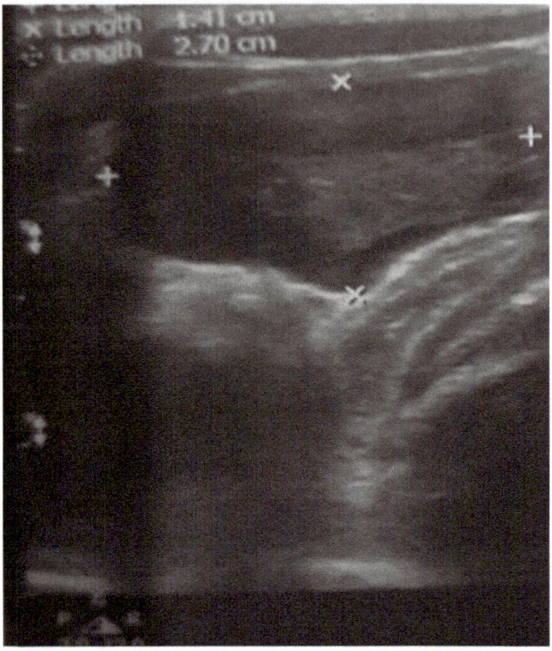

Fig. 5 USG pic showing a hypoechoic adenoma

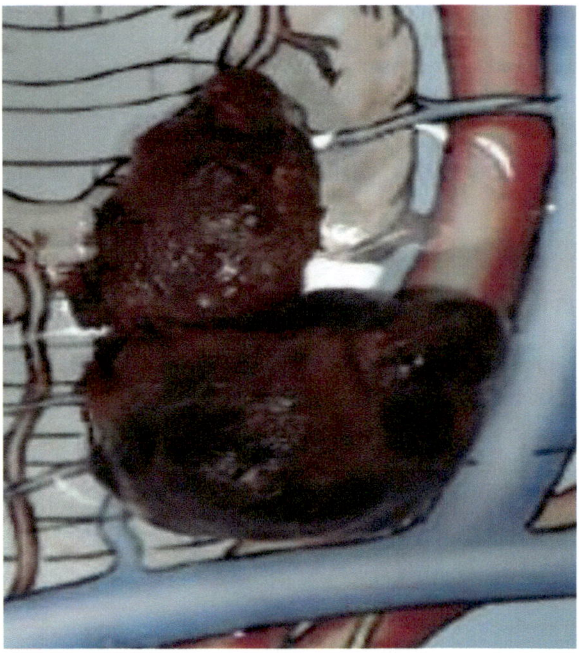

Fig. 6 Specimen of en-block hemithyroidectomy-parathyroid adenoma excision. Adenoma weighed 12 g (arrow)

Discussion

The differential diagnosis of a jaw tumor which has a ground-glass attenuation could be: **Ossifying fibroma, Brown tumor, Fibrous dysplasia, or Renal osteodystrophy.** In any such jaw swelling, the following four features should be noted:

1. Whether the swelling is tooth-related or osseous
2. Whether the appearance of lesion is ground-glass, sclerotic, lytic, or mixed sclerotic-lytic,
3. Whether the transition zone between normal and abnormal bone is narrow or wide
4. Whether the ground glass attenuation is diffuse (renal osteodystrophy, fibrous dysplasia), unifocal (seen in ossifying fibroma), or multifocal (brown tumors)

Ossifying Fibroma Associated with HPT-JT Syndrome

It is more common in women with peak incidence in the third and fourth decade of life. Their typical appearance is unifocal, unilocular expansile lesion with sharp margins and sclerotic rim, and low-attenuation halo. Ossifying fibromas of the jaw are benign lesions. However, they demonstrate locally invasive features, e.g., they may splay the teeth. They are expansile and can cause facial asymmetry. They can extend into the maxillary sinus or into the orbital floor where they may cause peri-orbital swelling or orbital pain. If left untreated, ossifying fibromas may continue to enlarge (usually >10 cm) and become severely disfiguring. It is usually associated with HPT-JT syndrome.

Fibrous Dysplasia

It is of three types and seen in association with Albright syndrome, cranio-fibrous dysplasia, and Lichtenstein-Jaffe fibrous dysplasia. At imaging, it is more likely than other lesions to have a ground glass appearance but with a wide and ill-defined transition zone and with a sclerotic and thick cortex unlike renal osteodystrophy which has a thin cortex. And unlike ossifying fibromas, the lesion of fibrous dysplasia expands more in the longitudinal direction.

Renal Osteodystrophy

Chronic renal failure may manifest two types of jaw tumors:

1. Cranio-facial bone lesions—when there are marked expansile facial deformities with macrognathia, cortial thickening and protrusion, and splaying of teeth (Saglikkar syndrome)

2. Benign fibro-osseous lesions which appear as areas of diffuse ground-glass attenuation and bone expansion of mandible/maxilla but with loss of definition of the cortex (a feature that differentiates it from the thick cortex seen in fibrous dysplasia)

Brown Tumors Associated with Sporadic PHPT

Usually associated with advanced PHPT but now rarely seen in developed countries. It is a lesion with multifocal ground-glass attenuation with thin cortex and sharp margins with hypoattenuation at the center. It is more lytic than ground glass (unlike the typical ground glass appearance of fibrous dysplasia) and lack the sclerotic rim associated with ossifying fibroma. The cornerstone of treatment of these lesions is reversal of hypercalcemia by parathyroidectomy. After treatment of the underlying metabolic disorder, brown tumors of jaw tend to become sclerotic and show regression Fig. 1 USG pic showing a hypoechoic adenoma.

Lithium-Induced Primary Hyperparathyroidism

Case
A 71-year-old male, who was suffering from bipolar disease, was treated with lithium therapy for many years. However, this therapy was discontinued, after he was found to have slightly raised adjusted calcium of 2.69 mmol/L, with a parathyroid hormone (PTH) of 14.3 pmol/L. About 2 years after cessation of therapy, he had developed osteoporosis, with calcium levels of 2.73 mmol/L and a PTH of 18.3 pmol/L.

As there had been no significant improvement since the cessation of his lithium, the patient was referred to the endocrine surgery department to discuss the option of surgical intervention. He underwent localization studies, which were negative. His ultrasound scan (US) only revealed a multinodular goiter, while the Technetium 99m Sestamibi (MIBI) did not show any avid lesions. Therefore, it was decided to perform a bilateral neck exploration, with inspection of all four parathyroid glands.

During this procedure, the right inferior and left superior gland were found to be enlarged, and were thus removed, while the other two parathyroid glands looked macroscopically normal in size and appearance and were left in situ. The final histology report showed that both removed glands were hyperplastic parathyroid glands. The patient is currently 2 years after his surgery, without any clinical or biochemical signs of recurrence, and has remained off his lithium therapy.

Discussion

Lithium is a mood stabilizer, mostly used as the first line treatment of bipolar disorder, as it is efficacious for both acute manic and depressive episodes, and also has long-term mood stabilizing effects [1]. Importantly, lithium has a narrow

Rajeev Parameswaran is the lead author of this chapter.

A. Agarwal et al., *Case Studies in Thyroid and Parathyroid Tumors*,
https://doi.org/10.1007/978-981-99-0938-4_14

therapeutic index, and has potential major adverse effects on the metabolic, renal, and endocrine systems, even at presumably safe therapeutic levels [2]. While most side effects are short-term and reversible after cessation of lithium, others are irreversible, such as lithium-induced hyperparathyroidism (LIH) [3]. LIH was first reported in 1973, but its exact pathophysiology as well as the appropriate management remain unclear. Although estimates vary widely, reported prevalence of LIH range from rare to almost 25% [4, 5].

It has been shown that lithium has the potential to increase the levels of serum calcium and PTH within weeks of initiation, but these do usually stay within the higher range of normal. The exact mechanisms of LIH remain to be elucidated, but it has been hypothesized that lithium can alter calcium metabolism in both acute and chronic ways [6]. According to the set-point hypothesis, lithium has the potential to directly antagonize the calcium-sensitive receptors (CaSR), thereby altering the set-point at which parathyroid glands react to plasma levels of calcium [7]. Others have postulated lithium to stimulate the development of parathyroid hyperplasia or adenoma [8], which could explain the relatively high rates of multi-glandular disease among lithium users. In clinical practice, 85–95% are caused by single gland disease, and multiglandular disease is seen in 5–10% of cases [9]. While a third hypothesis is based on the induction of hypocalcemia due to the inhibition of the intracellular second messenger cyclic adenosine monophosphate (cAMP) [8].

Also, there are no monitoring guidelines to help physicians screen patients for lithium-induced hyperparathyroidism. Guidelines on the management of patients for bipolar disorders proposed by the National Institute of Clinical Excellence guidelines in the UK [5] and the Royal Australian and New Zealand College of Psychiatrists [10] do not specifically mention the monitoring of calcium levels in patients treated with lithium. Some recommend that serum calcium level should be checked before commencing treatment with lithium and 6 monthly thereafter [11].

Prospective studies comparing different treatment pathways are currently lacking. There are generally four main strategies for the management of LIH. Firstly, lithium may be discontinued, since the acute effects of lithium are potentially reversible with cessation of therapy [12]. While normalization of calcium levels can occur within the first month in short-term users, it is unlikely in those having received lithium for more than a decade. Secondly, careful, but vigilant, surveillance may be an option for select patients. Thirdly, especially for those in whom cessation of therapy is no option, the use of calcimimetic therapy has been described [13], but not a definitive therapy. Fourthly, surgery can be considered, although there is an ongoing debate on the exact indications as well as the optimal surgical approach (i.e., four gland exploration versus focused parathyroidectomy).

Some groups have shown a focused approach to be beneficial, in a selected group of the patient in whom preoperative imaging demonstrates a single adenoma and when the use of intraoperative PTH monitoring is available [13]. However, LIH has a high chance of having multi-gland involvement, suggesting the need of an upfront bilateral neck exploration to reduce persistent or recurrent disease, as is the recommendation in the current guideline of the European Society of Endocrine Surgeons (ESES) [4]. Two published series from Australia and Sweden showed a recurrence rate of 16% and 42% following surgical intervention [14, 15]. To decrease the incidence of recurrence, it is therefore important to identify all glands and resect the diseased ones to achieve cure. Focused parathyroidectomy may be an option in patients where imaging is suggestive of single-gland disease but to rely on preoperative imaging alone may be unwise where the intention is to perform a focused parathyroidectomy [14].

References

1. Licht RW. Lithium: still a major option in the management of bipolar disorder. CNS Neurosci Ther. 2012;18(3):219–26.
2. McKnight RF, Adida M, Budge K, Stockton S, Goodwin GM, Geddes JR. Lithium toxicity profile: a systematic review and meta-analysis. Lancet. 2012;379(9817):721–8.
3. Bendz H, Sjödin I, Toss G, Berglund K. Hyperparathyroidism and long-term lithium therapy--a cross-sectional study and the effect of lithium withdrawal. J Intern Med. 1996;240(6):357–65.
4. Barczyński M, Bränström R, Dionigi G, Mihai R. Sporadic multiple parathyroid gland disease--a consensus report of the European Society of Endocrine Surgeons (ESES). Langenbeck's Arch Surg. 2015;400(8):887–905.
5. Awad SS, Miskulin J, Thompson N. Parathyroid adenomas versus four-gland hyperplasia as the cause of primary hyperparathyroidism in patients with prolonged lithium therapy. World J Surg. 2003;27(4):486–8.
6. Shapiro HI, Davis KA. Hypercalcemia and "primary" hyperparathyroidism during lithium therapy. Am J Psychiatry. 2015;172(1):12–5.
7. Nair CG, Menon R, Jacob P, Babu M. Lithium-induced parathyroid dysfunction: a new case. Indian J Endocrinol Metab. 2013;17(5):930–2.
8. Livingstone C, Rampes H. Lithium: a review of its metabolic adverse effects. J Psychopharmacol. 2006;20(3):347–55.
9. Sitges-Serra A, Bergenfelz A. Clinical update: sporadic primary hyperparathyroidism. Lancet. 2007;370(9586):468–70.
10. Malhi GS, Bell E, Boyce P, Bassett D, Berk M, Bryant R, et al. The 2020 Royal Australian and New Zealand College of psychiatrists clinical practice guidelines for mood disorders: bipolar disorder summary. Bipolar Disord. 2020;22(8):805–21.
11. Livingstone C, Rampes H. Lithium: a review of its metabolic adverse effects. J Psychopharmacol. 2005;20(3):347–55.
12. Mifsud S, Cilia K, Mifsud EL, Gruppetta M. Lithium-associated hyperparathyroidism. Br J Hosp Med (Lond). 2020;81(11):1–9.
13. Meehan AD, Udumyan R, Kardell M, Landén M, Järhult J, Wallin G. Lithium-associated hypercalcemia: pathophysiology, prevalence, management. World J Surg. 2018;42(2):415–24.
14. Norlén O, Sidhu S, Sywak M, Delbridge L. Long-term outcome after parathyroidectomy for lithium-induced hyperparathyroidism. Br J Surg. 2014;101(10):1252–6.
15. Järhult J, Ander S, Asking B, Jansson S, Meehan A, Kristoffersson A, et al. Long-term results of surgery for lithium-associated hyperparathyroidism. Br J Surg. 2010;97(11):1680–5.

Hyperparathyroidism with Femur Fracture

Severe morbidities of hyperparathyroidism like fractures, nephrolithiasis, or neuropsychiatric symptoms continue to remain prevalent in developing countries. A patient presenting with pathological femur fracture secondary to undiagnosed or in appropriately treated hyperparathyroidism lead to patient suffering in form of delayed or non-healing of fracture, malunion, limp discrepancies, and movement restrictions apart from other manifestations of HPT.

Case

A young female aged about 22 years presented with pain in right hip following a trivial trauma four months ago. The underlying femur fracture showed poor healing despite necessary orthopedic management. She had severe restriction of daily activities with her left lower limb externally rotated and shortened. A history of generalized weakness for the last 10 years, irritability compounded with forgetfulness, epigastric pain, and increased frequency of micturition for 2 months was elicited. She had undergone right nephrolithotomy and left PCNL 10 years back for kidney stones, Caldwell Luc Surgery for ossifying fibroma left cheek 4 years ago. Other family members did not have any similar complaints.

Biochemical evaluation revealed hypercalcemia [12.1 mg/dL (Total), normal range: 8.6–10.3 mg/dL, 7.29 mg/dl (Ionic), normal range:4.5–5.5 mg/dL], hypophosphatemia [2.12 mg/dL, normal range: 2.5–4.5 mg/dL] and hyperparathyroidism [843.50 pg/mL, normal range: 15–65 pg/mL], elevated serum alkaline phosphatase [617 IU/L, normal range:0–240 IU/L]. Vitamin D, serum Mg, s gastrin, and prolactin were within normal limits. Radiographic examination revealed left femur fracture with osteopenia and subperiosteal bone resorption (Fig. 1). DEXA scan had severe osteoporosis distal forearm [T-Score: -5.3], hip [T-Score: -2.7], and vertebrae [T-Score: -2.7].

Anand Mishra is the lead author of this chapter.

A. Agarwal et al., *Case Studies in Thyroid and Parathyroid Tumors*,
https://doi.org/10.1007/978-981-99-0938-4_15

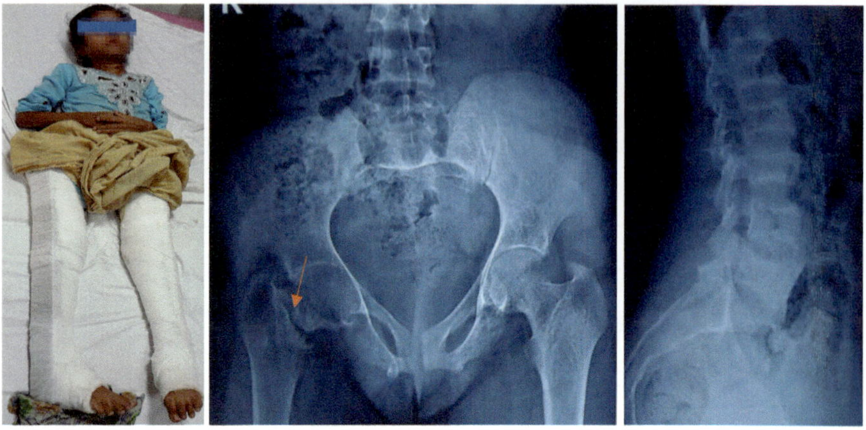

Fig. 1 PHPT patient with bilateral femur

MIBI scan and HRUSG neck were corroborating for right inferior parathyroid adenoma measuring 2.3 × 1.2 cm, however oval hypoechoic lesion (12 × 7 mm) adjacent to left carotid? ectopic parathyroid? lymph node.

She was optimized and underwent bilateral neck exploration and right inferior parathyroid adenectomy. A bilobed gland of size 2 × 2 cm, weighing 2.1 g, and retro esophageal extension of posterior limb was excised. Histopathological examination was suggestive of parathyroid adenoma. The perioperative period was uneventful.

Discussion

In developed countries, 80% patients of with PHPT are asymptomatic whereas the scenario is reversed in developing countries where 70% of the patients are symptomatic and present with fractures, nephrolithiasis or psychiatric symptoms even in young patients [1]. A high prevalence of vitamin D deficiency among the young population in developing countries may be the reason for significant skeletal manifestations [2]. Forearm, vertebral, and hip fractures are commoner in PHPT compared to matched population [3]. Misdiagnosis, inappropriate management at the first point of contact, and financial constraints lead to significant patient suffering. A patient presenting very late as femur fractures add to severe morbidity to the patient in form of delayed or non-healing, malunion, limb discrepancies, mobility restrictions of fracture sites, or multiple other bone fractures [4]. Only age and gender are significant predictors of fracture risk in HPT [5].

A patient's vague symptoms of weakness, myalgia, constipation, thirst, polyuria, depression, anxiety, anger, and sleep disturbances should be adequately evaluated for a timely diagnosis of HPT [6]. These patients merit proper immobilization and subsequent fixation of the fracture site after normalization of serum biochemical parameters post-parathyroid surgery [7].

Conclusion

Increased awareness and high index of suspicion by physicians' awareness can avoid various severe morbidities and long-term systemic dysfunctions of HPT.

References

1. Lin X, Fan Y, Zhang Z, Yue H, Brunetti G, Guarnieri V, et al. Clinical Characteristics of Primary Hyperparathyroidism: 15-Year Experience of 457 Patients in a. Single Center in China. Front Endocrinol. 2021;12:602221. Available from: www.frontiersin.org
2. Kumar Yadav S, Johri G, Ahmed Bichoo R, Kumar Jha C, Kintu-Luwaga R. Primary hyperparathyroidism in developing world: a systematic review on the changing clinical profile of the disease. Arch Endocrinol Metab. 2020;64(2):105–10. Available from: https://orcid.org/0000-0002-0682-4970
3. Ejlsmark-Svensson H, Rolighed L, Harsløf T, Rejnmark L. Risk of fractures in primary hyperparathyroidism: a systematic review and meta-analysis. Osteoporos Int. 2021;32(6):1053–60. https://doi.org/10.1007/s00198-021-05822-9. Epub 2021 Feb 1
4. Lewiecki EM, Miller PD. Skeletal effects of primary hyperparathyroidism: bone mineral density and fracture risk. J Clin Densitom. 2013;16(1):28–32.
5. Khosla S, Melton LJ 3rd, Wermers RA, Crowson CS, O'Fallon W, Bl R. Primary hyperparathyroidism and the risk of fracture: a population-based study. J Bone Miner Res. 1999;14(10):1700–7. https://doi.org/10.1359/jbmr.1999.14.10.1700.
6. Allerheiligen DA, Schoeber J, Houston RE, Mohl VK, Wildman KM. Hyperparathyroidism. Am Fam Physician. 1998;57(8):1795.
7. Tang F, Zhang W, Luo H, Wang Y, Tu C. Case Report Primary hyperparathyroidism presenting as bilateral femoral shaft fractures with severe bone mineral loss and normocalcemia in a young adult male: a case report. Int J Clin Exp Med. 2017;10:3787–93. Available from: www.ijcem.com/

Hypercalcemic Crisis

A hyperfunctioning parathyroid gland can occasionally present with elevations of serum calcium levels that can cause severe morbidity and occasionally result in loss of life. Hypercalcemic crisis though rare is an endocrine emergency that merits emergent measures and gives gratifying results.

Case
A healthy 31-year-old female presented with a sudden onset of generalized weakness, abdominal pain, and 1 episode of generalized tonic-clonic seizures. She was disoriented with raised blood pressure 170/100 at presentation. She was intubated and put on ventilatory support. Electrocardiogram showed sinus tachycardia, diffuse ST depressions, and prolonged QT interval. Bedside echocardiogram showed preserved ejection fraction and no wall motion abnormalities. Initial labs revealed severe hypercalcemia of 21.8 mg/dL with other parameters within the normal limits. Four liters of normal saline boluses were given in the initial 4 h followed by continuous forced saline diuresis and she was put on cerebro-protective strategy and other routine ICU care. Persistent hypercalcemia responded to Zolendronic acid infusion. HRUSG neck was done which showed 24 × 26 mm left inferior parathyroid lesion. PTH was more than 744 pg/mL (0–65). She was gradually weaned off the ventilator. BMD scan revealed osteoporosis at all distal forearm, femur neck, and vertebrae. MIBI scan and USG scan corroborated with each other. She was optimized and underwent an uneventful focused parathyroidectomy.

Discussion

Hypercalcemic crisis is life-threatening emergency clinical state characterized by progressive and markedly raised serum calcium levels. Patients often present with

Anand Mishra is the lead author of this chapter.

A. Agarwal et al., *Case Studies in Thyroid and Parathyroid Tumors*,
https://doi.org/10.1007/978-981-99-0938-4_16

profound anorexia, emesis, and altered mental status. They are severely dehydrated with occasionally compromised renal function and very likely to rapid deterioration and death if not treated appropriately [1, 2]. A cut-off serum calcium >14.5 mg/dL along with acute symptoms which reverses after lowering of calcium values is the generally accepted criterion for diagnosing hypercalcemia [3].

The incidence of hyperparathyroid-induced hypercalcemic crisis (HIHC) ranges from 1.6 to 6%. Primary hyperparathyroidism is responsible for more than 90% of outpatients evaluated for hypercalcemia. All age groups are susceptible though it more common during sixth decade and beyond. As for parathyroid carcinoma, HIHC is equally distributed among males and females [4].

An adenoma in one or more of the parathyroid glands is the commonest underlying cause in these cases. Parathyroid carcinoma though a rare cause of PHPT can be responsible for about 5% of HIHC [5]. Offending glands in HIHC may show areas of necrosis, fibrosis, hemorrhage micro cysts, and intra-cytoplasmic vacuoles which are not commonly seen in parathyroid lesions presenting without crisis [6].

Aggressive fluid replacement and diuresis is the cornerstone of management in emergent management of hypercalcemic crisis. This is attained by infusing isotonic saline at rates between 2 and 4 L/day depending upon the volume status or risk for precipitating circulatory compromise in the individual. Loop diuretics promotes calcium secretion, but its use should be curtailed to those in whom rehydration alone fails or precipitates cardiac compromise. Intravenous bisphosphonates like zolendronate decreases calcium levels within 24 h and falls to its nadir in 7 days in about 70 to 90% of patients. They act by inhibiting osteoclastic bone resorption and has been approved by Food and Drug Administration (FDA) as an agent of first choice [7]. Bisphosphonates can be used to buy time in patients unfit for surgery and its response may last from a week to months. Denosumab, a RANKL inhibitor though costly can be used in patients with renal compromise in whom bisphosphonates are contraindicated. Calcitonin also acts by inhibiting osteoclast function and can be used with other calcium-reducing measures. Though its effects are short-lived it can help in rapid reduction of calcium levels by more than 1 to 2 mg/dL.

Although immediate medical management and stabilization is very important in patients presenting with hypercalcemia, parathyroidectomy is the only curative modality. Though parathyroidectomy can be safely and effectively performed under local anesthesia in select cases, prompt medical management is the key to the successful management of hypercalcemic crisis.

Conclusion

Prompt recognition of HIHC and treatment with rehydration and forced saline diuresis along with bisphosphonates followed by a semi-emergent focused parathyroidectomy (when imaging is concordant) should be the standard of care in HIHC patients.

References

1. Wang CA, Guyton SW. Hyperparathyroid crisis: clinical and pathologic studies of 14 patients. Ann Surg. 1979;190(6):782–90.
2. Sarfati E, Desportes L, Gossot D. Acute primary hyperparathyroidism: experience of 59 cases. Dubost CBR J Surg. 1989;76(9):979–81.
3. Kebebew E, Clark OH. Parathyroid adenoma, hyperplasia, and carcinoma. Localization, technical details of primary neck exploration, and treatment of hypercalcemic crisis. Surg Oncol Clin North Am. 1998;7:721–48.
4. Fitzpatrick LA, Bilezikian JP. Acute primary hyperparathyroidism. Am J Med. 1987;82:2.
5. Gasparri G, Camandona M, Mullineris B, Raggio E, Vigna S, Dei Poli M. Acute hyperparathyroidism: our experience with 36 cases. Ann Ital Chir. 2004;75(3):321–4.
6. Starker LF, Björklund P, Theoharis C, Long WD 3rd, Carling T, Udelsman R. Clinical and histopathological characteristics of hyperparathyroidism-induced hypercalcemic crisis. World J Surg. 2011;35(2):331–5.
7. Stewart AF. Clinical practice. Hypercalcemia associated with cancer. N Engl J Med. 2005;352(4):373–9.

PHPT Presenting as Pancreatitis

Case 1: PHPT Presenting as Acute Pancreatitis

A 22-year-old boy, an engineer by profession, presented with a history of multiple episodes of non-bilious, non-projectile vomiting containing undigested food particles along with decreased appetite and generalized weakness since last 25 days. He also had abdominal pain for last 10 days which was sudden in onset, localized in epigastric region, severe in intensity, throbbing in nature, relieved on bending forwards, non-radiating, and non-migratory in nature. He had severe constipation for 7 days which was relieved with laxatives. On examination, he was sitting with forward bending. His biochemical profile was: S. Calcium (total): 14.7 mg/dL (9.0–11.0), S. Calcium (ionized): 2.06 mmol/L (1.15–1.33), S. Magnesium: 1.3 mg/dL (1.7–2.4), S. Alkaline phosphatase: 255, S. Amylase: 2240 (day 1), 409 (day 5), 277 (day 10), S. Lipase: 3510 (day 1), 475 (day 5), 146 (day 10), iPTH: 76.13 pmol/mL (1.6–6.9), S creatinine 1.48 mg/dL. Bone densitometry (DXA): Forearm- T score − 4.9, z score − 4.9. Ultrasonography whole abdomen showed mild hepatosplenomegaly, partially distended gall bladder, tail of pancreas obscured, no ascites, and Grade II medico-renal disease. CECT whole abdomen revealed acute pancreatic (Fig. 1) with cholelithiasis and bilateral enlarged kidneys. Ultrasonography neck and MIBI were concordant for left inferior parathyroid adenoma. He was optimized but his serum lipase and amylase remained elevated. Despite the ongoing process of pancreatitis he was taken up for surgery. He underwent focused left inferior parathyroidectomy and 1.5 × 1.0 cm adenoma was removed with curative fall in IOPTH(pmol/L):

- Pre – incision: 167.7 pmol/L.
- Pre – excision: 68.2 pmol/L.
- Post – excision (5 min): 32.66 pmol/L.
- Post – excision (10 min): 23.61 pmol/L.
- Post – excision (15 min): 18.29 pmol/L.

Amit Agarwal is the lead author of this chapter.

A. Agarwal et al., *Case Studies in Thyroid and Parathyroid Tumors*,
https://doi.org/10.1007/978-981-99-0938-4_17

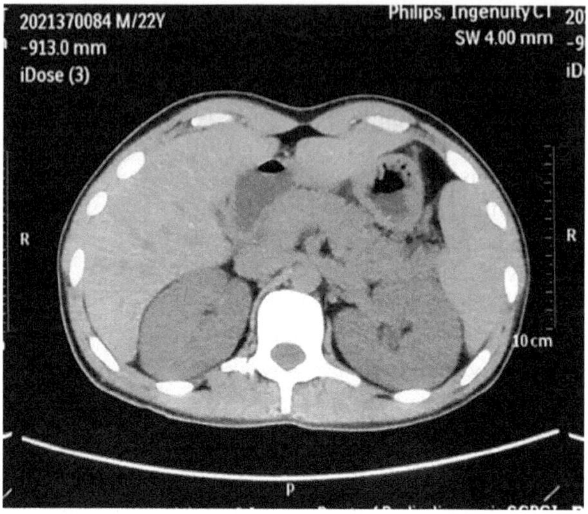

Fig. 1 CECT showing bulky pancreas with fat stranding suggestive of acute pancreatitis

In the postoperative period he did well and his serum amylase and lipase gradually came back to normal levels. During the one year of follow-up he did not experience further attack of pancreatitis and is eucalcemic.

Case 2: PHPT with Recurrent Acute Pancreatitis

A 40-year-old female was seen with severe pain abdomen × 1 day. Patient c/o severe acute onset pain in the epigastric region, radiating to back and associated with vomiting and obstipation. Pain was continuous and required iv analgesic. She was diagnosed as having acute pancreatitis with CT severity score of 6/10. Patient had similar pain 1 month ago and was diagnosed to have mild acute pancreatitis managed elsewhere conservatively and was relieved in 1 week. She also gave history of 5 such attacks of acute pancreatitis in last 5 years. She was found to be having elevated calcium and PTH (164.6 2) with low vit D (24.90). Both USG neck and parathyroid scan did not reveal any parathyroid adenoma. With a diagnosis of multiglandular hyperplasia she underwent bilateral exploration. All 4 glands were found to be enlarged (Figs. 2 and 3) and a 3 and half gland parathyroidectomy was done. It has been 10 years since her surgery and she is eucalcemic and did not have any attacks of acute pancreatitis during this period.

Case 3: PHPT with Chronic Pancreatitis

A 25 year-old female presented with a complaint of abdominal pain for 9 months. She gave a history of generalized body aches, generalized weakness, history of nausea and vomiting; history of amenorrhea for 6 months. No history of galactorrhea, recurrent fractures, renal stones, and headache. She was diagnosed as chronic pancreatitis since childhood and gave a history of repeated hospitalization. On examination patient was found to be emaciated (Fig. 4) and her systemic examination was unremarkable and there was no neck swelling. Her biochemistry and CECT confirmed the diagnosis of chronic pancreatitis (Fig. 5): serum amylase (79 u/L) and

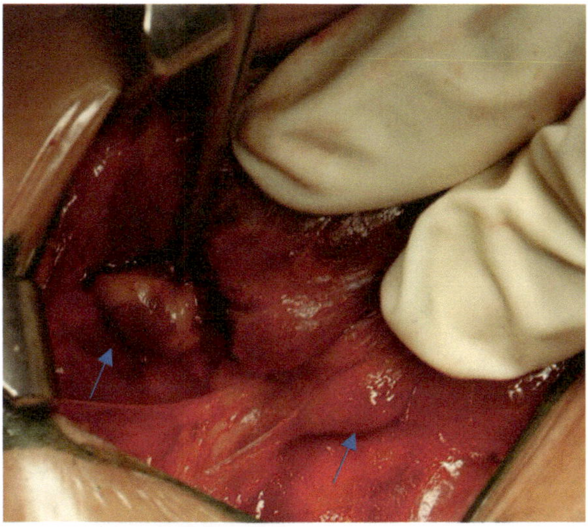

Fig. 2 Enlarged right glands(arrows)

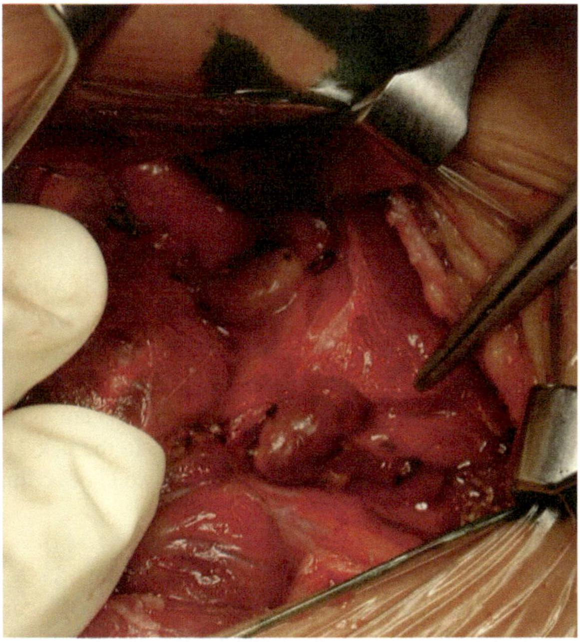

Fig. 3 Enlarged left parathyroid glands

serum lipase (46.6 u/L) were within normal limits. Anti-parietal cell antibody, anti-tissue transglutaminase antibody, and anti-nuclear antibody were all negative. Stool was negative for occult blood and stool fat examination showed 15 droplets/hpf. Red blood indices were: MCV:83.7, MCHC:33.2, and MCH: 27.8 with a reticulocyte count of <1% and Hb of 7.8% and Iron = 27.1, TIBC:107.5, Ferritin:234.4. CECT: multiple, hypodense foci within pancreatic parenchyma, MPD dilated.

Fig. 4 Emaciated patient of chronic pancreatitis

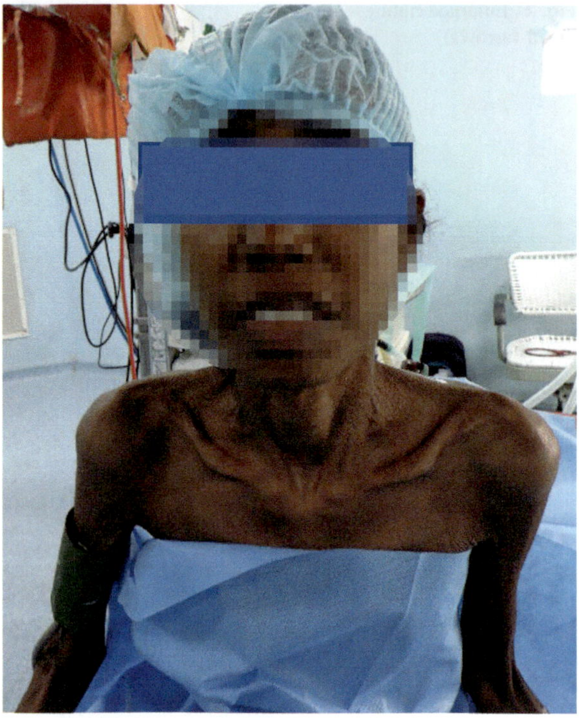

During the evaluation of chronic pancreatitis she was found to be having elevated calcium and subsequently elevated PTH. PTH – 68.73 pmol/L Ca(mg/dL): 11.4, 9.4, 11.1 ica (mmol/L): 1.8, 1.71 P: 3.0 25 OH Vitamin D: 37.7 nmol/mL. BMD showed osteoporosis with T score Spine −4.5, NOF -3.7 and forearm −5.9. With this imaging and biochemistry, a diagnosis of chronic pancreatitis with hyperparathyroidism was confirmed. USG Neck and MIBI were concordant for a left inferior parathyroid adenoma, measuring 1.4 × 1.4 × 3 cm. She underwent focused parathyroidectomy with curative fall in IOPTH. In the last 2 years of follow-up since her parathyroidectomy, there has been no episode of abdominal pain and she had since then gained weight.

Case 4: PHPT with Calcifying Pancreatitis

- A 38-year-old man presented with a history of recurrent renal stone for 15 years and had undergone open and ESWL nephrolithotomy on many occasions. He also gave a history of bone pains and weakness for 2 years. He had occasional upper abdominal discomfort but no acute attack of pancreatitis. X-ray KUB showed calcified pancreatitis (Figs. 6 and 7) along with renal calculi. His total serum calcium was high normal (10.7/10.8) but i Ca was elevated (1.52/1.43) (1.1–1.4 mmol/L). Subsequently, his iPTH was found to be very high: 741.3 pg/mL(9–55), with very low Vit D: 8.71 ng/mL. Hence a diagnosis of primary hyperparathyroidism was made. Both USG neck and MIBI were concordant for right inferior parathyroid adenoma. USG abdomen showed medullary nephro-

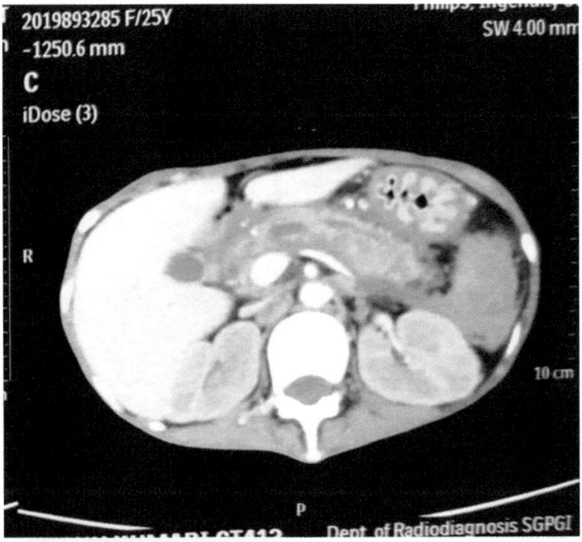

Fig. 5 CECT showing dilated MPD

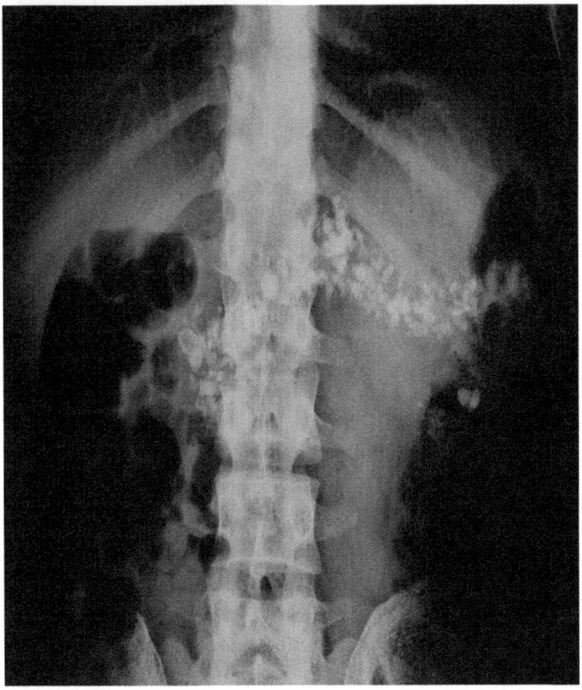

Fig. 6 X-ray showing opacities crossing midline suggestive of pancreatic calcification

calcinosis and CECT abdomen showed medullary nephrocalcinosis and nephrolithiasis and calcification throughout the parenchyma of the pancreas suggestive of chronic calcific pancreatitis. He underwent focused parathyroidectomy through endoscopic (chest wall approach) and parathyroid adenoma of size 3 × 1 × 1 cm was removed with curative fall in IOPTH.

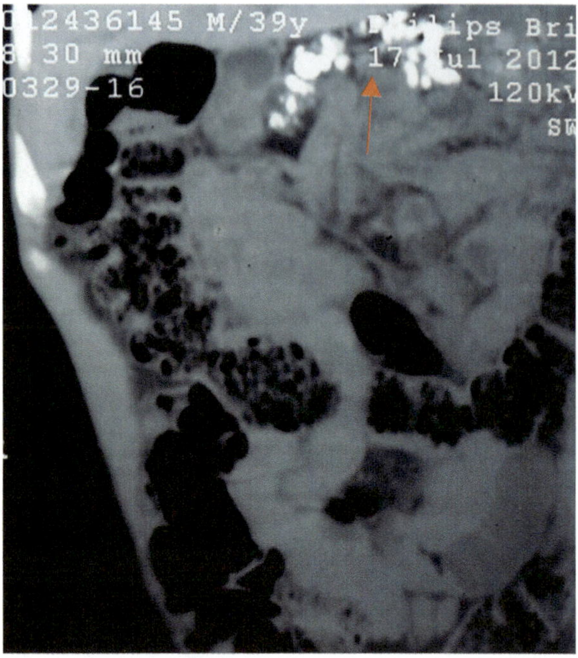

Fig. 7 CECT abdomen showing pancreatic parenchyma calcification (arrow)

Case 5: PHPT with Acute Necrotizing Pancreatitis

A 23-year-old student presented with complaints of sudden onset abdominal pain for 4 months associated with fever and vomiting. Pain was severe in intensity, sharp, and relieved on bending forward. He consulted a local physician and told to have acute pancreatitis and was managed conservatively. Similar episodes occurred 3–4 times over the last 3 months, all requiring hospitalization. Recent most episode was 10 days back for which he was admitted in an outside hospital. During evaluation for above symptoms, he was found to have raised serum calcium and PTH levels. He was then referred to SGPGI for further management. Initially, he was admitted under Gastromedicine dept. and was worked up. He was then referred to our dept. for surgical management. H/O fracture of distal phalanx of right fifth digit 2 years back. On general examination, he was found to be thin, frail, and febrile with pulse rate of 112 bpm. Investigations: USG Abdomen – Mild Hepato-splenomegaly, acute cholecystitis(no calculus, wall thickened), acute pancreatitis, minimal ascites, pancreatic collection (Vol 500 cm^3, bulky pancreas, shows multifocal small areas of necrotic changes suggestive of necrotizing pancreatitis. Large necrotic collection in peripancreatic region around pancreatic tail. MRI abdomen showed pancreatic tail is bulky and heterogenous with non-enhancing areas – acute necrotizing pancreatitis. CECT Abdomen showed atrophic pancreatic parenchyma with non-enhancing hypodense lesions (5.6 × 5 × 3.2 in tail, 8 × 6.8 × 7.1 cm in gastro splenic ligament) associated with peripancreatic soft tissue stranding and edema (Fig. 8). During evaluation, his biochemistry was found to be suggestive of primary hyperparathyroidism. Serum Ca 10., corrected Ca- 11.46 (Alb- 2.3); serum Phosphorous – 2.3; PTH – 35 pmol/L; Amylase – 76; Lipase – 55; Vit D- 137; Alk Phosphatase – 187. BMD – T score Spine −3.4 -, Femur -1.6, Radius -4.8. USG Neck and MIBI were concordant for left inferior parathyroid adenoma. He was started on IV antibiotics in view of sepsis and on NJ feeds (Fig. 9) for nutritional build-up. Then he underwent focused parathyroidectomy and a 5.6 g parathyroid adenoma was removed with curative fall in IOPTH (pmol/L): Pre-incision-146, Pre-excision -65, Post-excision (5 min)22.34, Post-excision (10 min), Post-excision (15 min)14.95. He had an uneventful operative and postoperative course, and remained free of any complications of anesthesia and surgery. Serial TLC showed decline as did the procalcitonin. Pancreatic collection was conservatively managed by the Gastromedicine team. He was given oral calcium carbonate and active vitamin D supplements starting post-op day one. He was discharged in a stable condition with NJ tube in situ. There has been no attack of pancreatitis in the 6 months of follow-up.

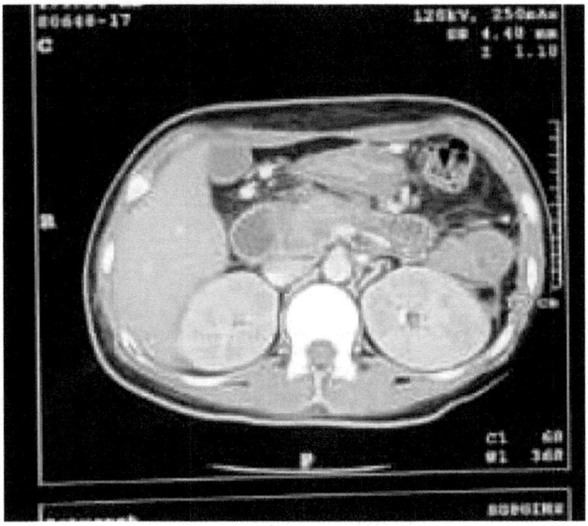

Fig. 8 CECT abdomen showing peripancreatic collections suggestive of necrotizing pancreatitis

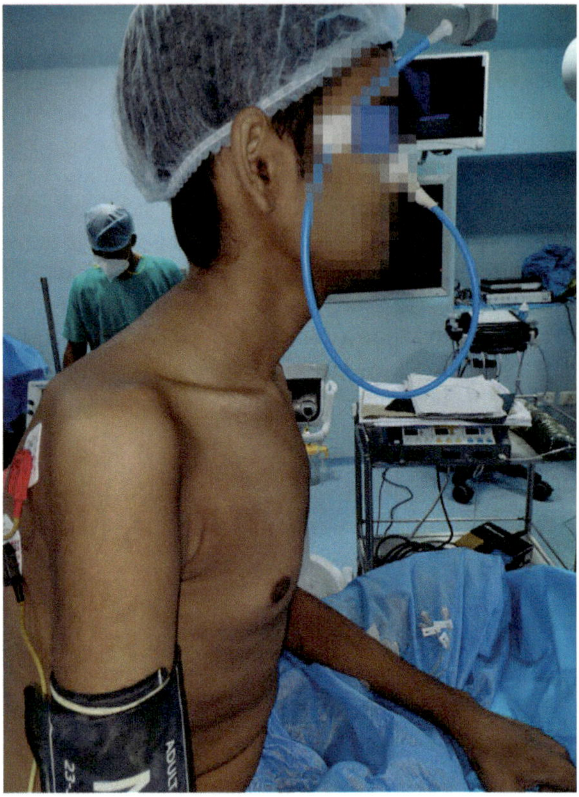

Fig. 9 The boy with NGT

Discussion

Metabolic causes of pancreatitis, although less common, constitute an important and treatable component of its etiologic actors. One of the metabolic causes is hypercalcemia and hyperparathyroidism. The prevalence of acute pancreatitis in PHPT has been estimated to be between 1.5% and 13% [1, 2]. PHPT can result in any one of the four forms of pancreatitis: (a) PHPT presenting as acute pancreatitis, (b) PHPT presenting as acute recurrent pancreatitis with no evidence of chronic pancreatitis, (c) PHPT presenting as chronic pancreatitis with or without pancreatic calcification, and (d) PHPT complicated by acute pancreatitis in the postoperative period. Unlike the classical PHPT the sex distribution in patients with pancreatitis showed a male preponderance with the male: female ratio being almost 2:1. Diagnosis of acute pancreatitis is usually based on any 2 of the following 3 criteria [3]:(1) abdominal pain (acute onset of a persistent, severe, epigastric pain, often radiating to the back); (2) serum lipase activity and/or serum amylase levels at least three times greater than the upper limit of normal; (3) characteristic findings of acute pancreatitis on imaging (contrast-enhanced computed tomography, magnetic resonance imaging, or transabdominal ultrasonography). The proposed mechanisms of hypercalcemia causing pancreatitis are: Hypercalcemia causes de novo activation of trypsinogen to trypsin, which results in acinar cell damage, autodigestion of the pancreas and, subsequently, pancreatitis [4]; secondly hypercalcemia can also lead to pancreatic calculi and protein plug formation by altering pancreatic secretion, resulting in ductal obstruction that leads to subsequent attacks of recurrent acute pancreatitis or chronic pancreatitis. Presence of acute pancreatitis as evidenced by elevated serum lipase and amylase should not be a deterrent to semi-emergent parathyroidectomy as this is the only way to ensure resolution of pancreatitis and prevent further attacks. Therefore, parathyroidectomy improves the clinical outcomes of PHPT and prevents further attacks of acute pancreatitis [5–7] In addition, the number of episodes and the severity of abdominal pain is reduced or completely abolished in patients with chronic pancreatitis.

References

1. Sitges-Serra A, Alonso M, de Lecea C, Gores PF, Sutherland DE. Pancreatitis and hyperparathyroidism. Br J Surg. 1988;75:158–60.
2. Carnaille B, Oudar C, Pattou F, Combemale F, Rocha J, Proye C. Pancreatitis and primary hyperparathyroidism: forty cases. Aust N Z J Surg. 1998;68:117–9.
3. Feldman M, Friedman LS, Brandt LJ. Sleisenger and Fordtran's gastrointestinal and liver disease E-book: pathophysiology, diagnosis, management, expert consult premium edition-enhanced online features. Amsterdam: Elsevier Health Sciences; 2010.
4. Kota SK, Krishna SV, Lakhtakia S, Modi KD. Metabolic pancreatitis: etiopathogenesis and management. Indian J Endocrinol Metab. 2013;17:799–805.
5. Diaconescu MR, Costea I, Glod M, Terinte R, Diaconescu S. Parathyroid adenomas in adults and adolescents. Critical appraisal and surgical strategy in 18 cases. Chirurgia (Bucur). 2017;112:18–24.
6. Aslam M, Talukdar R, Jagtap N, Rao GV, Pradeep R, Rao U, et al. Clinical profile and outcome of parathyroid adenoma-associated pancreatitis. Saudi J Med Med Sci. 2018;6:95–9.
7. Agarwal A, George RK, Gupta SK, Mishra SK. Pancreatitis in patients with primary hyperparathyroidism. Indian J Gastroenterol. 2003;22:224–5.

Part II

PHPT: Diagnostic Dilemma

Incidental Hyperparathyroidism

Case 1

A 65-year-old lady presented to us in the OPD with right solitary thyroid nodule measuring 4 × 3 × 2 cm with TIRADS 4. Fine needle cytology was suggestive of Bethesda 3 lesion. Hence after discussion with the patient she was planned for hemithyroidectomy. In preoperative evaluation, she was found to have high serum calcium levels. Hence, she was evaluated for primary hyperparathyroidism. Her intact PTH level was found to be high with normal creatinine and high alkaline phosphatase levels. Her BMD was found to be low. Her MIBI was suggestive of left superior parathyroid (Fig. 1). Repeat USG was done which showed 7 mm lesion near inferior pole of left lobe with right thyroid nodule in right lobe. Hence, we planned for bilateral exploration in view of thyroid nodule and left parathyroid discordant imaging. Left superior parathyroid was found to be enlarged (Fig. 2) and probably would have been missed if didn't have a preoperative diagnosis of primary hyperparathyroidism as the gland was superior and lateral to the upper pole. Left inferior gland was normal. Superior and inferior right parathyroid were normal. IOPTH was sent after removal of left superior gland and before proceeding to the right side. IOPTH showed a curative drop of more than 50% (Fig. 3). Histopathology turned out to be benign lesion for thyroid and parathyroid adenoma.

Roma Pradhan is the lead author of this chapter.

A. Agarwal et al., *Case Studies in Thyroid and Parathyroid Tumors*,
https://doi.org/10.1007/978-981-99-0938-4_18

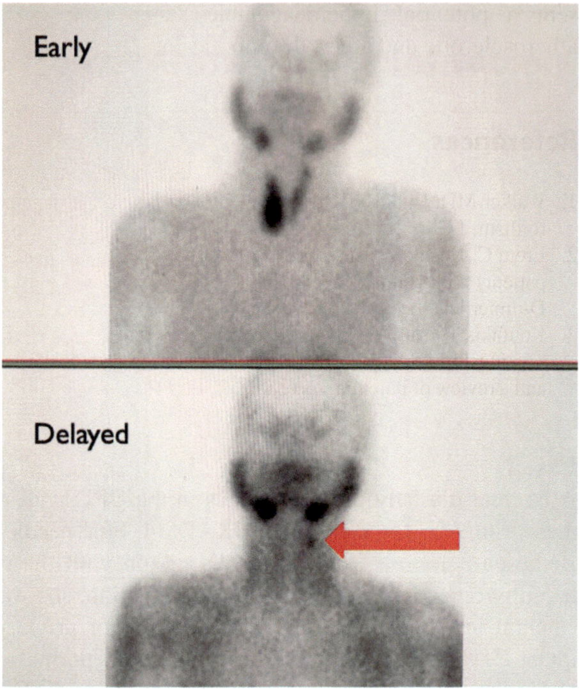

Fig. 1 MIBI with early delayed image with red arrow showing left superior gland

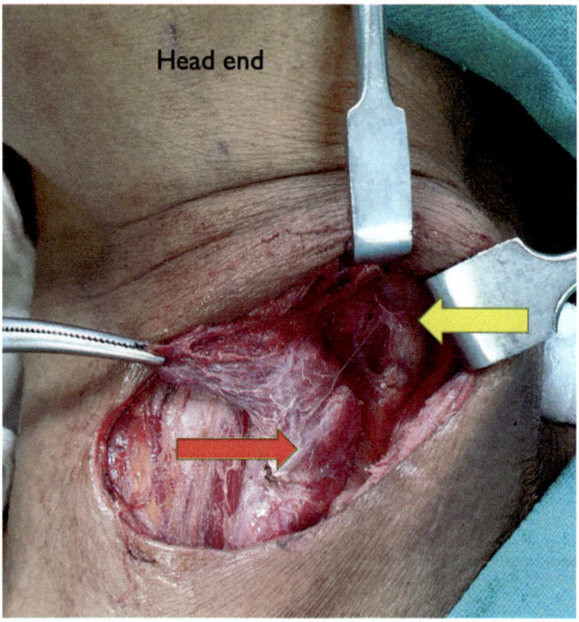

Fig. 2 Intraoperative picture showing superior parathyroid (yellow arrow) and thyroid (red arrow)

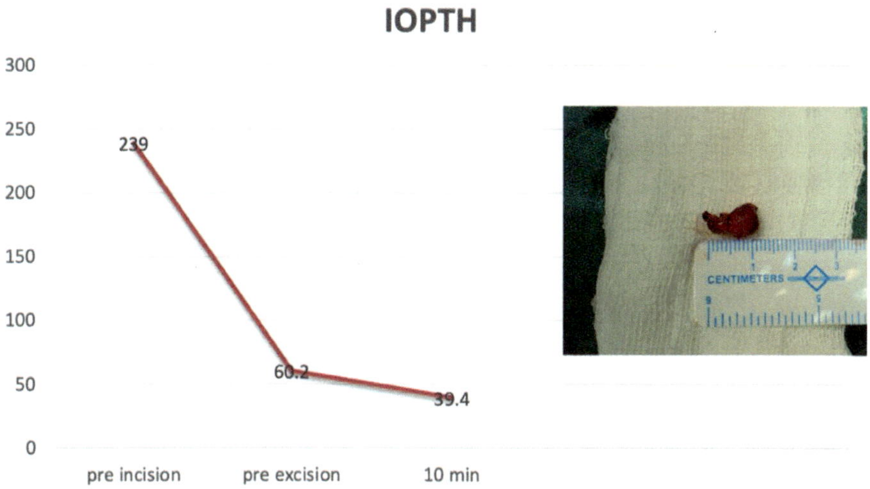

Fig. 3 IOPTH showing curative drop along with specimen

Discussion

Primary hyperparathyroidism patients are being diagnosed in the asymptomatic stage. The reasons for this are multifactorial and include sensitive parathyroid hormone assays and increased screening of patients with measurement of PTH and serum calcium. Investigation of thyroid disease often includes ultrasonography of the neck and diagnostic blood tests, and in some cases, coexistent thyroid and parathyroid disease may be noted. Patients with the suspicion of parathyroid disease should be fully investigated prior to their thyroid operation and if necessary have surgery to deal with both pathologies at the same time.

Parathyroid disease is often diagnosed when a raised calcium level is found on "routine" blood tests for other medical problems. Usually, these patients are asymptomatic or suffer from nonspecific symptoms of hypercalcemia such as fatigue, weakness, loss of appetite, nausea, and constipation. Less commonly nowadays, patients may present with significant renal and skeletal complications. Hence, we have an institute policy of getting serum calcium done for all thyroid cases we operate in a preoperative setting.

In some cases enlarged parathyroid may also be found during thyroid surgery as a surprise. In one such study [1] among 421 patients (355 who underwent thyroidectomy and 66 who underwent transhiatal esophagectomy), 5 cases of parathyroid incidentalomas (1.2%) were identified.

Studies have suggested that an enlarged parathyroid found during the course of a thyroid operation should always be removed [2–4] because the risk of developing into clinical hyperparathyroidism is considered to be unacceptable when compared with postoperative hypoparathyroidism, which is easily treated with calcium supplements. In such cases recurrent hyperparathyroidism or permanent hypoparathyroidism is also rare [3, 4].

References

1. Shroff P, McGrath GA, Pezzi CM. Incidentalomas of the parathyroid gland: multiple presentations, variable function, and review of the literature. Endocr Pract. 2005;11(6):363–9.
2. Katz AD, Kong LB. Incidental preclinical hyperparathyroidism identified during thyroid operations. Am Surg. 1992;58:747–9.
3. Carnaille BM, Pattou FN, Oudar C, Lecomte-Houcke MC, Rocha JE, Proye CA. Parathyroid incidentalomas in normocalcemic patients during thyroid surgery. World J Surg. 1996;20:830–4.
4. Prinz R, Paloyan E, Lawrence AM, Barbato A, Braithwaite S, Brooks M. Unexpected parathyroid disease discovered at thyroidectomy in irradiated patients. Am J Surg. 1981;142:355–7.

Negative Localization with USG and MIBI: Utility of 4D CT

Case

A 45-year-old lady was found to have hypercalcemia and raised PTH and renal stone during evaluation as a kidney donor. She gave a history of weakness in getting up for the last 8 months, history of constipation. Her biochemistry revealed elevated ionized calcium =1.53 mEq/L (1.13–1.32), S. Phosphorus: 3.1 mg/dL (3.5–5.5), S. Ipth:27.07 pmol/L (1.6–6.9), 25 OH Vit D: 26.20 nmol/L (50–250), S. ALP: 182 U/L (35–150), 24 h urine Creatinine: 0.192 g (1.0–2.0), 24 h urine Calcium: 196. BMD revealed osteoporosis with a T-score of −3.2 at forearm and −3.1 at femoral neck. USG Thyroid was negative for any parathyroid adenoma. MIBI and Tc subtraction scan were also negative for any parathyroid adenoma. 4D CT was suggestive of a well-defined lobulated lesion adjacent to the inferior pole of left thyroid lobe showing arterial phase enhancement and washout on delayed scans suggestive of a parathyroid adenoma (Fig. 1). We decided to do unilateral neck exploration. Left inferior adenoma was identified and removed. Left superior parathyroid gland was found to be normal and was preserved. The adenoma weighed: 0.9 g and measured 2 cm × 1 cm × 0.5 cm. There was curative fall in IOPTH: (pmol/L): Pre-incision: 28.6, Pre-excision: 32.02, Post-excision 5 min: 12.8, Post-excision 10 min: 8.9, Post-excision 15 min: 6.2. Postoperatively she developed clinical hypocalcemia on POD 1 and was given oral calcium carbonate and vitamin D supplements. HPE was reported as parathyroid adenoma.

Amit Agarwal is the lead author of this chapter.

A. Agarwal et al., *Case Studies in Thyroid and Parathyroid Tumors*,
https://doi.org/10.1007/978-981-99-0938-4_19

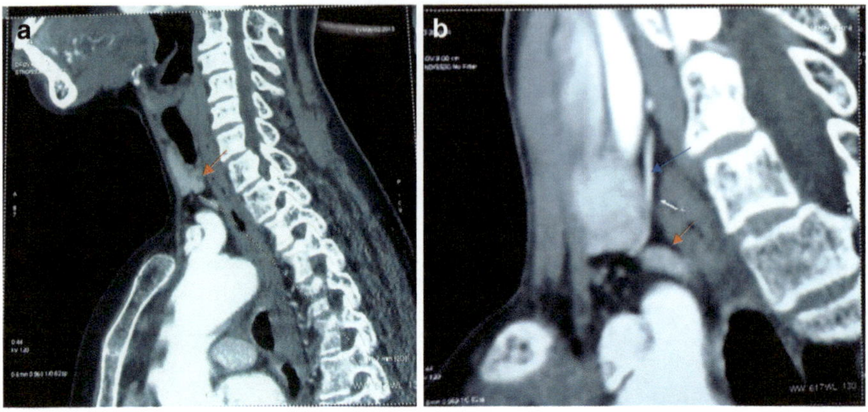

Fig. 1 (**a**, **b**) 4DCT showing parathyroid adenoma(orange arrow) just cranial to brachiocephalic trunk showing vivid arterial phase enhancement. The inferior thyroid artery (blue arrow) is seen coursing between the thyroid lobe and the adenoma

Discussion

Traditionally USG and MIBI scans are used as first-line localizing studies for hyperparathyroidism, especially if focused or target parathyroidectomy is planned. However, both these studies have some limitations and may result in false-negative localization. Ultrasonography remains operator dependent, requires an experienced technician, and has limited utility in the evaluation of substernal adenomas or in patients with large goiters. Nuclear medicine studies such as Sestamibi and single-photon emission computed tomography/computed tomography (SPECT/CT) are able to overcome some of the shortfalls of ultrasound, but these too have limitations of cost, and inability to precisely localize the site of the adenoma and inability to localize small adenoma. Multiphase(4 dimensional) 4DCT imaging was first described in 2006 and today is frequently used as either a second-line study after a non-localizing ultrasound or sestamibi scan or, increasingly, as a first-line study [1–3]. Presently, the most commonly used protocol involves 3 CT acquisitions of the neck and upper chest (non-contrast, arterial phase:30 s, and venous phase:60 s), with the fourth dimension referring to time. The fundamental principle of 4DCT is that the perfusion characteristics of parathyroid lesions are unique. The classic 4-D CT description of parathyroid adenoma is a lesion that is lower in attenuation than the normal thyroid gland on non-contrast images, exhibits attenuation greater than the thyroid on arterial phase images, and exhibits attenuation lower than the thyroid (washes out) on the venous or delayed phase images [4]. In patients with non-localizing, inconclusive, or discordant ultrasonography and sestamibi imaging outcomes, the sensitivity of 4D CT ranges from 67% to 89% and the PPV ranges from 65% to 87% [5, 6]. The advantages of 4-D CT include high-resolution anatomic information; short image acquisition; overall superior performance in most comparative studies; relative sensitivity for MGD; improved localization in the setting of mild hypercalcemia; ability to detect mildly enlarged glands; superior performance among patients with a previous failed operation; and ability to provide accurate localization in most patients with non-localizing, or discordant first-line imaging results. The disadvantages include relatively high radiation exposure and the need for iodinated contrast media administration.

References

1. Zafereo M, Yu J, Angelos P, et al. American head and neck society endocrine surgery section update on parathyroid imaging for surgical candidates with primary hyperparathyroidism. Head Neck. 2019;41(7):2398–409.
2. Rodgers SE, Hunter GJ, Hamberg LM, et al. Improved preoperative planning for directed parathyroidectomy with 4-dimensional computed tomography. Surgery. 2006;140(6):932–40. [discussion 940-931]
3. Suh YJ, Choi JY, Kim SJ, et al. Comparison of 4D CT, ultrasonography, and 99mTc sestamibi SPECT/CT in localizing single-gland primary hyperparathyroidism. Otolaryngol Head Neck Surg. 2015;152(3):438–43.
4. Paul M. Bunch preoperative imaging techniques in primary hyperparathyroidism a review. JAMA Otolaryngol Head Neck Surg. 2018;144(10):929–37.
5. Day KM, Elsayed M, Beland MD, Monchik JM. The utility of 4-dimensional computed tomography for preoperative localization of primary hyperparathyroidism in patients not localized by sestamibi or ultrasonography. Surgery. 2015;157(3):534–9.
6. Lubitz CC, Hunter GJ, Hamberg LM, et al. Accuracy of 4-dimensional computed tomography in poorly localized patients with primary hyperparathyroidism. Surgery. 2010;148(6):1129–37.

PHPT Diagnosed on MDP Bone

Case
A 65-year-old lady presented with complaints of generalized body ache for 4 years which was progressively increasing, and exacerbated over the past 3 months. She also gave a history of joint pains on b/l shoulder, elbows, knees, as well as a history of difficulty in climbing stairs for 6 months with h/o of epigastric pain and occasional constipation for 7 years, past history of pulmonary TB 20 years ago when she took ATT × 1 year O/E 2 × 2 cm firm nodule in right paratracheal region with restricted mobility. Serum calcium was found to be elevated on 2 occasions (14.2, 14.4 mg%), along with elevated PTH (349.1 pg/mL, ref range: 9–55 pg/mL), raised ALP (1495 IU/L), and insufficient vit D levels (28.59 ng/mL, ref. range: 9–7 ng/mL). Her bone scan done in another institution was reviewed and reported as showing diffusely increased tracer uptake at multiple sites:calvarium of the skull, mandible, sternum ('sternal tie sign'), long bones, multiple costochondral junction ('rachitic rosary sign'), and faint visualization of kidneys ('super scan') (Fig. 1). Skeletal survey revealed brown tumors (Fig. 2) in skull and ribs and BMD showed severe osteoporosis. So a working diagnosis of primary hyperparathyroidism with palpable parathyroid adenoma with severe bone disease was made. USG and MIBI localized a right superior parathyroid adenoma. She was taken up for focused parathyroidectomy and a 6 g adenoma was removed with curative fall in IOPTH. Histopathology was confirmatory of adenoma. Postoperatively she was put on prophylactic calcium and active vitamin D and was discharged on fourth postoperative day. She is eucalcemic on recent follow-up.

Amit Agarwal is the lead author of this chapter.

A. Agarwal et al., *Case Studies in Thyroid and Parathyroid Tumors*,
https://doi.org/10.1007/978-981-99-0938-4_20

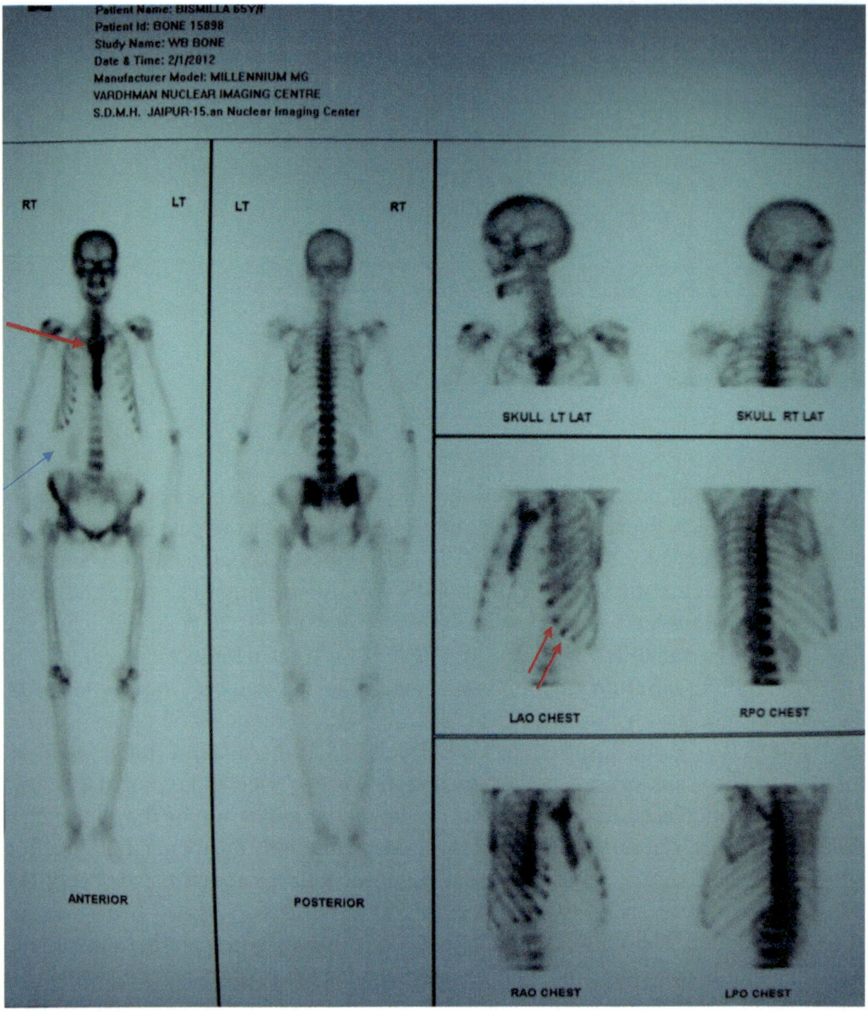

Fig. 1 MDP bone scan of a patient of PHPT, due to high turnover in certain bones and reduced kidney excretion, shows characteristic features: faint visualization of kidneys (super scan – long blue arrow), uptake in sternum (sternal tie sign – long red arrow) and uptake in costo-chondral junctions (rachitic rosary sign – short red arrows)

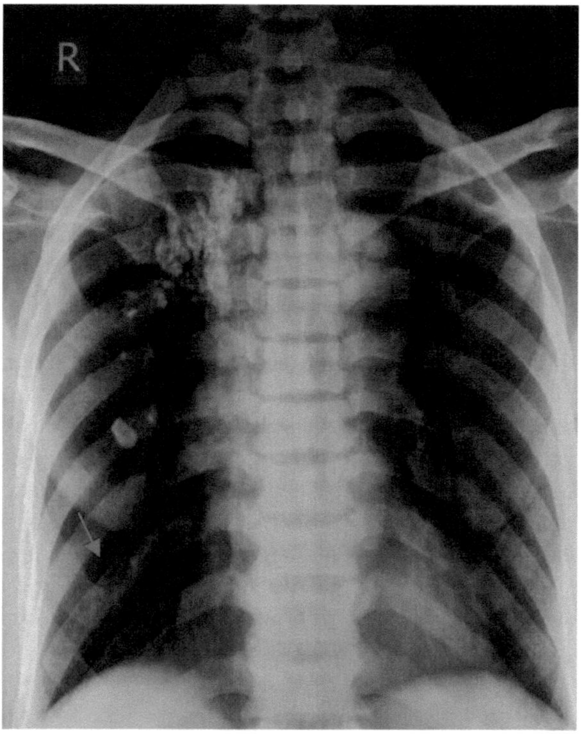

Fig. 2 X-ray chest showing brown tumors of ribs(arrows)

Discussion

The differential diagnosis of a bone scan suggestive of metabolic disease includes: Osteomalacia, Primary hyperparathyroidism, Renal Osteodystrophy, and Paget's disease.

A characteristic feature of Osteomalacia is Pseudo fracture (Looser's zone or milkman's fractures) which are often symmetric and perpendicular to the bone surface [1]. They are commonly found in the scapula, medial aspect of the femoral neck, pubic rami, ulna (proximal third), radius (distal third), ribs, clavicle, metacarpals, metatarsals, and phalanges. Pulsating vessels on the softened bone cortex have been suggested to be the origin of pseudo fractures. Pseudo fractures are most often seen in the ribs. The bone scan provides a sensitive means of identifying pseudo fractures, particularly in the ribs.

Another differential of a scan suggestive of metabolic bone disease is renal osteodystrophy which encompasses the changes in bone metabolism due to prolonged chronic renal disease. Most of the scan findings are due to increased bone turnover resulting from secondary hyperparathyroidism but 2 features help to differentiate from other metabolic diseases: one is absence of visualization of bladder and second in renal osteodystrophy bone scan uptake is usually diffuse and symmetric as opposed to advanced primary hyperparathyroidism where uptake is often asymmetric because of cystic lesions and brown tumors.

In advanced cases of primary hyperparathyroidism disease characteristic patterns of bone scan abnormality are commonly seen which includes [2, 3]: 'tie sternum' (due to a general increase of tracer uptake by the manubrium and, in the lateral borders of the body); beading of the costochondral junction ('rachitic rosary sign'); reduced renal activity, faint or absent kidney images (known as 'super scan' as a result of less tracer being available for excretion); increased tracer uptake in long bones; increased tracer uptake in axial skeleton; prominence of calvaria and mandible and increased tracer uptake in periarticular areas.

The bone scan in Paget's disease also shows markedly increased uptake of tracer throughout most or all of the affected bone but lesions in Paget's disease may be clearly identified(hot spots) because of the clear differentiation between normal and abnormal bones. Paget's disease usually affects transverse spinous processes of the vertebrae which has a typical appearance that has been described as a "Mickey Mouse" sign because of the inverted triangular uptake distribution or it may show uptake in mandible described as the "black beard" sign (monostotic mandible disease) and the "short pants" sign (spine, pelvis, and upper femoral disease).

The bone scan in our patient was thus diagnostic of a metabolic bone disease showing specific signs of primary hyperparathyroidism.

References

1. Hain SF, Fogelman I. Nuclear medicine studies in metabolic bone disease. Semin Musculoskelet Radiol. 2002;6(4):323–9.
2. Chakraborty PP, Bhattacharjee R, Mukhopadhyay S, Chowdhury S. 'Rachitic rosary sign' and 'tie sign' of the sternum in tumour-induced osteomalacia. BMJ Case Rep. 2016;2016:bcr2016214766.
3. Sood A, Agarwal K, Shukla J, et al. Bone scintigraphic patterns in patients of tumor induced osteomalacia. Indian J Nucl Med. 2013;28:173–5.

Discordant Ultrasound Scan and Technetium ^{99}m Sestamibi Scan

Case

A 66-year-old female presented to the endocrinology department with Hashimoto's thyroiditis and subclinical hypothyroidism, for which she was already started 50 µg of Thyroxin. During her work-up, she was noted to have raised calcium levels. She denied any complaints, specifically no constipation or abdominal pain, no excessive fatigue or low mood, no muscle weakness, and no increased thirst or nocturia. She had no history of kidney stones, but she had been found to be osteoporotic on a recent DEXA scan, for which she was started on Denosumab injection.

Upon physical examination, no abnormalities were noted. Her laboratory results showed an adjusted calcium of 3.08 mmol/L, with a parathyroid hormone (PTH) of 41.8 pmol/L and vitamin D of 20.6 µg/L. Her calcium: creatinine clearance ratio was 0.0235, excluding familial hypocalciuric hypercalcemia (FHH). With the diagnosis of primary hyperparathyroidism (PHPT) made, she subsequently underwent dual localization studies. Her Technetium ^{99}m sestamibi (MIBI) scan did not reveal a MIBI-avid lesion to suggest a parathyroid adenoma or hyperplasia (Fig. 1). Conversely, on her ultrasound scan (US), an extra-thyroidal lesion measuring 2.5 cm in maximum diameter cranial to the right thyroid lobe was demonstrated. This scan also showed parenchymal findings in keeping with her known Hashimoto's thyroiditis.

She was advised to drink up to 3 L of plain water a day, which resulted in normalization of her adjusted calcium levels to 2.49 mmol/L, and she was referred to the endocrine surgery department, where she was counseled for an urgent parathyroidectomy. This was performed as a unilateral neck exploration. The right-sided superior gland was found to be enlarged at about 2.7 cm and subsequently removed (Fig. 2), while the right inferior gland was normal in size and appearance.

Rajeev Parameswaran is the lead author of this chapter.

A. Agarwal et al., *Case Studies in Thyroid and Parathyroid Tumors*,
https://doi.org/10.1007/978-981-99-0938-4_21

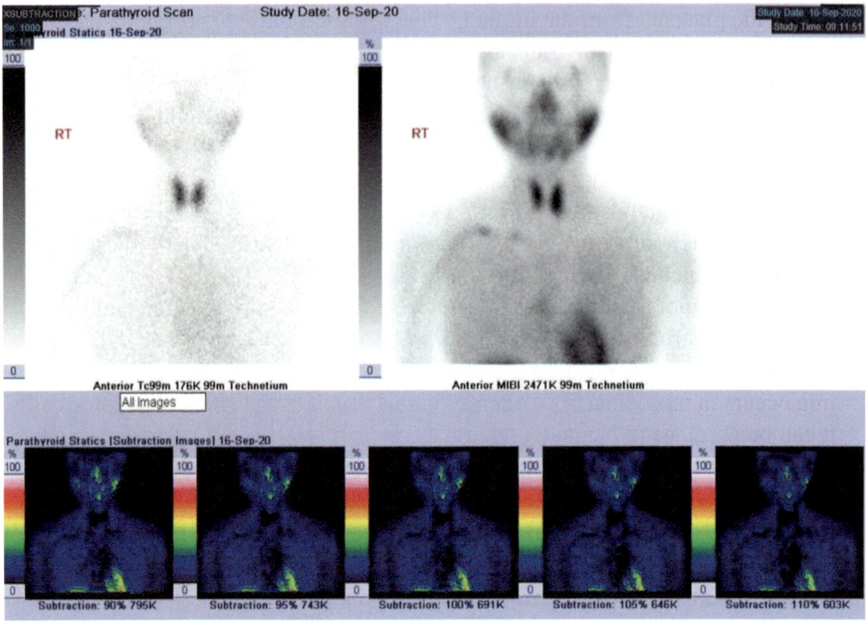

Fig. 1 Sestamibi scan showing no uptake of the parathyroid in both early and delayed phase

Fig. 2 Excised right superior parathyroid gland

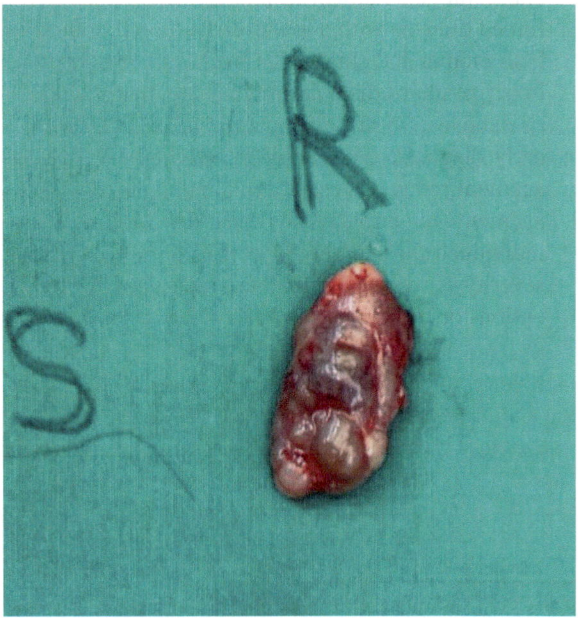

On the first postoperative day, her PTH had normalized to 9.2 pmol/L, while her calcium dropped to the low-normal at 2.18 mmol/L. She was discharged on the second postoperative day, with calcium carbonate 1250 mg TD and calcitriol 0.5 μg BD, expecting a further drop in her calcium level. Her histology report described a parathyroid gland measuring 2.8 × 1.6 × 0.9 cm and weighing 2.4 g, with features compatible with a parathyroid adenoma.

During her postoperative clinic visit, she was doing well and had no issues regarding her scar or voice. Her calcium levels had dropped somewhat (nadir 2.08 mmol/L), so she was kept on her calcium and vitamin D replacements. She is currently under follow-up by our endocrine medicine department, aiming to taper her supplements, while also managing her osteoporosis.

Discussion

Primary hyperparathyroidism (PHPT) is a biochemical diagnosis, based on an elevated serum calcium concentration combined with a PTH level that is either elevated or inappropriately normal [1]. Surgical intervention is indicated for all patients with symptomatic PHPT (nephrolithiasis, fractures, symptomatic hypercalcemia) or those diagnosed at 50 years or younger [2]. The decision to obtain imaging studies should only be made after biochemical confirmation of PHPT, and after an indication for surgery is set, as the predominant use of imaging is to aid in planning the operative approach [3].

As PHPT is a functional disease, functional imaging using a tracer, in the form of MIBI (^{99m}Tc-MIBI), has been included in the work-up [4]. However, due to various aspects, a negative MIBI occurs in about 15–25% of patients with PHPT. One of the factors increasing the risk of a negative MIBI is the presence of thyroiditis [5] – as was the case with our patient. Moreover, MIBI does not provide any additional details regarding possible concurrent thyroid disease. Therefore, US is another imaging modality often used, being highly sensitive in experienced hands, inexpensive, non-invasive, and able to assess any concurrent thyroid pathology [4].

While influenced by several confounding factors, combining MIBI with US has been reported to provide a high sensitivity (up to 95%) for localizing single-gland disease [4]. However, a work-up consisting of two imaging modalities could result in discordant outcomes. And while this finding will impact the operative planning and decision-making, importantly, discordant imaging does not provide a reason not to operate. It has been shown that for patients with thyroiditis and discordant imaging results, US is correct more often [5]. Conversely, this same group reported that without thyroiditis, MIBI had a greater sensitivity in predicting the correct laterality of the adenoma [5], underlining the strength of a dual imaging work-up.

Generally, while a bilateral neck exploration (NE) has been the golden standard regarding efficacy and safety in the definitive treatment of PHPT, a minimally invasive procedure (MIP) can be performed for the subgroup with concordant imaging.

For those with discordant imaging, a planned unilateral of bilateral NE should be considered, also depending on available intraoperative adjuncts such as intraoperative PTH measurements [2]. The introduction of several emerging techniques, such as 4D-computed tomography (CT) [6] or PET-choline (i.e., positron emission tomography (PET) using the tracer fluorine 18 (18F) choline) [7], will likely further alter the decision-making algorithm for surgery in PHPT in the near future.

References

1. Bilezikian JP. Primary Hyperparathyroidism. J Clin Endocrinol Metab. 2018;103(11):3993–4004. https://doi.org/10.1210/jc.2018-01225.
2. Wilhelm SM, Wang TS, Ruan DT, et al. The American Association of endocrine surgeons guidelines for definitive management of primary hyperparathyroidism. JAMA Surg. 2016;151(10):959–68. https://doi.org/10.1001/jamasurg.2016.2310.
3. Bunch PM, Kelly HR. Preoperative imaging techniques in primary hyperparathyroidism: a review. JAMA Otolaryngol Head Neck Surg. 2018;144(10):929–37. https://doi.org/10.1001/jamaoto.2018.1671.
4. Patel CN, Salahudeen HM, Lansdown M, Scarsbrook AF. Clinical utility of ultrasound and 99mTc sestamibi SPECT/CT for preoperative localization of parathyroid adenoma in patients with primary hyperparathyroidism. Clin Radiol Apr. 2010;65(4):278–87. https://doi.org/10.1016/j.crad.2009.12.005.
5. Beck AC, Kashyap AK, Lal G, et al. Discordant findings on preoperative imaging for primary hyperparathyroidism and thyroid disease: choosing the path to follow. Surgery. 2019;166(4):678–85. https://doi.org/10.1016/j.surg.2019.05.057.
6. de Jong MC, Jamal K, Morley S, et al. The use of computed tomography as a first-line imaging modality in patients with primary hyperparathyroidism. Hormones (Athens). 2021;20(3):499–506. https://doi.org/10.1007/s42000-020-00205-x.
7. Kluijfhout WP, Pasternak JD, Drake FT, et al. Use of PET tracers for parathyroid localization: a systematic review and meta-analysis. Langenbeck's Arch Surg. 2016;401(7):925–35. https://doi.org/10.1007/s00423-016-1425-0.

Familial Isolated Hyperparathyroidism with CDC73 Mutation

Case

A 26-year-old woman with a history of uterine fibroid and menorrhagia underwent health screening and biochemistry showed elevated calcium (2.88 mmol/L) and parathyroid hormone (22.7 pmol/L) levels. She was referred to the endocrine clinic for further work up. On further enquiry, it was revealed that her first cousin had parathyroid surgery with a history of renal stones. One of her uncles also had parathyroid surgery in his 20s and her grandmother underwent 2 neck surgeries to treat a "tumor," the details of which were unclear. The family pedigree is shown in Fig. 1. Imaging investigations in the form of ultrasound scan of the neck showed the presence of a double adenoma and Sestamibi scanning showed similar uptake bilaterally in the superior poles. The patient underwent a bilateral neck exploration under general anesthesia and the adenomas were resected. Histology confirmed the presence of a double adenoma. In the postoperative phase, patient experienced symptoms of hypocalcemia, which was corrected with oral calcium and magnesium replacement. Genetic mutation analysis showed the presence of CDC73 gene with no mutations of MEN-1, FHH, and HPT-JT gene.

Rajeev Parameswaran is the lead author of this chapter.

A. Agarwal et al., *Case Studies in Thyroid and Parathyroid Tumors*,
https://doi.org/10.1007/978-981-99-0938-4_22

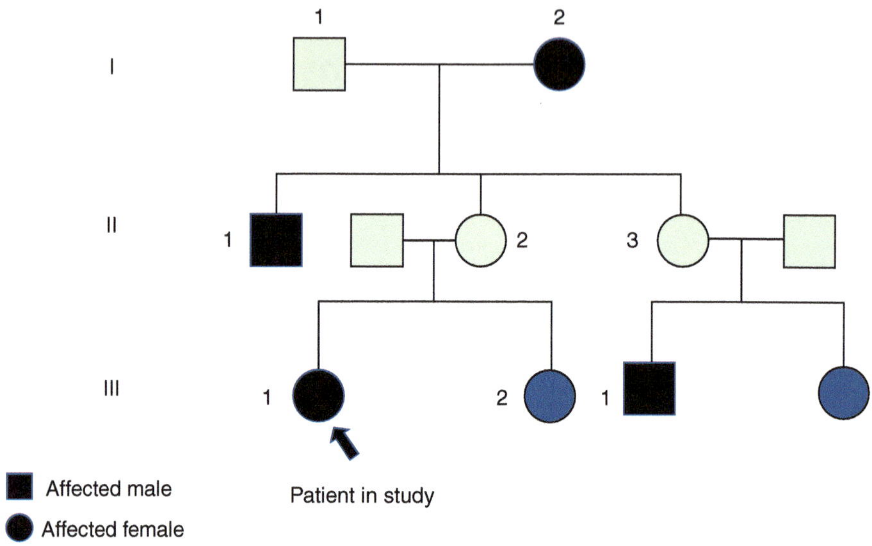

Fig. 1 Pedigree chart

Discussion

Familial isolated hyperparathyroidism (FIHPT) is a diagnosis of exclusion, and it represents kindreds with incomplete expression or specific features associated with syndromes such as MEN 1, MEN 2A, HPT-JT, or FHH [1–4]. However, in a fraction of FIHPT cases, germline mutations of MEN1, CDC73, and CaSR genes have been reported, although the exact mechanisms determining the phenotypical expression is less well understood [5, 6]. A recent germline mutation which has been discovered in about 20% of families with FIHPT, is a mutation in GCM2, a nuclear transcription factor required for parathyroid gland organogenesis [7]. It has recently been shown that a positive family history is strongly predictive of a pathogenic germline variant in a susceptibility gene, while age at diagnosis and the presence of multiple gland disease were not [8].

FIHPT can occur as genetic or sporadic entity (where there is a coincidental clustering of sporadic cases among close relatives in the absence of any defined mutations). In the genetic type, the diagnosis of hyperparathyroidism is usually made at a later age and associated with symptomatic disease [7]. The diagnosis and management of FIHPT relies on clinical and biochemical findings, as well as on any histological results available. A careful examination of the family is also essential, as a negative genetic test cannot fully exclude a diagnosis of FIHPT [9].

It has been suggested up to one-in-ten primary hyperparathyroidism cases can be classified as familial, which may only rise once more mutations are established [10]. Currently no mutation can be identified in the majority of FIHPT cases, forcing a diagnosis based on clinical and biochemical investigations. In terms of familial implications, among those families with multiglandular disease, genetic analysis of MEN1 should be offered, while for those with solitary adenoma or parathyroid carcinoma, HPT-JT syndrome should be considered.

The indications for surgery among those with FIHPT are similar as for patients with sporadic forms of hyperparathyroidism, and the goal is to achieve and maintain a normocalcemic state for the longest period possible, while avoiding hypoparathyroidism or other complications [11, 12]. Additionally, any future surgery for recurrent disease should also be facilitated [13]. For patients with familial hypocalciuric hypercalcemia (FHH), surgery is not the treatment of choice.

A preoperative diagnosis of FIHPT has therapeutic consequences concerning the extent of parathyroid surgery performed. However, the exact surgical strategy for this kind of PHPT remains controversial for the group of FIHPT as a whole, as guidelines are based on limited data [14]. There is a wide heterogeneity of the disease, and thus interventions should be individualized in FIHPT. Generally, for all patients with a preoperative diagnosis of FIHPT, a bilateral neck exploration is advised. For those with FIHPT linked to mutations in the MEN1-gene, the extent of parathyroidectomy should be in concordance with current guidelines, i.e., by performance of a subtotal (three and one-half glands) parathyroidectomy or a total parathyroidectomy with auto-transplantation) [15]. A recent series on GCM2-associated hyperparathyroidism showed that there was a substantial rate of multiple gland disease and a relatively lower chance of biochemical cure [16], suggesting the management of FIHPT linked to GCM2-mutation to therefore be similar to that in MEN1 [15]. Conversely, for those with FIHPT linked to other, thus far identified, disorders such as HPT-JT syndrome (CDC73/HRPT2), or mutations in the CaSR-gene, recommendations on the extent of parathyroidectomy are still being developed. Some support the performance of a selective parathyroidectomy in this group, i.e., resection of only grossly enlarged parathyroid glands, unless parathyroid cancer is suspected [13]. However, based on the substantial overall risk of recurrence, as well as the incidence of parathyroid cancer among those with HPT-JT, others advice treating all patients with FIHPT with a (sub)total parathyroidectomy [17, 18].

Although clinical data are scarce, the medical treatment of FIHPT in patients who are poor surgical candidates, is similar as for sporadic disease, by using calcimimetics [9].

References

1. Simonds WF, James-Newton LA, Agarwal SK, Yang B, Skarulis MC, Hendy GN, et al. Familial isolated hyperparathyroidism: clinical and genetic characteristics of 36 kindreds. Medicine. 2002;81(1):1–26.
2. Simonds WF, Robbins CM, Agarwal SK, Hendy GN, Carpten JD, Marx SJ. Familial isolated hyperparathyroidism is rarely caused by germline mutation in HRPT2, the gene for the hyperparathyroidism-jaw tumor syndrome. J Clin Endocrinol Metabol. 2004;89(1):96–102.
3. Warner J, Epstein M, Sweet A, Singh D, Burgess J, Stranks S, et al. Genetic testing in familial isolated hyperparathyroidism: unexpected results and their implications. J Med Genet. 2004;41(3):155–60.

4. Starker LF, Åkerström T, Long WD, Delgado-Verdugo A, Donovan P, Udelsman R, et al. Frequent germ-line mutations of the MEN1, CASR, and HRPT2/CDC73 genes in young patients with clinically non-familial primary hyperparathyroidism. Horm Cancer. 2012;3(1): 44–51.
5. Cristina E-V, Alberto F. Management of familial hyperparathyroidism syndromes: MEN1, MEN2, MEN4, HPT-jaw tumour, familial isolated hyperparathyroidism, FHH, and neonatal severe hyperparathyroidism. Best Pract Res Clin Endocrinol Metab. 2018;32(6):861–75.
6. Blau JE, Simonds WF. Familial hyperparathyroidism. Front Endocrinol (Lausanne). 2021;12:623667.
7. Guan B, Welch JM, Sapp JC, Ling H, Li Y, Johnston JJ, et al. GCM2-activating mutations in familial isolated hyperparathyroidism. Am J Hum Genet. 2016;99(5):1034–44.
8. Mariathasan S, Andrews KA, Thompson E, Challis BG, Wilcox S, Pierce H, et al. Genetic testing for hereditary hyperparathyroidism and familial hypocalciuric hypercalcaemia in a large UK cohort. Clin Endocrinol. 2020;93(4):409–18.
9. Pontikides N, Karras S, Kaprara A, Anagnostis P, Mintziori G, Goulis DG, et al. Genetic basis of familial isolated hyperparathyroidism: a case series and a narrative review of the literature. J Bone Miner Metab. 2014;32(4):351–66.
10. Miedlich S, Krohn K, Paschke R. Update on genetic and clinical aspects of primary hyperparathyroidism. Clin Endocrinol. 2003;59(5):539–54.
11. Bilezikian JP, Brandi ML, Eastell R, Silverberg SJ, Udelsman R, Marcocci C, et al. Guidelines for the management of asymptomatic primary hyperparathyroidism: summary statement from the fourth international workshop. J Clin Endocrinol Metabol. 2014;99(10):3561–9.
12. Bilezikian JP. Primary hyperparathyroidism. J Clin Endocrinol Metab. 2018;103(11): 3993–4004.
13. Stålberg P, Carling T. Familial parathyroid tumors: diagnosis and management. World J Surg. 2009;33(11):2234–43.
14. Marx SJ. New concepts about familial isolated hyperparathyroidism. J Clin Endocrinol Metab. 2019;104(9):4058–66.
15. Thakker RV, Newey PJ, Walls GV, Bilezikian J, Dralle H, Ebeling PR, et al. Clinical practice guidelines for multiple endocrine neoplasia type 1 (MEN1). J Clin Endocrinol Metab. 2012;97(9):2990–3011.
16. El Lakis M, Nockel P, Guan B, Agarwal S, Welch J, Simonds WF, et al. Familial isolated primary hyperparathyroidism associated with germline GCM2 mutations is more aggressive and has a lesser rate of biochemical cure. Surgery. 2018;163(1):31–4.
17. Sarquis MS, Silveira LG, Pimenta FJ, Dias EP, Teh BT, Friedman E, et al. Familial hyperparathyroidism: surgical outcome after 30 years of follow-up in three families with germline HRPT2 mutations. Surgery. 2008;143(5):630–40.
18. VanderWalde LH, Haigh PI. Surgical approach to the patient with familial hyperparathyroidism. Curr Treat Options in Oncol. 2006;7(4):326–33.

Double Parathyroid Adenomas

Case

A 58-year-old patient was evaluated by Neurologist for the complaint of low back ache and proximal muscle weakness of the lower limbs for the past 2 years. As he had a past history of Pulmonary Kochs and preliminary X-rays of the spine showed a lytic lesion destroying L1 vertebrae, a provisional diagnosis of Potts' spine was made. On examination, there was tenderness at L1 level and 2 nodules that moved with deglutition detected in the neck (left side 4 × 3 cm and right side 2 × 2 cm). Serum Chemistry revealed elevated calcium (13.5 mg/dL) and PTH (760 pg/mL). X-ray KUB revealed bilateral nephrocalcinosis. Bone scan revealed diffuse uptake in the calvaria, left and right 6–9 ribs, ASIS, upper ends of tibia and L1 vertebra. USG of the neck revealed enlarged right and left parathyroid glands and these were confirmed by CT scan (Fig. 1) of the neck. However, MIBI scan revealed increased uptake in the region of the parathyroid on the right side only. He underwent bilateral exploration and a left superior parathyroid adenoma measuring 4 × 4 × 1.5 cm, weighing 9.5 g and a right Inferior parathyroid adenoma measuring 1 × 0.8 cm, weighing 0.1 g were excised. Postoperative period was uneventful and he was discharged with calcium and vitamin D supplements. He has been maintaining eucalcemia for the last 13 years.

Amit Agarwal is the lead author of this chapter.

A. Agarwal et al., *Case Studies in Thyroid and Parathyroid Tumors*,
https://doi.org/10.1007/978-981-99-0938-4_23

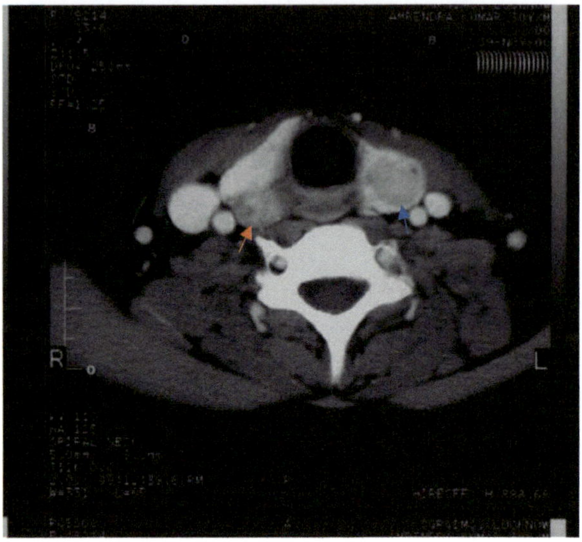

Fig. 1 CECT neck showing right inferior and left superior parathyroid adenomas

Discussion

Multiglandular diseases of parathyroid include double or triple adenomas and hyperplasia of all parathyroid glands. It has been a matter of intense debate whether double adenomas represent a form of asynchronous four-gland hyperplasia. However, considering the high long-term cure rate of two-gland resection equivalent to uniglandular disease is the best evidence of double adenoma as a separate disease. The reported incidence of double adenomas varies between 1.9% and 12% in different series [1–3]. Double adenomas were most likely to be found in a crossed configuration affecting a superior parathyroid gland on one side and the inferior parathyroid gland on the opposite side [4] (laryngoscope). The accuracy of preoperative localization tests like USG and MIBI unfortunately is much lower for patients with multiple abnormal parathyroid glands. The rate of concordance of these tests for identifying double adenomas is very low, approximately only 10%. This observation suggests that when preoperative localization tests are discrepant, multiple abnormal parathyroid glands are more likely. Multiglandular diseases, including double adenomas, are an important factor in operations that are unsuccessful. The inability to distinguish adenoma from hyperplasia on histologic grounds has resulted in different recommendations about the appropriate surgical management of primary hyperparathyroidism. In the absence of firm evidence, some authors favor subtotal parathyroidectomy [5] 2 of laryngoscope) In one series [6] (kandil), of the 47 patients of double adenomas, 46 (98%) remained normocalcemic after surgery and remained so for at least 6 months. In their series all 47 patients were approached with targeted parathyroidectomy for presumed single-gland disease. However, in cases in which IOPTH levels did not decrease to the normal range, the surgeon continued to look for a second adenoma. If a second adenoma was found and the IOPTH level decreased to normal, the search for additional glands to rule out hyperplasia ended at that point. Only 1 patient was still hypercalcemic after surgery and was treated with medication. Therefore, the authors concluded that IOPTH monitoring is a very useful tool to predict a durable biochemical resolution of hyperparathyroidism in patients with DA.

References

1. Tezelman S, Shen W, Shaver JK, et al. Double parathyroid adenomas; clinical and biochemical characteristics before and after parathyroidectomy. Ann Surg. 1993;218:300–9.
2. Milas M, Wagner K, Easley KA, et al. Double adenomas revisited: nonuniform distribution favors enlarged superior parathyroids(fourth pouch disease). Surgery. 2003;134:995–1004.
3. Bartsch D, Nies C, Hasse C, et al. Clinical and surgical aspects of double adenoma in patients with primary hyperparathyroidism. Br J Surg. 1995;82:926–9.
4. Abboud B, Sleilaty G, Helou E, Mansour E, Tohme C, Noun R, Sarkis R. Existence and anatomic distribution of double parathyroid adenoma. Laryngoscope. 2005;115:1128–31.
5. Bergson EJ, Heller KS. The clinical significance and anatomic distribution of parathyroid double adenomas. J Am Coll Surg. 2004;198:185–9.
6. Kandil E, Alabbas HH, Bansal A, Islam T, Tufaro AP, Tufano RP. Intraoperative Parathyroid Hormone Assay in Patients With Primary Hyperparathyroidism and Double Adenoma. Arch Otolaryngol Head Neck Surg. 2009;135(12):1206–8.

Sporadic Multi-glandular Disease

Case

A 40-year-old male patient with recurrent lower abdominal pain and renal colic for the last 5 years, having undergone endoscopic removal of bladder stone and ESWL thrice, was referred to this hospital for further management. He was found to have hypercalcemia. However, he had no history of bone pains or muscle weakness. His evaluation results were as follows:

S. Ca	10–11.3 mg/dL
S. Phosphorus	1.6 mg/dL
ALP	235 U/L
S. Creat	1.1 mg/dL
25 OH vit D	24.49 ng/mL
PTH	135 pg/mL
Usg neck	Right inferior(2.6 × 1.58 cm) and left Inferior parathyroid (1 × 0.5 cm) lesion
MIBI neck	Right superior and left inferior parathyroid Adenomas

With a discordant imaging suggestive of multiglandular disease he was taken up for bilateral parathyroid exploration. At the operation all 4 glands were found to be enlarged, so a 3 and half gland excision was done. The glands sizes were as follows: Rt inf gland: 3.8 g, 3 × 2.5 × 1.5 cm, Lt sup. Gland: 0.5 g, 1.2 × 0.8 cm, Lt inf gland: 1.5 g, 1.5 × 1.4 × 0.8 cm while the right superior gland was most normal looking (Figs. 1 and 2). IOPTH showed curative fall (Fig. 3). Postoperative period was uneventful and histopathology was suggestive of parathyroid hyperplasia.

Amit Agarwal is the lead author of this chapter.

A. Agarwal et al., *Case Studies in Thyroid and Parathyroid Tumors*,
https://doi.org/10.1007/978-981-99-0938-4_24

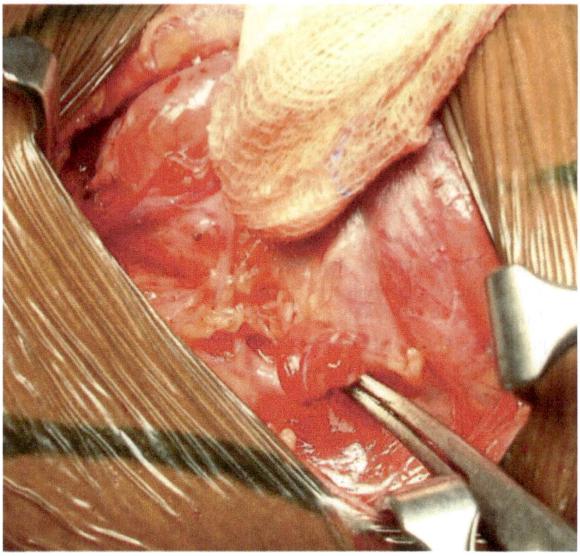

Fig. 1 Hyperplastic parathyroid gland

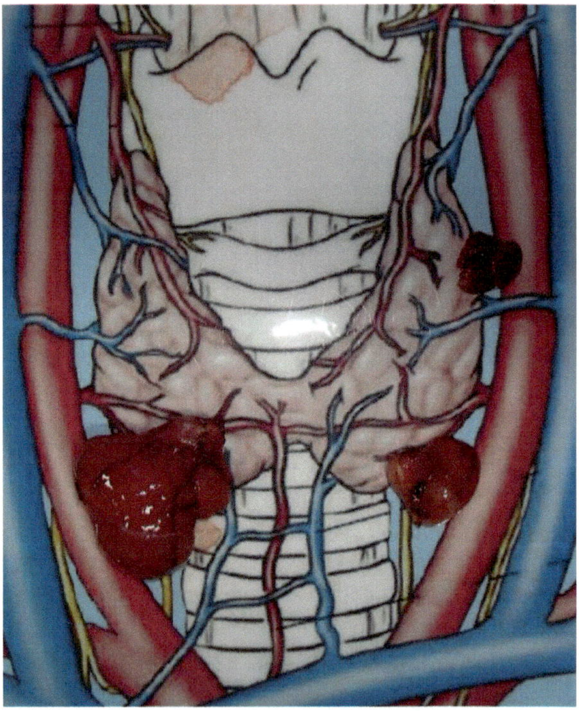

Fig. 2 Specimen picture of sub-total parathyroidectomy

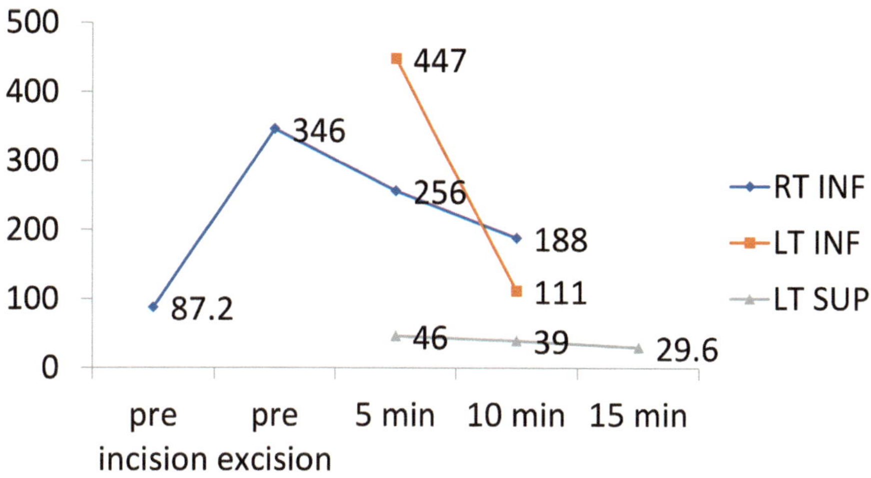

Fig. 3 IOPTH values after each parathyroid gland removal

Discussion

Sporadic primary hyperparathyroidism (pHPT) is caused by a single-gland adenoma in 70–80% ofpatients while the incidence of multiglandular disease (MGD) has been shown to vary in the range of 7–23% [1]. Patients with MGD, especially with ectopic parathyroid adenomas, have an increased risk for persistence/recurrence after surgery. Hence, to counsel patients about the risks and benefits of surgery for pHPT, and to plan the extent of operation, it would be of great benefit to predict MGD preoperatively. However, it is very difficult to predict the MGD in a given patient even though concordant ultrasonographic and scintigraphic results are highly predictive for solitary adenomas whereas negative localization studies are predictive of MGD. In one study negative sestamibi scintigraphy, diabetes, and elevated osteocalcin levels were predictors of MGD [2]. Some groups have reported higher serum calcium and intact PTH levels in patients with SGD compared to MGD [3, 4] while others could not confirm these findings. The cure rate of surgery for multiglandular disease can be increased with the use of IOPTH. However, IOPTH in MGD will be useful only if a stricter criterion of IOPTH is followed. Requiring both a 50% decrease in IOPTH over 15 min and normalization of the post-excisional value would increase the sensitivity of IOPTH in predicting cure in cases of MGD [5].

References

1. Barczynski M, et al. Sporadic multiple parathyroid gland disease—a consensus report of the European Society of Endocrine Surgeons (ESES). Langenbeck's Arch Surg. 2015;400:887–905.
2. Their M, Daudi S, Bergenfelz A, Almquist M. Predictors of multiglandular disease in primary hyperparathyroidism. Langenbeck's Arch Surg. 2018;403:103–9.
3. Kebebew E, Hwang J, Reiff E, Duh QY, Clark OH. Predictors of single-gland vs multigland parathyroid disease in primary hyperparathyroidism: a simple and accurate scoring model. Arch Surg. 2006;141(8):777–82.
4. Mazeh H, Chen H, Leverson G, Sippel RS. Creation of a " Wisconsin index" nomogram to predict the likelihood of additional hyperfunctioning parathyroid glands during parathyroidectomy. Ann Surg. 2013;257(1):138–41.
5. Bhangu JS, Riss P. The role of intraoperative parathyroid hormone (IOPTH) determination for identification and surgical strategy of sporadic multiglandular disease in primary hyperparathyroidism (pHPT). Best Pract Res Clin Endocrinol Metab. 2019;33(5):101310.

Ectopic Locations

Case

A 55-year-old lady presented with symptoms of generalized aches and pains and lethargy. There was no family history of relevant disorders. Biochemical investigations showed elevated serum calcium (2.84 mmol/L) and elevated PTH at 16.4 pmol/L. Urine investigations in the form of calcium:creatinine clearance ratio ruled out familial hypocalciuric hypercalcemia (FHH). DEXA scan of her skeletal system showed moderate osteoporosis with T-score of −2.5 at hip and spine. Imaging to localize her parathyroid glands was discordant with Technetium ^{99}m Sestamibi (MIBI) scan showing a MIBI-avid lesion to suggest a parathyroid adenoma or hyperplasia at the left superior pole. However, the US scan did not reveal any obvious lesion.

She underwent an open parathyroidectomy under general anesthesia. On exploration on the left side a normal parathyroid was found in the superior position posterior to the thyroid gland but no inferior gland was found in conventional positions. Exploration of the left side continued to the carotid sheath and retro-esophageal and retro-tracheal areas. *A palpable nodular lesion measuring about 1.6 cm was found in the carotid sheath at the level of bifurcation of the carotids.* This was excised and IOPTH done as per Miami criteria, and the PTH dropped to 2.4 pmol/L, confirming cure. Her postoperative period was uneventful and was discharged home the following day. Histology confirmed the presence of parathyroid adenoma measuring 1.5 × 1.2 cm and weighing about 2.1 g.

Discussion

The parathyroid glands were first identified in the Indian Rhinoceros in 1850 [1], and were subsequently recognized in humans about thirty years later [2]. Typically,

Rajeev Parameswaran is the lead author of this chapter.

A. Agarwal et al., *Case Studies in Thyroid and Parathyroid Tumors*,
https://doi.org/10.1007/978-981-99-0938-4_25

there are two superior and two inferior parathyroid glands, immediately posterior to the thyroid gland. The parathyroid glands arise from endodermal epithelial cells. As the superior parathyroid glands are derived from the fourth branchial pouch, these have a short line of embryologic descent and are closely associated with the lateral lobes of the thyroid [3]. Conversely, the inferior parathyroid glands, which are derived from the third branchial pouch, have a longer line of embryologic descent, leading to more variability in their anatomic position [3].

Parathyroid glands in ectopic positions have a reported frequency of 5–20% [4], and they could be one of the four parathyroid glands, or a supernumerary gland. Overall, ectopic parathyroid glands can be found in numerous locations between mouth and diaphragm, such as in the mediastinum or intra-thyroidal (as shown in Table 1) [5]. The inferior glands are more frequently ectopic when compared to the superior glands due to the more extensive migration during the embryological descent [6]. Ectopia in the carotid sheath is reported in less than 2% of cases, and usually concerns an undescended inferior parathyroid gland [7]. In our own institution, we have only encountered 1 case of carotid sheath parathyroid adenoma (0.2%) in 447 parathyroidectomies performed. The challenge is, that the presence of an ectopic parathyroid adenoma often poses diagnostic difficulties, while it is also a common reason for failed initial parathyroid surgery.

Most of the cases reported on a parathyroid adenoma in the carotid sheath required multiple surgeries to obtain cure [8]. Generally, when a parathyroid adenoma is not to be found in the normal position, a meticulous systematic dissection should be undertaken, including all possible locations of ectopic parathyroid glands. The option of an undescended gland in the carotid sheath should also be considered, although the majority of the adenomas uncovered in this location are found posterior of the vascular trunks, and thus require extensive dissection even after opening of the carotid sheath [8].

Apart from the possible lack of awareness of the carotid sheet as a potential location of a parathyroid adenoma, there could also be a reduced sensitivity of traditional isotope studies, for instance due to overlapping submandibular activity [9], or due to not including the high cervical region in the field [10]. While ^{18}F-fluorocholine positron emission tomography-computed tomography (^{18}F-PET/CT) has been shown to have a high diagnostic accuracy in the detection of ectopic parathyroid adenoma [11]. Combining ultrasound of the neck with dual-phase 99mTc-sestamibi/99mTcO4 planar scintigraphy and SPECT has shown to raise sensitivity to 96% in successfully detecting parathyroid lesions [12]. Conversely, ectopic

Table 1 Location of ectopic parathyroids

Superior parathyroids	Inferior parathyroids	Rare locations
Tracheoesophageal groove	Thymus gland	Carotid bifurcation
Retroesophageal region	Thyroid gland	Posterior triangle of the neck
Posterosuperior mediastinum	Thyrothymic ligament	Within the vagus nerve
Paraesophageal region	Submandibular area	Within the hypoglossal nerve
Thyroid gland		Pericardium
Carotid sheath		Right dome of diaphragm

parathyroid adenoma within the carotid sheath has also been reported to mimic other lesions, such as a carotid body tumor [13].

References

1. Professor Owen FRS, F, c. III. On the anatomy of the Indian rhinoceros (Rh. Unicornis, L.). Trans Zool Soc London. 1852;4(2):31–58.
2. Seipel C. On a new gland in man and several mammals (glandulae parathyroideae) by Ivar Sandström (English translation). Baltimore: Johns Hopkins Press; 1938.
3. Bliss RD, Gauger PG, Delbridge LW. Surgeon's approach to the thyroid gland: surgical anatomy and the importance of technique. World J Surg. 2000;24(8):891–7.
4. Roy M, Mazeh H, Chen H, Sippel RS. Incidence and localization of ectopic parathyroid adenomas in previously unexplored patients. World J Surg. 2013;37(1):102–6.
5. Noussios G, Anagnostis P, Natsis K. Ectopic parathyroid glands and their anatomical, clinical and surgical implications. Exp Clin Endocrinol Diabetes. 2012;120(10):604–10.
6. Mariani G, Gulec SA, Rubello D, Boni G, Puccini M, Pelizzo MR, et al. Preoperative localization and radioguided parathyroid surgery. J Nucl Med. 2003;44(9):1443–58.
7. Eslamy HK, Ziessman HA. Parathyroid scintigraphy in patients with primary hyperparathyroidism: 99mTc sestamibi SPECT and SPECT/CT. Radiographics. 2008;28(5):1461–76.
8. Chopra A, Bansal R, Sharma N, Kulshreshtha B. Parathyroid adenoma within the carotid sheath. Acta Endocrinol (Buchar). 2020;16(4):497–500.
9. Mahajan S, Schoder H. Ectopic undescended parathyroid adenoma-SPECT/CT avoids false-negative interpretation on 99mTc-MIBI dual-phase scintigraphy. Clin Nucl Med. 2018;43(3):199–200.
10. Ezzine A, Ben FM, Azzabi A, Talmoudi A, Sahtout W, Boukadida R, et al. Undescended parathyroid gland mimicking salivary gland uptake. J Nephrol Ther. 2016;6(268):2161.
11. Boccalatte LA, Higuera F, Gómez NL, de la Torre AY, Mazzaro EL, Galich AM, et al. Usefulness of 18F-fluorocholine positron emission tomography–computed tomography in locating lesions in hyperparathyroidism: a systematic review. JAMA Otolaryngol Head Neck Surg. 2019;145(8):743–50.
12. Ansquer C, Mirallié E, Carlier T, Abbey-Huguenin H, Aubron F, Kraeber-Bodéré F. Preoperative localization of parathyroid lesions. Value of 99mTc-MIBI tomography and factors influencing detection. Nuklearmedizin. 2008;47(4):158–62.
13. Libé R, Calvani J, Cottereau AS, Connan TL, Gaujoux S, Groussin L, et al. An ectopic parathyroid adenoma mimicking a carotid body paraganglioma. J Endocr Soc. 2020;4(12):bvaa143.

Mediastinal Parathyroid Adenomas

Case 1
A 52-year-old woman presented with a history of bony pain and proximal muscle weakness for 1.5 years with no history of renal colic or recent bony fractures. On evaluation she was found to have raised Calcium and PTH.

Test	Value
S.Calcium Total: Ionic:	12.0 mg/dL 5.2 mg/dL
S.Phosphorus	2.2 mg/dL
S.ALP	156 U/L
S.Creatinine	0.9 mg/dL
S.PTH	528 pg/mL
S.Vit D	25.7 ng/mL

USG neck was negative for any parathyroid adenoma in the neck. SPECT-MIBI revealed an ectopic parathyroid in the mediastinum. CECT showed parathyroid adenoma in the anterior mediastinum in the pre-vascular space (Fig. 1). She underwent focused Parathyroidectomy and a 3.0 × 1.5 × 0.3 cm maroon-colored adenoma was found embedded in the thymus. The adenoma was delivered through the cervical incision after pulling up the thymic limb. The specimen weighed 2.6 g. The IOPTH was suggestive of cure: **IOPTH values**: Pre-incision: 404, Pre-excision: 235, Post-excision 5 min: 111, Post-excision 10 min: 74, Post-excision 15 min: 42.

Case 2
A 58-year-old woman presented with complaints of proximal muscle weakness and easy fatigability × 2 months. She gave a history of having sustained a fracture of the left leg following trivial trauma – 4 years back which was treated by screw and plate.

Roma Pradhan is the lead author of this chapter.

A. Agarwal et al., *Case Studies in Thyroid and Parathyroid Tumors*,
https://doi.org/10.1007/978-981-99-0938-4_26

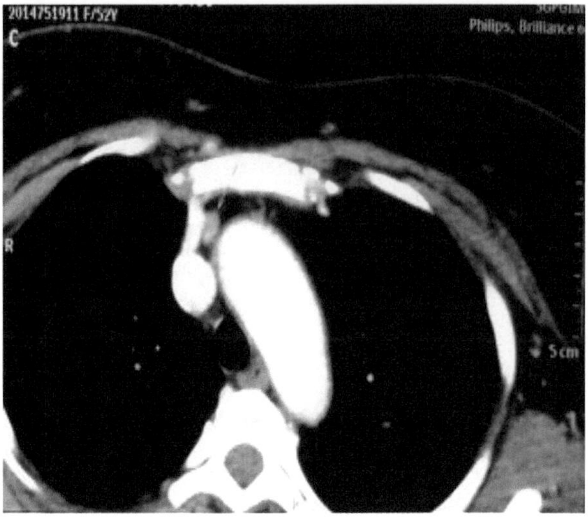

Fig. 1 CECT of case 1 showing the adenoma in the anterior mediastinum in the pre-vascular space (arrow)

On evaluation her biochemistry was as follows: Calcium: 12.0, 11.6, 11.6 mmol/L (8.5–10.5), Ionic calcium: 1.59, 1.50 mEq/mL, s. Phosphorous: 2.9 mg/dL (2.5–4.5), s. albumin: 4.2 g/dL (3.5–5.5), s. PTH: 234 226 pg/mL (9–55), ALP: 53 IU/dL (55–150), 25 hydroxy vitamin D: 51.8 ng/mL (9–47), BMD (T score): −2.1 (spine), −1.5 (hip), −2.5 (radius). USG neck did not reveal any parathyroid adenoma in the neck. Tc99m-Sestamibi-Scan delayed images and SPECT showed tracer concentration in mediastinum (Fig. 2) on the right side suggestive of a mediastinal parathyroid adenoma. CECT Thorax showed a well-defined homogenously intensely enhancing oval mass lesion in the anterior mediastinum (Fig. 3), anterior to junction of ascending aorta and arch of aorta, at the level of T6/T7 level and sternal angle s/o – Mediastinal ectopic parathyroid gland enlargement. We decided to do a partial sternotomy since the adenoma was near the sternal angle (Fig. 4). At operation a single ovoid maroon-colored mediastinal parathyroid just inferior to Rt Innominate vein in the anterior mediastinum was found. There was more than 50% fall in IOPTH.

Time	Pre-incision	Pre-excision	5 min after excision	10 min after excision	15 min after excision
PTH(pg/mL)	782	336	277	143	91.3

Case 3

A 51-year-old lady presented to the dental OPD with maxillary swelling, a biopsy was done which was suggestive of brown tumor, hence the patient was sent to endocrine surgery OPD for further evaluation. Biochemical investigations were suggestive of primary hyperparathyroidism with hypercalcemic crisis (S. calcium 15.2 mg/dL Normal: 8.8–10.6, iPTH 1650 pg/mL Normal: 11–67 pg/mL).

The patient was then lost to follow-up and attended our OPD after 2 months. She got admitted with complaints of vomiting, and pain in the abdomen. Hence a clinical diagnosis of hypercalcemic crisis with acute pancreatitis was made. Her calcium was 20 and serum creatinine was 2.2 mg/dL and hence patient planned for dialysis

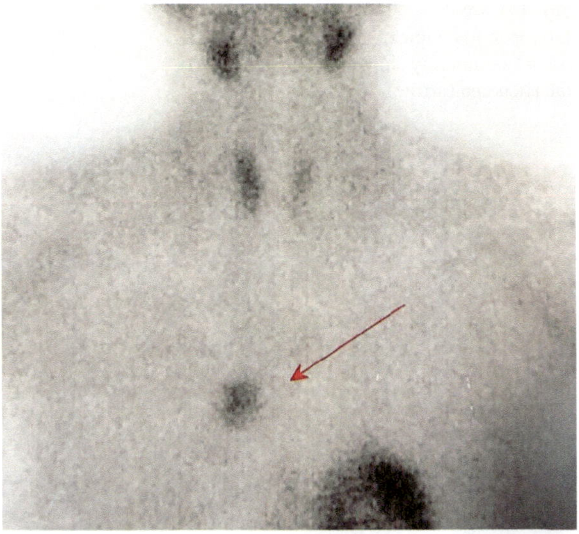

Fig. 2 Case 2: MIBI scan showing the ectopic MIBI avid parathyroid adenoma in the mediastinum

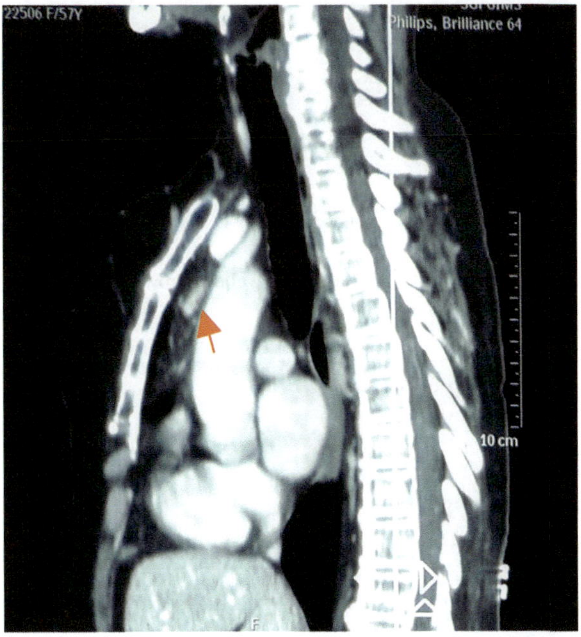

Fig. 3 Case 2: CECT showing parathyroid adenoma in anterior mediastinum at the level of sternal angle (arrow)

to manage this acute crisis. This was confirmed with increase in serum amylase and lipase. The patient was managed conservatively. Her pain was excruciating and was managed with epidural. While being managed for pancreatitis, she developed spontaneous clavicular fracture which was managed conservatively. Her localizing investigations (CT Neck, sestamibi, and SPECT CT scan) pointed toward a right parathyroid adenoma extending posteriorly into the mediastinum (Fig. 5a, b and c). NCCT was done as the patient had deranged renal parameters. Surgical approach depends on the part of the mediastinum the adenoma is localized (Fig. 6). We

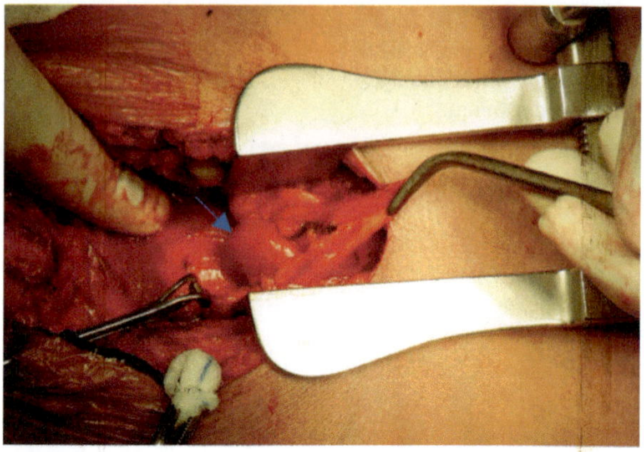

Fig. 4 Case 2: Intraoperative view of partial sternotomy showing the adenoma (arrow)

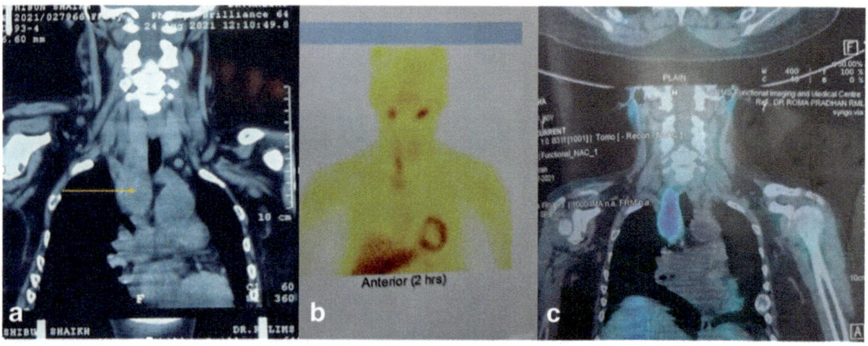

Fig. 5 (**a**) CT Neck with adenoma (yellow arrow), (**b**) MIBI delayed images, (**c**) SPECT CT image

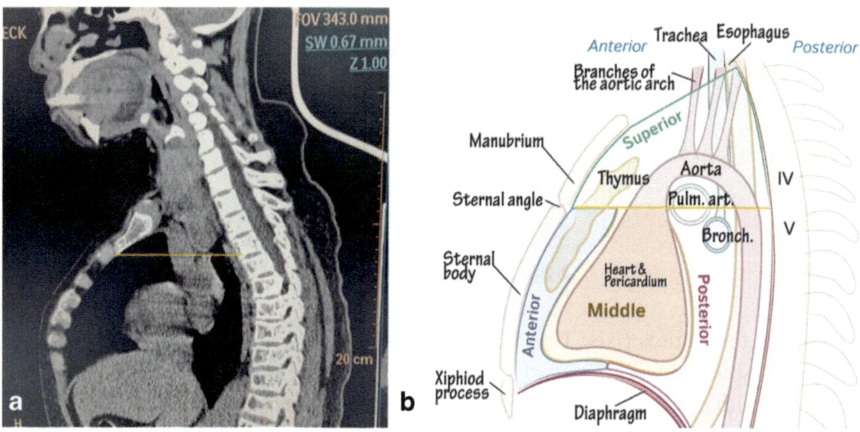

Fig. 6 (**a**) CT sagittal section of a patient with yellow line drawn at the level of sternal angle, (**b**) Image showing various divisions with corresponding yellow line at sternal angle

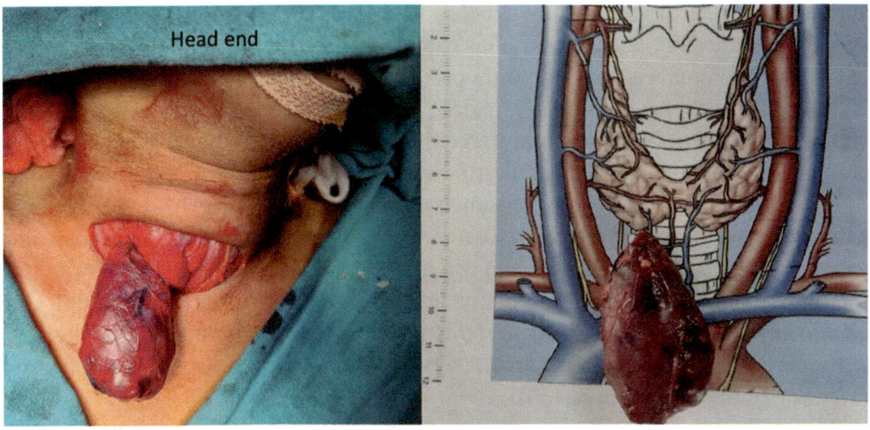

Fig. 7 Specimen weighing 36 g

planned for the removal of the adenoma via cervical incision. The adenoma was found extending in the posterior part of the superior mediastinum behind the brachiocephalic vein (Fig. 7). IOPTH showed more than 50% drop. The weight of the adenoma was 36 g and measured 6 × 3.5 × 3 cm.

Learning point in the case: Venous supply to the gland should be done at last after the arterial supply or else the gland swells up and there are chances of capsule rupture while delivering the gland from the mediastinum.

Discussion

A mediastinal parathyroid is defined as a parathyroid found completely below the level of the clavicle. Mediastinal parathyroid adenomas have been reported to be associated with more severe clinical manifestations of primary hyperparathyroidism, along with high calcium levels and bone disease [1]. The probable reason is delay in diagnosis and localization.

Churchill was the first to recognize hyperfunctioning ectopic parathyroid glands in 1932. The patient, Captain Charles E. Martell, underwent six prior unsuccessful cervical explorations and had severe osteitis fibrosa cystica until the ectopic gland was removed by a transsternal approach [2]. Majority of mediastinal parathyroid adenomas can be removed by cervical incision while 1–2% cases may need sternotomy, thoracotomy, or VATS. surgical excision should be planned based on thorax CT and parathyroid scintigraphy findings. The difficulty lies in determining the best approach for each patient. This was explained by Iihara et al. [3] in their retrospective analysis of 14 patients. They suggested the level of the aortic arch on the horizontal chest CT should be used as a landmark for guiding a suitable surgical approach. Those adenomas found above the aortic arch in the superior mediastinum can be treated successfully by a transcervical approach while those found in the anterior or posterior mediastinum below the level of the aortic arch should be approached transthoracic (Fig. 3). This can be understood by our patient images. In case 1 the adenoma was in the anterior part of the superior mediastinum so could be delivered from the neck. Similarly, in case 2 the adenoma was at the junction of the superior and anterior mediastinum so required partial sternotomy to deliver the adenoma. In the third patient the parathyroid extended to the posterior part of the superior mediastinum, hence could be delivered through the neck. However, the only caution that needs to be followed is extreme careful handling of the gland and avoiding rupturing of the capsule which may lead to parathyromatosis.

Inferior parathyroid glands normally descend into the anterior mediastinum. Our case is rare owing to its size, much of this inferior adenoma prolapsed into the posterior part of the superior mediastinum, a possibility in the case of large non-thymic inferior parathyroid adenomas [4].

Mediastinal parathyroid adenomas are separate clinical entities in primary hyperparathyroidism where difficulties lie in preoperative diagnosis and surgical approach to such cases. Nevertheless, the advances in imaging modalities available and surgical techniques have led to proper management on these cases.

References

1. Mendoza V, Ramírez C, Espinoza AE, et al. Characteristics of ectopic parathyroid glands in 145 cases of primary hyperparathyroidism. Endocr Pract. 2010;16:977–81.
2. Liman ST, Topcu S, Dervisoglu E, Gorur GD, Elicora A, Burc K, et al. Excision of ectopic mediastinal parathyroid adenoma via Para- sternal videomediastinoscopy. Ann Thorac Cardiovasc Surg. 2014;20:67–9.
3. Iihara M, Suzuki R, Kawamata A, Horiuchi K, Okamoto T. Thoracoscopic removal of mediastinal parathyroid lesions: selection of surgical approach and pitfalls of preoperative and intraoperative localization. World J Surg. 2012;36(6):1327–34.
4. Miller BJ, Isaacs K, Khan E, et al. Transcervical excision of a giant mediastinal parathyroid adenoma. BMJ Case Rep. 2019;12:bcr-2018-228292.

Part III

PHPT: Surgical Challenges and Conundrum

Bilateral Exploration in Non-localized PHPT

Case

A 56-year-old man, a known case of single left functioning kidney underwent left ESWL for left renal stone in 2001. During evaluation he was detected to have hyperparathyroidism with elevated PTH levels and was referred to us for definitive management. His biochemistry was as follows: serum ionized calcium: 1.51, iPTH:599.1 pg/mL. Both neck USG and Tc99Mmibi did not reveal any parathyroid avid tumor. So a decision for bilateral neck exploration was taken. At operation, right inferior parathyroid gland was found to be enlarged (Fig. 1) while the rest of the parathyroid glands were normal looking. A 1.9 × 0.7 × 0.5 cm, maroon-colored,

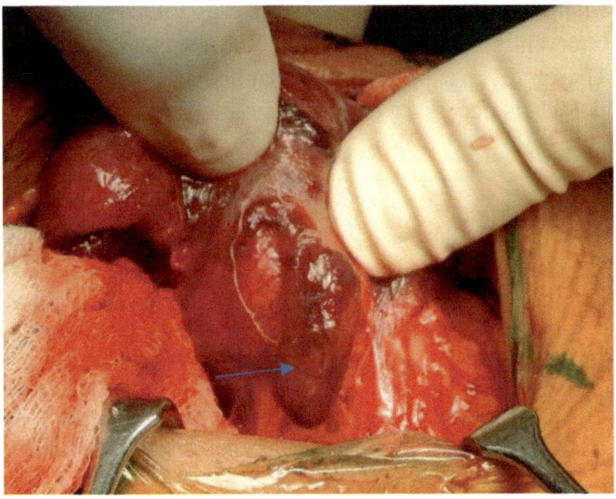

Fig. 1 Solitary adenoma in a non-localized case of PHPT

Amit Agarwal is the lead author of this chapter.

A. Agarwal et al., *Case Studies in Thyroid and Parathyroid Tumors*,
https://doi.org/10.1007/978-981-99-0938-4_27

ovoid parathyroid adenoma was removed and it weighed 700 mg. There was curative fall in IOPTH as per Miami criteria: IOPTH values (pg/mL)-Pre-incision – 351, Pre-excision – 217, Post-excision 5 min – 102, Post-excision 10 min – 70.2, Post-excision 15 min – 58.4. The HPE was reported as parathyroid adenoma.

Discussion

Few studies have evaluated the best course of action for patients with PHPT whose disease fail to localize on a MIBI scan and USG. It is unclear whether these patients should undergo further imaging with multiphasic CT scan. It is also uncertain whether the surgeon should proceed directly with a bilateral neck exploration or whether continued observation be considered. Reasons for failure to localize radiographically include multiglandular disease, ectopic location, associated nodular thyroid disease, and inadequate sestamibi uptake by parathyroid tissue in cases of small adenomas and oxyphill adenomas [1–4]. Patients with negative MIBI scans have statistically significant lower serum calcium, urinary calcium, and phosphate levels. There may be a correlation between these values and the lack of avid uptake on MIBI scan because it may represent an earlier stage of disease. A recent study by Bergenfelz et al. [5] examined 984 patients with preoperative localization with both sestamibi and US and found that when both studies were negative before operative intervention, the failure rate of surgery approached 18%. The lower cure rate for patients with 1HPT and a negative MIBI scan is likely related to multiglandular disease and difficulty identifying abnormal parathyroid glands when they are smaller in size. However, the use of IOPTH may aid in the success of operative intervention as well as visualization of glands and number of parathyroids excised. Therefore, if exploration is planned in a non-localized case of PHPT, the use of IOPTH is necessary to reduce failure rates.

References

1. Howson P, Kruijff S, Aniss A, Pennington T, Gill AJ, Dodds T, Delbridge LW, Sidhu SB, Sywak MS. Oxyphil cell parathyroid adenomas causing primary hyperparathyroidism: a Clinico-pathological correlation. Endocr Pathol. 2015;26:250–4.
2. Khorasani N, Mohammadi A. Effective factors on the sensitivity of preoperative sestamibi scanning for primary hyperparathyroidism. Int J Clin Exp Med. 2014;7(9):2639–44.
3. Isik S, Akbaba G, Berker D, Tutuncu YA, Ozuguz U, Aydin Y, Peksoy I, Guler S. Thyroid-related factors that influence preoperative localization of parathyroid adenomas. Endocr Pract. 2012;18(1):26–33.
4. Harari A, Mitmaker E, Grogan RH, Lee J, Shen W, Gosnell J, Clark O. Quan-Yang duh primary hyperparathyroidism patients with positive preoperative Sestamibi scan and negative ultrasound are more likely to have posteriorly located upper gland adenomas (PLUGs). Ann Surg Oncol. 2011;18:1717–22.
5. Bergenfelz AO, Wallin G, Jansson S, et al. Results of surgery for sporadic primary hyperparathyroidism in patients with preoperatively negative sestamibi scintigraphy and ultrasound. Langenbeck's Arch Surg. 2011;396:83–90.

Difficult Parathyroidectomy

Case

A 59-year-old male presented with a history of acute, intermittent abdominal. During evaluation, on USG, the patient was found to have bilateral renal calculi which was managed conservatively. During this period he developed episode of headache, sweating, and syncope and was found to be having rhythm problems and so pacemaker implantation (Fig. 1) was done. He also underwent cardiac angiography which showed mild LAD 50%, Lcx plaquing, mild RCA and angioplasty was done and was discharged on antiplatelet drugs. During evaluation he was found to be having elevated calcium and low phosphorous: 12/2.0. Subsequently, he was found to be having elevated PTH: 89.43 pmol/L, low Vit D – 19.01 nmol/L, and high ALP: 427u/L. NCCT neck showed a well-defined soft tissue lesion measuring 18.7 × 13 × 25 mm isodense lesion in the left cervical region. USG Neck showed a well-defined solid hypoechoic lesion 17 × 12 mm along the left lobe of thyroid, medial to left CCA and abutting the left thyroid suggestive of parathyroid adenoma. Tc 99m MIBI Parathyroid scan revealed MIBI avid tumor suggestive of parathyroid adenoma in the neck superior and posterior to left thyroid lobe. NCCT KUB showed B/L renal calculi, no hydronephrosis, pancreas atrophic, with dilated PD and multiple calculi were seen in pancreatic parenchyma and main pancreatic duct largest measuring 10 mm in main pancreas. BMD revealed severe osteoporosis with T score of −5.1 at forearm. 2 D ECHO showed concentric LVH with diastolic dysfunction. The patient was admitted and optimized for surgery. Antiplatelets were stopped prior to surgery and cardiology clearance was taken. Pacemaker mode was changed to non-sensing mode (VOO) and the patient was operated.: Focussed left superior parathyroidectomy was done and a 4 × 1.5 × 1 cm large, maroon-colored adenoma (Fig. 2) weighing 6.2 g was removed with curative fall in IOPTH. He had an uneventful intraoperative and postoperative course with normalized calcium

Amit Agarwal is the lead author of this chapter.

A. Agarwal et al., *Case Studies in Thyroid and Parathyroid Tumors*,
https://doi.org/10.1007/978-981-99-0938-4_28

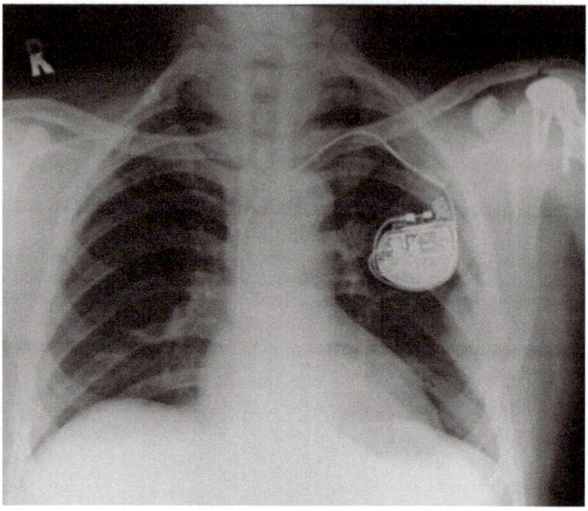

Fig. 1 Chest x-ray showing the implantable pacemaker

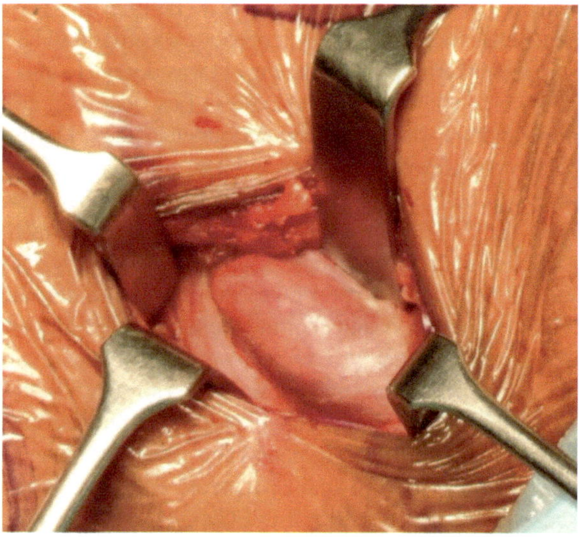

Fig. 2 Intraoperative view of the parathyroid adenoma

values and iPTH levels. No evidence of biochemical or clinical hypocalcemia was noted. The patient was advised to restart antiplatelets on POD 3 and Pacemaker Mode was switched back to sensing (VII).

Discussion

The use of anticoagulant and/or antiplatelet medications is expanding in our aging population. These medications are designed to prevent platelet aggregation or clot formation, both of which are crucial for hemostasis after any operation and their continued use may result in postoperative hematoma with its serious consequences. At the same time, however, the indications for antiplatelet and anticoagulant use can be equally critical in preventing embolic or thrombotic events and discontinuation may lead to stroke, heart attack, or pulmonary embolism. The impact of antiplatelet and anticoagulant therapies on postoperative hemostasis is not equal. Antiplatelet therapies are often provided to prevent in-stent thrombosis in patients who have undergone previous percutaneous coronary or other vascular intervention, and they are less problematic for many surgical procedures Anticoagulant therapy poses a much larger problem. One study [1] has demonstrated hematoma rates of 2.2 and 10.7%, respectively, for those patients receiving particular antiplatelet or anticoagulant therapies, which is significantly higher than the overall POH rate of 0.5%. The sub-group analysis of this study had the following results: Rates of POH in patients receiving <325 mg ASA or not receiving any form of antiplatelet medication (0.1 and 0.5%, respectively) were low, while patients receiving >325 mg ASA (0.8%) and clopidogrel (2.2%) had higher rates of POH ($p = 0.045$). Patients not receiving any form of anticoagulation had low POH rates (0.4%), but oral anticoagulation increased POH rates 5.5-fold (2.2%) and injectable anticoagulant increased POH rates 26.8-fold (10.7%, $p < 0.001$). Use of a single agent (either antiplatelet or anticoagulant) resulted in a slight increase in POH rate (0.8%), whereas the use of both increased POH over sevenfold (2.3%, $p = 0.033$). Also, rates of postoperative hematoma are much higher after thyroidectomy as compared to parathyroidectomy. Despite their infrequent use, anticoagulants have a strong association with increased rates of hematoma formation in both parathyroid and thyroid surgery, even if stopped 5–7 days before surgery. Injectable anticoagulants in particular increase the odds of hematoma formation 29-fold.

The practice advisory clearly delineates that pacemaker-dependent patients or those with implantable cardioverter-defibrillators (ICDs) should have those devices altered to suspend pacemaker sensing or ICD anti-tachycardia therapy for monopolar electrosurgery superior to the umbilicus. In patients requiring the use of monopolar cautery and surgical site is within 6 in. of PM, the pacemaker should be re-programmed to asynchronous mode and should be programmed back to baseline settings before discharge [2].

References

1. Oltmann SC, Alhefdhi AY, Rajaei MH, Schneider DF, Sippel RS, Chen H. Antiplatelet and anticoagulant medications significantly increase the risk of postoperative hematoma: review of over 4500 thyroid and parathyroid procedures. Ann Surg Oncol. 2016;23(9):2874–82.
2. Hunter CBG, Chen TH. An attractive shift in polarity: a new algorithm for the perioperative management of cardiac implantable electronic devices (CIEDs). J Clin Anesth. 2021;70:110161.

Intra-Thyroidal Parathyroid Adenoma

Case 1

A 63-year-old lady presented with fever and swelling over face which was progressive along with raised creatinine levels. She was diagnosed with chronic kidney disease with bilateral renal calculi in the nephrology department. The patient then underwent left-sided percutaneous nephrostomy in urology and was found to have high serum calcium and PTH level, hence referred to Endocrine surgery. Localizing investigations were done. MIBI was suggestive of left inferior parathyroid lesion (Fig. 1). USG neck shows a 2.3 cm lesion in the left lobe with increased vascularity (TIRADS 5). Surgeon performed ultrasound showed a lesion posteriorly to the thyroid with no definite planes with thyroid (Fig. 2), hence planned for unilateral exploration. Intraoperatively superior parathyroid gland was normal, no inferior gland was seen therefore a decision of left hemithyroidectomy (Fig. 3) was taken. Specimen was bisected and showed parathyroid lesion (Fig. 4) which was confirmed on frozen. IOPTH showed more than 50% drop (Miami's criteria).

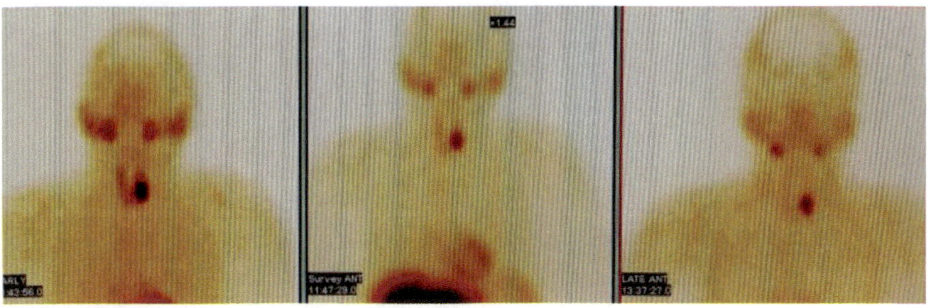

Fig. 1 MIBI suggestive of left inferior parathyroid

Roma Pradhan is the lead author of this chapter.

A. Agarwal et al., *Case Studies in Thyroid and Parathyroid Tumors*,
https://doi.org/10.1007/978-981-99-0938-4_29

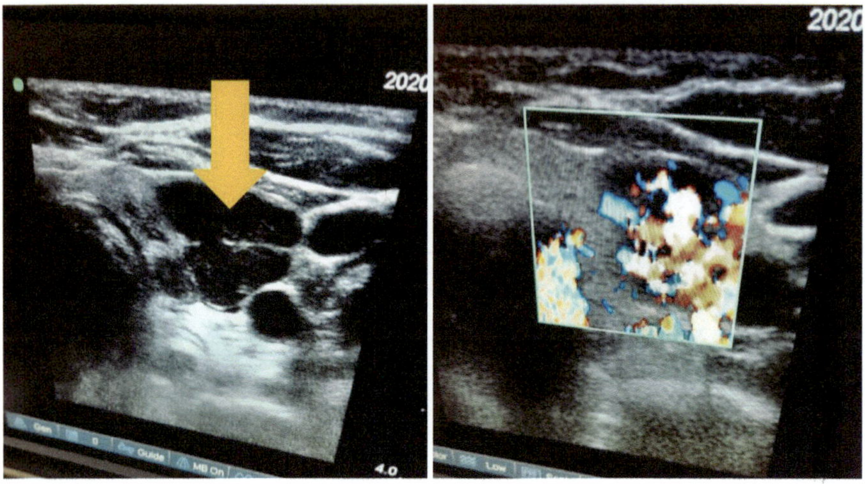

Fig. 2 Surgeon performed USG showing parathyroid lesion (orange arrow)

Fig. 3 Hemithyroid specimen

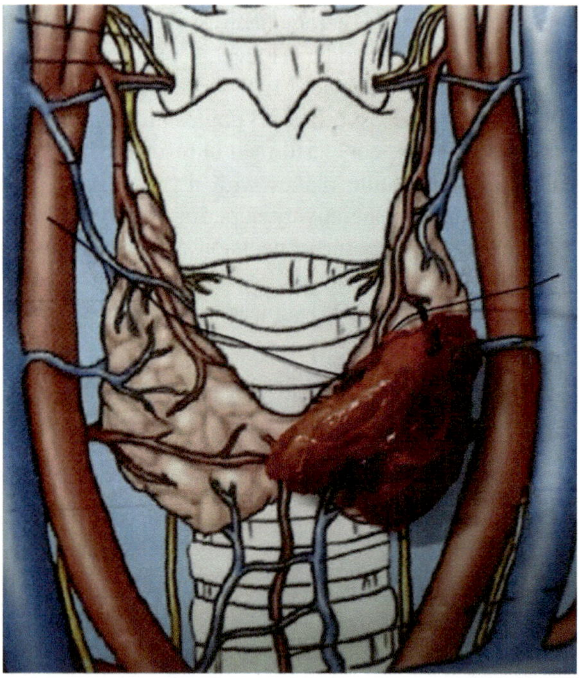

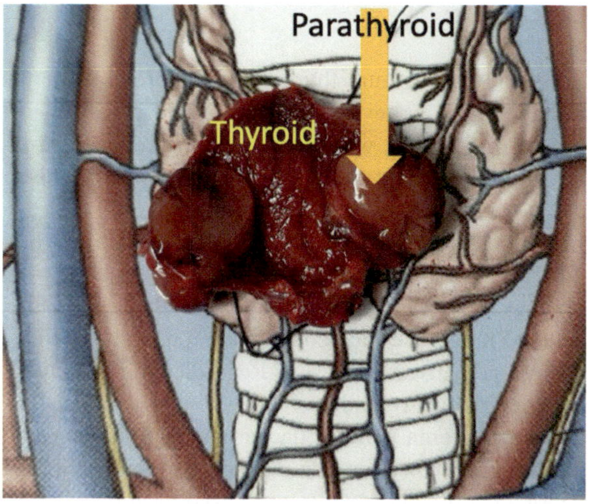

Fig. 4 Bisected specimen showing parathyroid lesion(orange arrow)

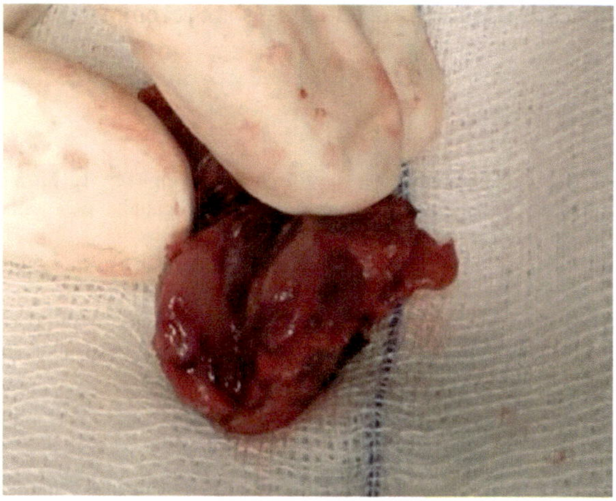

Fig. 5 Bisected hemithyroidectomy specimen showing the intra-thyroid parathyroid adenoma

Case 2

A 25-year-old girl was evaluated for loin pain and was found to be having elevated serum calcium and PTH. With suspicion of PHPT, USG neck was done which revealed a small rounded, hypoechoic lesion inferior to the left lobe of the thyroid. MIBI scan was negative for any MIBI avid lesion in the neck or mediastinum. In view of discordant imaging, unilateral exploration was done and the lesion inferior to the left lobe of the thyroid was excised and sent for frozen section which was reported as lymph node tissue; IOPTH also did not show curative fall at 15 min (pre-excision: 19.19 while post-excision at 15 min:19.14). A decision for left hemithyroidectomy was taken and the cut-section revealed a 1 × 1 cm lesion in the inferior pole of the thyroid (Fig. 5) which was reported as parathyroid tissue on frozen section and there was curative fall of IOPTH (Post-excision 10 min: 2.2). HPE was reported as an intra-thyroidal parathyroid adenoma.

Discussion

The incidence of Intra-thyroidal parathyroid adenoma ranges from 1.3% to 6.7%. Some authors believe that intra-thyroid parathyroid tumors are mainly superior parathyroid glands, whereas others believe the intra-thyroid lesions mainly involve the inferior parathyroid glands [1]. The rarity of this entity makes the preoperative diagnosis elusive. Intrathyroidal PAs have no specific sonographic features, apart from the hypoechoic appearance and the abundant blood supply. Even so, they are difficult to be distinguished from thyroid nodules, which may exhibit similar morphology. On functional imaging with 99mTc sestamibi scan, both thyroid nodules and PAs may be visualized and therefore, the presence of tracer accumulation is not always indicative of a PA [2]. Regardless of its rarity, however, a surgeon operating for primary hyperparathyroidism should be cognizant of its possibility when a parathyroid adenoma is not found in its usual location. Though conventional teaching has been that when performing a parathyroid exploration, if a missing gland cannot be found, it may lie in an intra-thyroid location and performing a thyroid lobectomy is appropriate. However, thyroid lobectomy for a missing parathyroid adenoma is typically unsuccessful and thus is not recommended [3].

References

1. Bahar G, Feinmesser R, Joshua BZ, Shpitzer T, Morgenstein S, Popovtzer A, et al. Hyperfunctioning intrathyroid parathyroid gland: a potential cause of failure in parathyroidectomy. Surgery. 2006;139:821–6.
2. Chen J, Ma Z, Jianchun Y. Diagnostic pitfalls in a cystic ectopic intrathyroidal parathyroid adenoma mimicking a nodular goiter: A care-compliant case report. Medicine. 2019;98(5):e14351.
3. Goodman A, Politz D, Lopez J, Norman J. Intrathyroid parathyroid adenoma: incidence and location—the case against thyroid lobectomy. Otolaryngol Head Neck Surg. 2011;144:867–71.

Parathyroid Cyst

Case

A 35-year-old woman presented with complaints of anterior neck swelling for 15 months which was painless and gradually progressive. She had a history of primary hypothyroidism and was on thyroxine, 75 mcg since 5 years. On examination of neck she had 8.4 × 6.2 cm firm nodule arising from the left lobe of the thyroid (Fig. 1). USG neck revealed a well-defined cystic lesion with internal echoes and septations measuring 3.4 × 8.6 cm arising from the left lobe of thyroid (Fig. 2) with relatively preserved medial part of the left thyroid lobe. The right lobe was normal with the impression of left colloid goiter. Guided FNAC showed few clusters as well as singly scattered population of benign thyroid follicular cells and cystic macrophages with abundant colloid in the background with a final impression of Colloid nodule with cystic degeneration. Her thyroid function profile was normal. She was taken up for a hemithyroidectomy. Intra-operatively a cystic mass in the region of the left lobe of the thyroid was found but the left lobe of the thyroid and isthmus were not seen (Fig. 3). Also, the left superior and inferior parathyroid glands were not seen while the right lobe of the thyroid was normal. The specimen measured 7 × 6 × 3 cm, was cystic and weighed 50 g. Cut section showed a thin-walled cyst, filled with brown fluid with 1.5 × 1 cm growth in the inferior wall. Post-operatively she developed symptomatic hypocalcemia (positive T-sign) within 18 h of surgery and required IV calcium infusion for 4 days after which she was kept on oral calcium and vitamin D supplements which were continued for 3 months. The histopathology was suggestive of parathyroid cyst-sections from the cyst wall showed fibro-collagenous wall lined by multilayered clear epithelium cells along with nests of normal parathyroid tissue.

Amit Agarwal is the lead author of this chapter.

A. Agarwal et al., *Case Studies in Thyroid and Parathyroid Tumors*,
https://doi.org/10.1007/978-981-99-0938-4_30

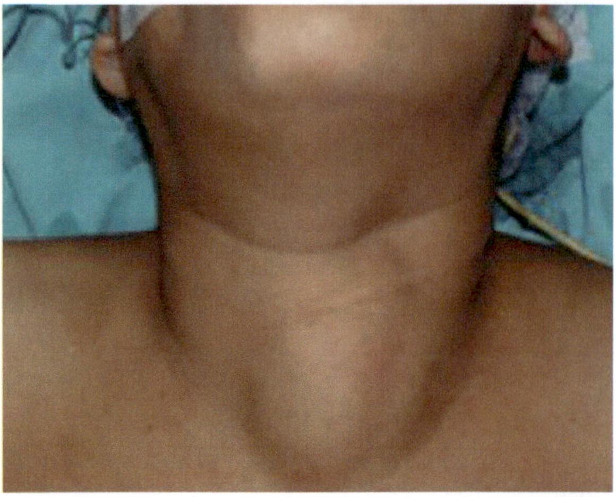

Fig. 1 Patient presented with a solitary thyroid nodule

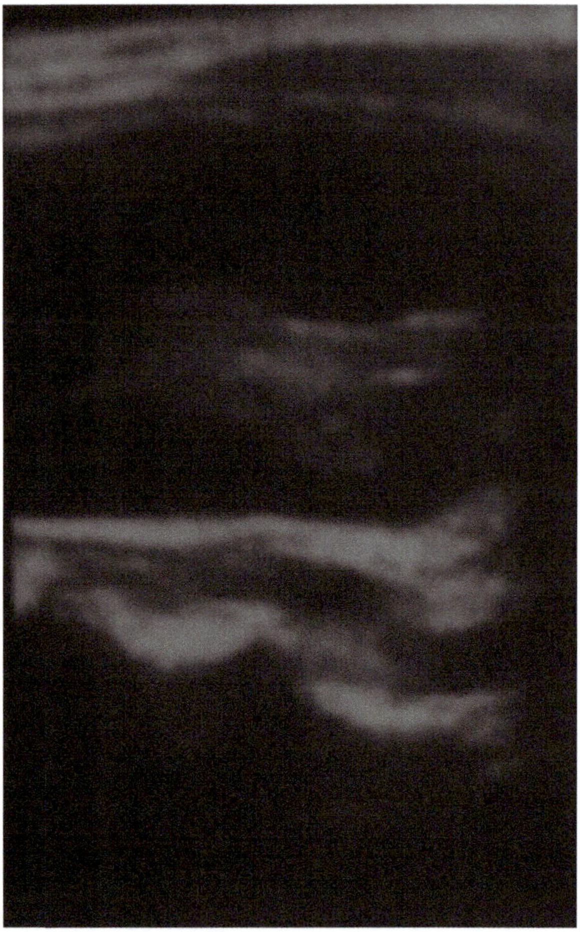

Fig. 2 USG showed a well-defined cystic lesion with internal echoes and septations

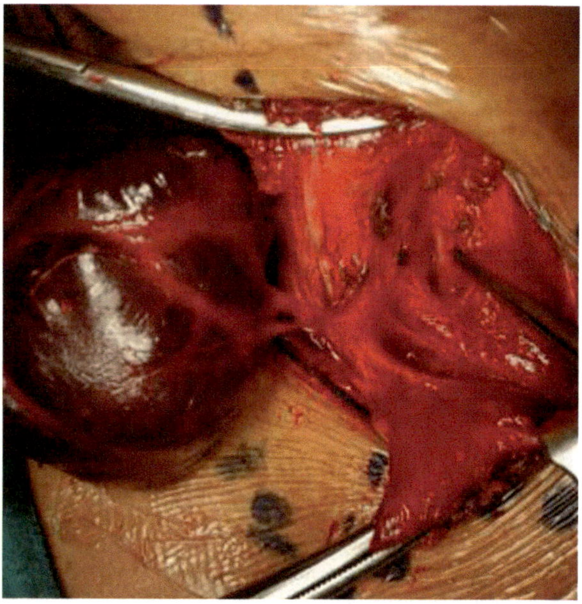

Fig. 3 Intra-operative view of the cyst

Discussion

Parathyroid cyst is an uncommon entity with just 300 cases being reported in the world literature so far. It accounts for 0.5% of the parathyroid diseases and 1% of all cystic lesions of the neck [1]. There is a female predilection with female:male ratio of 2.5:1. It usually occurs in the fourth–fifth decades of life and can be found anywhere from the mandible to the mediastinum. Most common location is the cervical region, with left inferior parathyroid is the most common gland to be affected [2]. It is thought to arise from embryologic remnants of the third and fourth pharyngeal pouches or might result from the coalescence of pre-existing microcysts which might enlarge due to retention of cyst fluid; or it might result from cystic degeneration of a parathyroid adenoma due to partial infarction as the gland outgrows its blood supply. On histopathology the cysts are usually lined by a solitary layer of compressed cuboidal or columnar epithelium which stains positive for glycogen. Presence of parathyroid tissue within the cyst wall is diagnostic. It typically presents as asymptomatic neck mass but may uncommonly cause dysphagia, hoarseness, pain, neck mass, and tracheal or esophageal compression and in mediastinum, can cause recurrent laryngeal nerve paralysis. Usually presents as apparent thyroid nodule and moves on swallowing and hence correct diagnosis is usually made intra-operatively. Differential Diagnosis includes: Thyroid cyst/Thyroglossal duct cyst(usually in the midline and move with deglutition), Branchial cleft cyst, Thyroid adenoma, Parathyroid carcinoma, Cystic papillary cancer, esophageal duplication cysts. The intra-operative appearance is a smooth, shiny, semi-transparent thin cyst loosely attached to the thyroid but easily dissected free from the thyroid and surrounding structures. FNAC is suggestive if it reveals crystal clear, colorless, acellular fluid with elevated PTH levels in the cystic fluid which is confirmatory. A minimum of 1 mL of aspirate is needed for the assays [3–5]. On imaging, USG neck will show a solitary pure cyst located usually posterior to thyroid lobe and thyroid scan will show a cold nodule. Treatment modalities include: Aspiration, Sclerotherapy and Surgery. USG-guided aspiration is the initial treatment as it is safe, easy and repeatable. Reports of sclerotherapy with ethanol or tetracycline as the sole treatment for non-functioning parathyroid cysts are there but it may result in damage to the recurrent laryngeal nerve. If repeated aspirations fail or if the cyst is functional with high serum PTH levels then surgical excision is the treatment of choice.

References

1. Ippolito G, Palazzo FF, Sebag F, Sierra M, De Micco C, Henry JF. A single-institution 25-year review of true parathyroid cysts. Langenbeck's Arch Surg. 2006;391(1):13–8.
2. Ihm PS, Dray T, Sofferman RA, Nathan M, Hardin NJ. Parathyroid cysts: diagnosis and management. Laryngoscope. 2001;111(9):1576–8.
3. Cao H, Lai CK, Head CS, Sercarz JA. Cystic parathyroid presenting as an apparent thyroid goiter. Eur Arch Otorhinolaryngol. 2008;265(10):1285–8.
4. Ujiki MB, Nayar R, Sturgeon C, Angelos P. Parathyroid cyst: often mistaken for a thyroid cyst. World J Surg. 2007;31(1):60–4.
5. Layfield LJ. Fine needle aspiration cytology of cystic parathyroid lesions. Acta Cytol. 1991;35:447–50.

Parathyroidectomy Under Regional Anesthesia

Case

A 24-year-old young man presented with chief complaints of fever for 1 year, loss of weight, bone pains, generalized weakness for 1 year. He had sustained repeated fractures of right tibia, right radius & ulna, and left humerus. He also had a history of renal stones, constipation, proximal muscle weakness, nausea & vomiting. At presentation he had plaster cast in both arms and a splint in the right lower limb (Fig. 1a, b, c). He was bedridden and was also found to be having bilateral femoral neck fractures (Fig. 1d and e). He was found to be in hypercalcemic crisis with serum calcium of 15.9 mg/dL. His PTH values were extremely high: 2398 pg/mL and very low vit D levels: 2.5 ng/mL with hemoglobin of 5.6 g/dL. He was put on forced saline diuresis and was given blood transfusions. Both USG and MIBI were concordant for a left superior parathyroid gland. In view of poor anesthetic risk, it was decided to operate upon him as a semi-emergent case under cervical block (Fig. 1f). Focused parathyroidectomy was done and an enlarged left sup parathyroid gland, measuring 3 × 2 × 1 cm (Fig. 1g) and weighing 5.5 g, was excised in weight.

Amit Agarwal is the lead author of this chapter.

A. Agarwal et al., *Case Studies in Thyroid and Parathyroid Tumors*,
https://doi.org/10.1007/978-981-99-0938-4_31

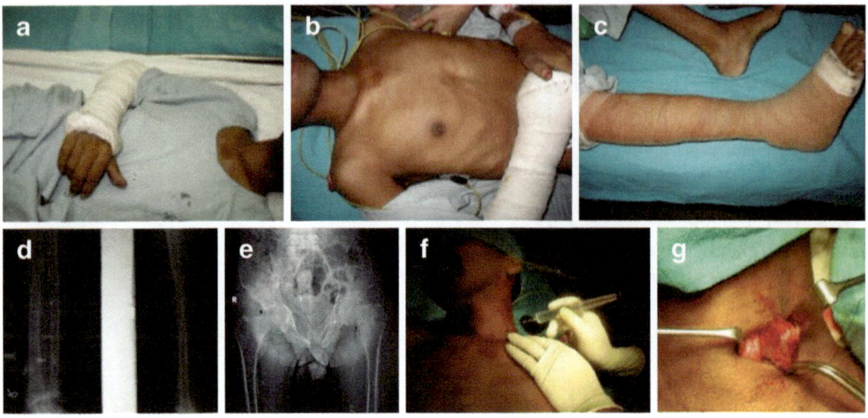

Fig. 1 (**a–g**) Showing the multiple fractures including bilateral FNF, superficial cervical plexus block being initiated and the intra-operative picture of adenoma being removed through a small unilateral incision

Discussion

Minimally invasive parathyroidectomy can be performed with cervical plexus block (CPB) due to the limited unilateral incision. Regional anesthesia avoids complications associated with general anesthesia, including endotracheal intubation, which has been reported to cause vocal cord changes in up to 5% of patients [1]. The patients experience return of energy level to normal more quickly and return to work sooner after surgery under regional anesthesia. The two common techniques that are employed are the superficial cervical block or a combination of superficial and deep cervical block [2]. All blocks should be performed by an anesthetist who is experienced in this technique. During block placement, patients usually lie supine with their heads slightly extended and rotated to the lateral side opposite to the block. The superficial cervical block (SCB) is administered after local skin infiltration with 2 mL of 2% lidocaine at the midpoint of the posterior border of the sternocleidomastoid (SCM) muscle using a 22-gauge needle, which is followed by an injection of 0.5% levobupivacaine subcutaneously along the posterior border of the muscle in cranial and caudal directions and deeper, on the medial surface of the muscle (beneath the muscle) with the total dosage of 0.35 mL/kg. The combined CPB is started by a deep block using a single injection technique at the C3 vertebral level. After palpating the transverse process (next to the posterior border of SCM muscle) and local skin infiltration with 2 mL of 2% lidocaine, a 24-gauge needle is introduced perpendicularly in a slightly caudal direction until the transverse process is located in the depth of 2–3 cm followed by an injection of 0.2 mL/kg of 0.5% levobupivacaine after negative aspiration for blood and/or cerebrospinal fluid. This is followed by the superficial CPB as mentioned. During block placement and throughout surgery, patients can be sedated, if needed, with IV midazolam. In most tertiary care endocrine centers, regional block is usually surgeon administered [3]. Many studies have shown that adding deep CPB to the superficial does not increase the efficacy and success rate of CPB in patients undergoing MIP. In fact, deep CPB has been reported to be associated with complications like phrenic nerve block and hemidiaphragmatic paresis in up to 61% of patients [3–5]. Even RLN palsy has been associated with deep CPB. Thus, the technique of choice is superficial CPB.

References

1. Stojadinovic A, Shaha A, Orlikoff R, et al. Prospective functional voice assessment in patients undergoing thyroid surgery. Ann Surg. 2002;236:823–32.
2. Pintaric TS, Hocevar M, Jereb S, Casati A, Novak JV. A prospective, randomized comparison between combined (deep and superficial) and superficial cervical plexus block with levobupivacaine for minimally invasive parathyroidectomy. Anesth Analg. 2007;105(4):1160–3.
3. Miccoli P, Barellini L, Monchik JM, Rago R, Berti PF. Randomized clinical trial comparing regional and general anaesthesia in minimally invasive videoassisted parathyroidectomy. Br J Surg. 2005;92:814–8.
4. Lo GP. Loco-regional anesthesia for thyroidectomy: evaluation as an outpatient procedure. Surgery. 1998;124:975–9.
5. Pandit JJ, Bree S, Dillon P, Elcock D, McLaren ID, Crider B. A comparison of superficial versus combined (superficial and deep) cervical plexus block for carotid endarterectomy: a prospective, randomized study. Anesth Analg. 2000;91:781–6.

Secondary Hyperparathyroidism (SHPT)

Case

A 49-year-old woman was referred from Nephrology. She was a known case of CKD (hypertensive origin?) for the last 5 years and was on continuous ambulatory peritoneal dialysis (CAPD) for 2 years. She had developed bone pains and was found to be having elevated PTH (2536 pg/mL) and was put on oral calcium, vit D and cinacalcet (30 mg BD). Subsequently, her PTH reduced to only 1203 pg/mL (9–55). She continued to have severe bone pains, progressive proximal muscle weakness and could not do her daily activities. Her biochemistry revealed: Calcium-7.2, 9.0, 9.4 mmol/L (8.5–10.5), serum phosphorous: 6.2, 5.3, 5.3 mg/dL (2.5–4.5), iPTH:1203 pg/mL (9–55), ALP;553 IU/dL (55–150), S. creatinine: 7.30 mg/dL, 25 hydroxy vitamin D: 20.1 ng/mL (9–47),. BMD (T score): −2.3 (spine), −2.4 (femur neck), −4.4 (forearm). USG neck showed bilateral inferior parathyroid enlargement: Rt – 0.9 × 1.5 cm, left – 0.6 × 1.6 cm. Tc 99m-MIBI SPECT scan revealed only left inferior parathyroid enlargement. She underwent bilateral exploration with 3 gland parathyroidectomy as right superior gland was not visualized (Fig. 1). Cervical thymectomy was added.

	Wt	Size
Left superior gland	0.4 g	1.4 × 1 × 0.6 cm
Left inferior	0.7 g	1.6 × 1.1 × 0.8 cm
Rt inferior	0.9 g	1.6 × 1.8 × 0.7 cm

IOPTH

Time	Pre-incision	Pre-excision	5 min after excision	10 min after excision	15 min after excision
PTH(pg/mL)	>1440	456	387	158	43.6

Amit Agarwal is the lead author of this chapter.

A. Agarwal et al., *Case Studies in Thyroid and Parathyroid Tumors*,
https://doi.org/10.1007/978-981-99-0938-4_32

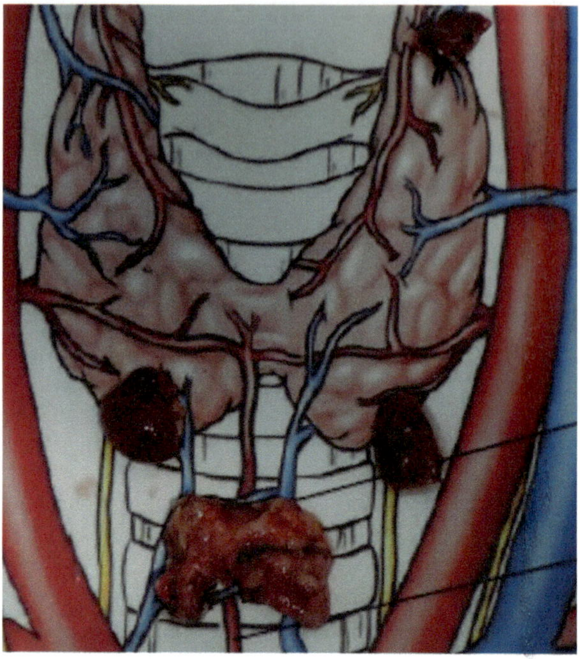

Fig. 1 Specimen of 3-gland parathyroidectomy

Discussion

Secondary HPT occurs most commonly "secondary" to chronic renal failure (CRF). For this reason, secondary HPT is frequently referred to as renal HPT. Estimates report that as many as 90% of patients with CRF develop this disease by the time hemodialysis is initiated [1]. Other causes of secondary HPT include osteomalacia, rickets, and malabsorption. The pathophysiology of SHPT results from prolonged hypocalcemia which causes parathyroid hyperplasia and increased secretion of PTH. Elevated PTH results in skeletal and other target organ abnormalities. Hypocalcemia results from elevated phosphate levels (due to abnormalities in renal tubular reabsorption of phosphate) and reduced intestinal absorption of calcium (due to Impaired renal conversion of 25-hydroxycholecalciferal to 1,25-dihydroxycholecalciferol (vitamin D, calcitriol). Most patients of SHPT may be asymptomatic and may just show abnormal laboratory findings such as hypocalcemia/normocalcemia, hyperphosphatemia, and low vitamin D levels. However, untreated SHPT may lead to progressive bone disease, osteitis fibrosa cystica, and soft-tissue calcifications resulting in intractable bone pain or fractures, pruritis, nephrolithiasis, pancreatitis, soft tissue or vascular calcifications, and mental status changes. Skeletal survey and 3-site BMD may reveal severe osteoporosis.

Management of patients with secondary HPT is predominantly medical aiming to lower phosphate level into the normal range and keep PTH levels between two and nine times of the upper normal range of intact PTH in dialysis patients. The

National Kidney Foundation of the USA proposed for renal HPT patients on dialysis in the Kidney Disease Outcomes Quality Initiative (K/DOQI) a serum calcium level between 8.4 and 9.5 mg/dL, serum phosphate level of 3.5–5.5 mg/dL, calcium/phosphorus product of <55 mg^2/dl^2, and intact PTH (iPTH) of 150–300 pg/mL [2]. Supplementation with calcium and active vitamin D is usually sufficient to manage PTH levels in patients with CRF and secondary HPT. To treat patients with secondary HPT who become refractory to replacement of calcium and vitamin D, several alternative therapies have become available over the last 10 to 15 years which include calcimimetics, such as Cinacalcet (which alter calcium receptor sensitivity of parathyroid glands and kidneys, thus reducing PTH secretion and restoring calcium-phosphorus homeostasis), new phosphate binders, and vitamin D analogs that are less likely to result in hypercalcemia. For avoiding the risk of hypercalcemia with calcitriol, parathyroid VDR-specific VDRAs (vitamin D receptor activators) are now widely used for SHPT treatment. These agents are designed to bridge patients to renal transplant, the optimal treatment for secondary HPT [3]. However, a small proportion of patients of SHPT, about 1–2%, will require parathyroidectomy each year. Surgical treatment is now favoredas it proficiently and quickly lowers calcium, PTH and phosphorus levels and also aims to prevent cardiovascular complications and ectopic calcifications, reducing morbidity and mortality in CRF patients. The indications for parathyroidectomy in SHPT are [4]:

1. Calciphylaxis.
2. Patient preference.
3. Medical observation not possible.
4. Failure of maximal medical management (active vitamin D and/or cinacalcet for at least 3 months) with:
   (a) Hypercalcemia.
   (b) Hypercalcuria.
   (c) PTH >800 pg/mL.
   (d) When the volume of at least one hyperplastic gland is 500 mm^3 (gland >1 cm).
   (e) Hyperphosphatemia (with calcium×phosphorus >70).
   (f) Osteoporosis.
   (g) Symptoms: pruritis, pathologic bone fracture, ectopic soft tissue calcifications, severe vascular calcifications, or intractable bone pain.
   (h) Intolerance to Cinacalcet (severe hypocalcemia, digestive intolerance).

Pre-operative localizing studies, like USG and MIBI scan, are not recommended except in re-operative cases because the underlying pathology in SHPT is a 4-gland hyperplasia. However, sometimes imaging studies may be helpful in picking up an ectopic gland. Most patients on dialysis with secondary hyperparathyroidism have multiple enlarged parathyroid glands, for which the surgical options are subtotal or total parathyroidectomy. The primary goal of surgery for renal HPT is the elimination of the PTH excess with prevention of persistent/recurrent disease and avoidance of postoperative permanent hypoparathyroidism. The selection of a specific operative approach will be mainly directed by prospective time on dialysis and realistic prospect of kidney transplantation, as well as the target range of iPTH between 150 and 300 pg/mL for patients on permanent dialysis according to the KDOQI guidelines, should guide the surgical strategy. There are four different approaches for the surgical treatment of renal HPT: (1) subtotal PTX with bilateral cervical thymectomy (3.5 parathyroid gland resection; subtotal PTX), (2) total PTX (TPTX) with autotransplantation of parathyroid tissue and bilateral cervical thymectomy (TPTX+AT), (3) TPTX without autotransplantation and without thymectomy, and (4) TPTX without autotransplantation and with bilateral cervical thymectomy (TPTX+BCT). Most experts recommend subtotal PTX and TPTX+AT as standard procedures [5]. Resection of less than 3.5 parathyroid glands in renal HPT patients may not be considered an adequate option due to the high risk of persistence/recurrence. There is controversy regarding the utility of IOPTH in surgery for SHPT. Application of the customary criteria of 50% IOPTH decline determining the success of PTX in primary HPT may result in low specificity in renal HPT. Hence, a 70% decline from baseline is recommended to declare biochemical cure in surgery of renal HPT [6].

References

1. Levin A, Bakris GL, Molitch M, Smulders M, Tian J, Williams LA, Andress DL. Prevalence of abnormal serum vitamin D, PTH, calcium, and phosphorus in patients with chronic kidney disease: Results ofthe studyto evaluate early kidney disease. Kidney Int. 2007;71:31–8.
2. Kidney Foundation. K/DOQI clinical practice guidelines for bone metabolism and disease in chronic kidney disease. Am J Kidney Dis. 2003;42(S1):S1–201.
3. Tonbul HZ, Solak Y, Atalay H, et al. Efficacy and tolerability of intravenous paricalcitol in calcitriol-resistant hemodialysis patients with secondary hyperparathyroidism: 12-month prospective study. Ren Fail. 2012;34:297–303.
4. Cunningham J, Locatelli F, Rodriguez M. Secondary hyperparathyroidism: pathogenesis, disease progression, and therapeutic options. Clin J Am Soc Nephrol. 2011;6:913–21.
5. Schneider R, Bartsch DK. Role of surgery in the treatment of renal secondary hyperparathyroidism. Br J Surg. 2015;102(4):289–90.
6. Freriks K, Hermus AR, de Sévaux RG, Bonenkamp HJ, Biert J, den Heijer M, et al. Usefulness of intraoperative parathyroid hormone measurements in patients with renal hyperparathyroidism. Head Neck. 2010;32(10):1328–35.

Tertiary Hyperparathyroidism Requiring Parathyroidectomy

Case

A 36-year-old male with diagnosis of obstructive uropathy having undergone DJ stenting for bilateral renal stones, and hypertension and CKD having undergone renal transplant 2 years back referred to our institution for post-transplant follow-up. He was found to have raised serum calcium and PTH, and referred for further management to Endocrine surgery. He has no history of bony pains, proximal muscle weakness, fractures, or mood disturbances. He has past history of bilateral renal calculi, post PCNL, URS, ESWL, and HTN on hemodialysis. Also gave a history of h/o renal stones in his brother. On evaluation he was found to have low serum Phosphorous: 1, 9, 2, 0, 1, 9, elevated serum calcium:11.1, 11.3, 14.7, 14.0 mg/dL and elevated PTH: 518.8 pg/mL, with low 25(OH) levels: 14.7. Thus, a diagnosis of tertiary hyperparathyroidism was made. USG neck showed 1.4 cm well-defined lobulated hypoechoic lesion at the lower pole of the left lobe of the thyroid which was confirmed by MIBI scan. He had severe osteoporosis at the forearm with a T-score of −5.2. Indications for parathyroidectomy in him included persistent hypercalcemia even after 2 years of medical treatment, very high PTH > 500 pm/L, USG: parathyroid >1 cm(500 mg) and hypophosphatemia. Bilateral Neck Exploration with 3 gland parathyroidectomy with intraoperative parathyroid hormone (IOPTH) monitoring was done. Findings included: 1.5 × 1.5 cm maroon-colored nodule, posterior to the lower pole of the left lobe of the thyroid, anterior to left RLN (Fig. 1), left superior parathyroid not seen. Right superior (Fig. 2) and inferior parathyroid glands (Fig. 3) were identified. There was a curative fall in IOPTH. IOPTH values (pmol/l) – Pre-incision – 57.5 Pre-excision – 21.1, Post-excision 5 min: 12.8, Post-excision 10 min –10.2, Post-excision 15 min 7.64 Gross: Left Inferior: Weight- 0.4 g 1.5 × 1.5 cm Right Superior: Weight- 0.1 g Size 0.5 × 0.5 cm Right Inferior: Weight- 0.1 g Size- 0.5 × 0.5 cm. He is eucalcemic on 2 years follow-up.

Amit Agarwal is the lead author of this chapter.

A. Agarwal et al., *Case Studies in Thyroid and Parathyroid Tumors*,
https://doi.org/10.1007/978-981-99-0938-4_33

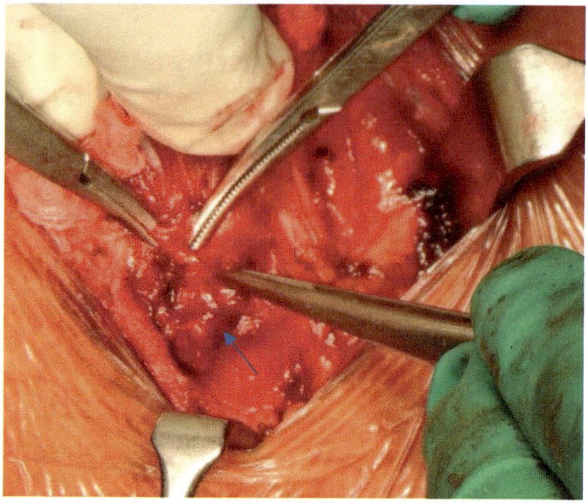

Fig. 1 Hyperplastic left inferior parathyroid gland

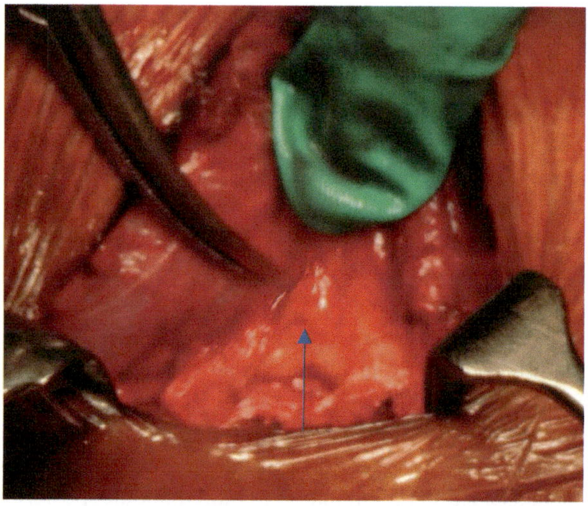

Fig. 2 Hyperplastic right superior gland

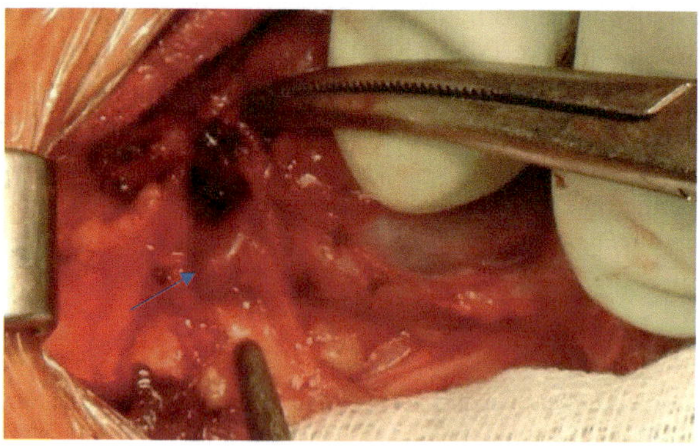

Fig. 3 Hyperplastic right inferior gland

Discussion

For most patients with end-stage renal disease (ESRD), kidney transplantation is the treatment of choice as it will improve patient survival while increasing quality of life compared to remaining on dialysis. Allograft survival has improved over the decades, and the one-year allograft survival has now reached over 93% for first-time transplant recipients, and over 72% for five-year allograft survival [1]. While patients benefit from improved allograft survival, they are burdened with the lasting effects of their chronic kidney disease (CKD). Even after kidney transplantation, recipients can continue to have elevated parathyroid hormone (PTH) levels. Several studies have evaluated the levels of PTH post-kidney transplantation showing an initial decrease in the PTH levels within the first 12 months post-transplant. Hence, most transplant physicians will allow up to 12 months posttransplant for normalization of PTH. Past this point, a PTH level greater than two times normal (>130 pg/mL) is consistent with persistent post-transplant hyperparathyroidism (PT-HPT) and this is known as TERTIARY HPT. Other lab abnormalities such as hypercalcemia, hypophosphatemia, and an elevated alkaline phosphatase, can be associated with persistent PT-HPT. With the onset of severe CKD, overt hyperphosphatemia, low levels of 1,25(OH)2D lead to progressive SHPT and PT hyperplasia. FGF23 levels continue to increase due to hyperphosphatemia. Thus, at the time of kidney transplant, patients commonly have SHPT and enlarged PT glands, hyperphosphatemia, low 1,25(OH)2D levels, and elevated FGF23. Within the first 3 months post-transplant, mild to profound hypophosphatemia may develop, and appears due to the combined phosphaturic actions of PTH and FG23. Hypophosphatemia is a short-lived event in most patients and improves over the course of the first-year post-transplant. However, the improvement in hypercalcemia is incremental; by 12 months post-transplant there are 11% of patients in the low PTH group and 25% of patients in the high PTH who continued to have hypercalcemia. Levels of 1,25(OH)2D increased in both groups through to 12 months post-transplant. Despite the improvement in FGF23, phosphate and vitamin D levels after a kidney transplant, there is a subset of patients that maintain a persistently high PTH level as well as hypercalcemia in some cases. One of the main drivers of persistent SHPT is the enlarged PT glands due to hyperplasia that has occurred during the longstanding SHPT. As a result of the ongoing stimulation of parathyroid tissue by the dysregulation in metabolic bone mineral parameters, the parathyroid tissue first undergoes diffuse hyperplasia, and in some patients develops into nodular hyperplasia. These nodules exhibit characteristics of autonomous adenomas seen in patients with primary hyperparathyroidism, with a marked reduction in expression of CaSR and Vitamin D receptors, rendering them less responsive to elevation in serum calcium and 1,25(OH)2D levels. As mentioned above, spontaneous regression of glandular hyperplasia may take 6–12 months; thus, it is prudent to wait 12 months post-transplantation before considering PTX. The prevalence of post-transplant PTX varies between 1 and 5.6%. Indications for parathyroidectomy in patients with tertiary HPT include: severe hypercalcemia (serum calcium >11.5 or 12 mg/dL), persistent hypercalcemia (serum calcium >10.2 mg/dL more than three months to one year after surgery) despite medical treatment, severe osteopenia (low bone mineral density), renal phosphorous wasting and hypophosphatemia, elevated ALP indicating high bone turnover, parathyroid gland weight more than 500 mg on USG(>1 cm), symptomatic hyperparathyroidism with fatigue, pruritis, bone pain or pathologic bone fracture, peptic ulcer disease, and mental status changes. Given the lack of best practice guidelines, the specific surgical technique used depends more on surgeons' preferences rather than patients' characteristics. Surgical techniques include subtotal PTX, or total PTX with or without autotransplantation. In the rare event of a parathyroid adenoma, targeted PTX is also an option. Subtotal PTX involves leaving a small remnant from the most normal appearing hyperplastic gland. This technique has the benefit of fewer hypocalcemia complications but a higher incidence of treatment failure -(5–30%) requiring repeated neck surgery [2]. Total PTX with auto-transplantation involves creating a parathyroid gland autograft, which is usually placed in the non-dominant forearm. Potential additional sites for implantation include the sternocleidomastoid muscle or subcutaneous abdominal adipose tissue. This is the preferred technique for patients with strong reasons to avoid repeated neck surgeries [3]. This technique has also the potential of treatment failure if the implant hypertrophies and becomes autonomous. However, the implants are usually more surgically accessible than parathyroid remnants, making the repeated surgery easier to accomplish. On the other hand, total PTX with auto-transplantation may cause severe hypocalcemia if the implant fails. In this setting, the availability of tissue cryopreservation conveys the advantage of repeat auto-transplantation at a later time if needed. Total PTX without auto-transplantation is not recommended in the kidney transplant population as the subsequent hypocalcemia becomes difficult to control for patients of dialysis [4]. Controversy persists regarding the usefulness of intraoperative PTH (ioPTH) monitoring. As opposed to primary HPT where established protocols exist for ioPTH monitoring, no such protocols have been validated for ESRD-related HPT. This may be in part related to delayed renal clearance of PTH in the ESRD population. Intact PTH (iPTH) assays cross-react with PTH fragments, which can experience reduced clearance leading to an overestimation of PTH concentration. Whole PTH (wPTH) assays cross-react with 1–84 PTH molecules only, thus providing more accurate data. A small study of 42 patients undergoing PTX found that IOPTH at 30 min post-excision was very accurate at predicting the persistence of SHPT. A 30-min IOPTH level >12% from baseline and a concentration >166 pg/mL predicted persistent SHPT with a sensitivity of 100%, specificity 71%, and a negative predictive value of 100%. As far as medical treatment of THPT is concerned studies have shown that parathyroidectomy for tertiary hyperparathyroidism is associated with lesser rates of renal allograft failure compared with cinacalcet management [5]. Patients with inadequate parathyroid hormone control on cinacalcet at 1 year posttransplant should be considered for parathyroidectomy to prevent potential allograft failure [6].

References

1. Evenepoel P, Claes K, Kuypers D, et al. Natural history of parathyroid function and calcium metabolism after kidney transplantation: a single-Centre study. Nephrol Dial Transplant. 2004;19(5):1281–7.
2. Pitt SC, Sippel RS, Chen H. Secondary and tertiary hyperparathyroidism, state of the art surgical management. Surg Clin North Am. 2009;89(5):1227–39.
3. Triponez F, Clark OH, Vanrenthergem Y, et al. Surgical treatment of persistent hyperparathyroidism after renal transplantation. Ann Surg. 2008;248(1):18–30.
4. Triponez F, Kebebew E, Dosseh D, et al. Less-than-subtotal parathyroidectomy increases the risk of persistent/recurrent hyperparathyroidism after parathyroidectomy in tertiary hyperparathyroidism after renal transplantation. Surgery. 2006;140(6):990–7. discussion 997–9
5. Serra AL, Schwarz AA, Wick FH, et al. Successful treatment of hypercalcemia with cinacalcet in renal transplant recipients with persistent hyperparathyroidism. Nephrol Dial Transplant. 2005;20(7):1315–9.
6. Finnerty BM, Chan TW, Jones G, Khader T, Moore M, Gray KD, Beninato T, Watkins AC, Zarnegar R, Fahey TJ 3rd. Parathyroidectomy versus cinacalcet in the management of tertiary hyperparathyroidism: surgery improves renal transplant allograft survival. Surgery. 2019;165(1):129–34.

Surgery in MEN-1

Case

A 23-year-old man was referred to the endocrine surgery department with primary hyperparathyroidism (pHPT) and a suspicion of multiple endocrine neoplasia type 1 (MEN1). He had recently undergone a distal pancreatectomy for a neuroendocrine tumor, which was incidentally discovered during workup of ureteric colic.

He was subsequently found to have a raised corrected calcium (cCa) of 3.01 mmol/L [2.15–2.55], with an intact parathyroid hormone (PTH) of 13.9 pmol/L [1.3–7.6]. His calcium: creatinine clearance ratio was 0.031, excluding familial hypocalciuric hypercalcemia as a cause of his high serum calcium.

After this biochemical diagnosis of primary hyperparathyroidism, he underwent localization studies. Technetium ^{99}m Sestamibi (MIBI) scanning showed a lesion adjacent to the left lower pole of the thyroid, and a smaller, less intense lesion adjacent to the right lower pole. Ultrasound scan (US) was concordant, revealing lesions inferior to both lobes of the thyroid, suggestive of double parathyroid adenomas.

As a clinical diagnosis of MEN-1 was made, the patient was referred for genetic counseling. While these results were pending, he underwent all appropriate screening. His prolactin was markedly elevated at 1018 mIU/L [80–390], and a magnetic resonance imaging (MRI) scan of his pituitary gland was suggestive of a pituitary microadenoma. Moreover, while his initial computed tomography (CT) scan revealed bilateral adrenal incidentalomas, his phaeochromocytoma screen was unremarkable. Ultimately, genetic testing confirmed the patient to be a MEN-1 mutation carrier.

To treat his pHPT, a bilateral neck exploration with removal of all four parathyroid glands and a thymectomy was undertaken. Both inferior parathyroid glands were found to be enlarged, while the superior glands appeared normal in size. No ectopic glands were found. The right superior parathyroid gland, i.e., a normal-appearing gland, was partially transplanted into the patient's deltoid muscle after confirmation on the frozen section.

Rajeev Parameswaran is the lead author of this chapter.

A. Agarwal et al., *Case Studies in Thyroid and Parathyroid Tumors*,
https://doi.org/10.1007/978-981-99-0938-4_34

Histology showed diffuse and focal nodular proliferations in all the parathyroid glands. The patient developed no complications and was discharged on day two after surgery. After a short period on calcium-supplements, his PTH stabilized at 6.9 pmol/L, with a cCa of 2.53 mmol/L. He remains under stringent follow-up.

Discussion

Multiple endocrine neoplasia type 1 (MEN-1) is an autosomal-dominant disorder, associated with a triad of primary hyperparathyroidism (pHPT), anterior pituitary tumors, and pancreaticoduodenal endocrine tumors (PET) – thus, the mnemonic of the 3 Ps. MEN-1 should be clinically suspected when a patient has two or more MEN-1-associated tumors. Moreover, genetic screening is indicated in case of: [1].

- A clinical diagnosis of MEN-1.
- A suspicion of MEN-1, including those who develop parathyroid adenomas before the age of 30; patients with a gastrinoma or multiple pancreatic PETs at any age; or patients who have two or more MEN-1-associated tumors that are not part of the previously described triad.
- All first-degree relatives of known MEN-1 mutation carriers.

Among those with a mutation in their MEN-1-gene, pHPT has 90–100% penetrance and pHPT is frequently the initial presenting symptom of MEN1. The age of onset of MEN-1-associated pHPT is more than three decades earlier than in sporadic disease, and the female-to-male ratio is equal, whereas in sporadic disease it favors females [2]. While monitoring and surveillance can be undertaken immediately if MEN-1 is expected, there is no yield in screening before the age of five, as the mutation is non-penetrant before this age [1]. Screening specific to pHPT should include serum-corrected calcium and PTH, while it should also include components for non-parathyroid disease [1].

Among those with known or presumed MEN-1, the indications for surgery for pHPT are similar to those in patients with sporadic disease. A MEN-1-specific indication for parathyroidectomy is the presence of severe peptic ulcer disease or other symptoms caused by a gastrinoma (the Zollinger-Ellison syndrome), as hypercalcemia tends to worsen hypergastrinemia. In asymptomatic patients, surgery may be considered, although conservative management is also an option [1].

The majority of patients with pHPT in the setting of MEN-1 have multiglandular disease, necessitating an upfront bilateral neck exploration to attempt to localize all glands. Thus, the added value of preoperative localization studies (e.g., US or MIBI) is debatable for those who did not undergo prior surgery. Conversely, before reoperation in patients with recurrent or persistent disease, the performance of localization studies is recommended.

The optimum extent of the parathyroidectomy procedure remains controversial. In general, persistent disease is known to be more common among those treated with less than a subtotal parathyroidectomy, thus the recommendation is to remove at least three and one-half glands [1]. As a total parathyroidectomy without autotransplantation will render 100% of patients permanently dependent on calcium-supplements, this is currently not considered an option, with respect to the patient's quality of life [2]. Options therefore include a more aggressive procedure, in order to reduce the risk of persistent or recurrent disease, by performance of a complete parathyroidectomy and transplantation of a small parathyroid autograft [3]. However, there incorporates a risk of long-term or permanent hypoparathyroidism if the graft does not function. A more commonly chosen option therefore is a less extensive procedure, by performance of a subtotal parathyroidectomy, involving removal of three and one-half parathyroid glands. This procedure does carry a risk of recurrence of disease, at a rate significantly higher than in non-familial (sporadic) pHPT [1]. It is paramount that surgery for MEN-1 carriers should only be performed by surgeons who are highly experienced in parathyroid surgery.

It is also generally recommended to perform a bilateral thymectomy, as thymic tissue is known to harbor parathyroid tissue [2, 4]. Moreover, there is an association between MEN-1 and thymic carcinoma, [5] although data to support the performance of a prophylactic thymectomy to reduce the risk of development of a thymic carcinoma is scarce. For those patients in whom surgery is contraindicated or with multiple recurrent disease, calcimimetic such as cinacalcet have been used to treat hyperparathyroidism [1].

References

1. Thakker RV, Newey PJ, Walls GV, Bilezikian J, Dralle H, Ebeling PR, et al. Clinical practice guidelines for multiple endocrine neoplasia type 1 (MEN1). J Clin Endocrinol Metabol. 2012;97(9):2990–3011.
2. Iacobone M, Carnaille B, Palazzo FF, Vriens M. Hereditary hyperparathyroidism—a consensus report of the European Society of Endocrine Surgeons (ESES). Langenbeck's Arch Surg. 2015;400(8):867–86.
3. Tonelli F, Marcucci T, Fratini G, Tommasi MS, Falchetti A, Brandi ML. Is total parathyroidectomy the treatment of choice for hyperparathyroidism in multiple endocrine neoplasia type 1? Ann Surg. 2007;246(6):1075–82.
4. Powell AC, Alexander HR, Pingpank JF, Steinberg SM, Skarulis M, Bartlett DL, et al. The utility of routine transcervical thymectomy for multiple endocrine neoplasia 1-related hyperparathyroidism. Surgery. 2008;144(6):878–83; discussion 83–4
5. de Laat JM, Pieterman CR, van den Broek MF, Twisk JW, Hermus AR, Dekkers OM, et al. Natural course and survival of neuroendocrine tumors of thymus and lung in MEN1 patients. J Clin Endocrinol Metab. 2014;99(9):3325–33.

Surgery in MEN-2A

Case
A 25-year-old female was referred to our endocrine surgery clinic with a suspicion of MEN-2A syndrome. She had presented earlier with severe muscle aches and general weakness. Her work-up revealed an adjusted calcium of 2.75 mmol/L, with a parathyroid hormone (PTH) of 148.3 pmol/L, leading to the diagnosis of primary hyperparathyroidism (PHPT). Her Technetium ^{99}m sestamibi (MIBI) showed a possible left inferior parathyroid adenoma, which was corroborated by her ultrasound scan (US). However, this latter scan also revealed a suspicious thyroid nodule in her right thyroid lobe, which – after further evaluation with fine needle aspiration (FNAC) – was found to be a medullary thyroid cancer (MTC). Her calcitonin at the time of diagnosis was 235 pg/mL; with a CEA of 9.1 μg/L.

In view of the concurrent primary hyperparathyroidism and MTC, screening for a pheochromocytoma was undertaken, and revealed raised 24 h urinary epinephrine, metanephrine, and normetanephrine, with the remaining results within the normal limits. The subsequently conducted CT-abdomen showed bilateral adrenal nodules (right: 2.0 × 1.2 cm and left: 1.6 × 1.2 cm), suggestive of bilateral pheochromocytomas.

She was thus referred to our endocrine surgery clinic, with PHPT, MTC with a raised calcitonin, and bilateral pheochromocytomas, for which she was on α- and β-blockade. After her ^{68}Ga-DOTANOC PET-CT-scan did not reveal any other sites of disease, she underwent an uneventful bilateral retroperitoneal endoscopic adrenalectomy, during which three nodules (medial limb, genu, lateral limb) were appreciated in the left adrenal gland, and one in the medial limb of the right adrenal gland, without histological signs of malignancy.

Her genetic testing, which had been pending at the time of adrenalectomy, revealed a RET Cys634Arg mutation, confirming MEN-2A syndrome. About one

Rajeev Parameswaran is the lead author of this chapter.

A. Agarwal et al., *Case Studies in Thyroid and Parathyroid Tumors*,
https://doi.org/10.1007/978-981-99-0938-4_35

month after her bilateral adrenalectomy, she underwent a total thyroidectomy with bilateral central and lateral neck dissection for her MTC, as well as a total parathyroidectomy and thymectomy, with autotransplantation of frozen section proven parathyroid tissue into her right sternocleidomastoid muscle for her PHPT. Her histology revealed multifocal, bilateral MTC, with one out of 34 lymph nodes involved by metastatic medullary thyroid carcinoma. Her tumour markers returned to the normal range following surgery.

The histology of her parathyroid glands revealed four-gland hyperplasia, with one notably larger gland. Her post-operative PTH dropped to within the normal range (2.2 pmol/L) and has remained so, and while she initially was dependent on calcium and vitamin D supplements, her latest adjusted calcium is also normal at 2.25 mmol/L. The patient is currently four years after her surgeries without any clinical or biochemical signs of recurrence.

Discussion

Among MEN-2A carriers, the overall pooled risk of developing primary hyperparathyroidism (PHPT) lies between 5–20%, and once PHPT does develop, its nature is often mild and asymptomatic [1, 2]. As the mean age of onset of PHPT is in the fourth decade of life, it usually only presents after diagnosis and treatment of MTC. However, there seems to be a codon-dependent difference, not only in the risk of developing PHPT, but also in its presentation. Specifically, a mutation in codon 634 has been associated with a higher penetrance of PHPT (up to 30%), compared with mutations in codons 609, 611, 618, and 620 (penetrance between 2% and 12%) [3, 4]. Moreover, it is thought to be highly probable that the activating mutations of the codon 634 generate or predispose to hyperplasia of parathyroid tissue, instead of the formation of a single adenoma [5].

For those patients who do not have signs of PHPT at the time of surgery for their MTC, performance of a systematic prophylactic parathyroidectomy is not recommended [6], but all patients should undergo pre-operative screening to allow for curative management of PHPT simultaneously [4]. Moreover, annual screening for PHPT is also advised by the ATA-guidelines, with a differentiated starting age based on the affected codon, i.e. at 11 for those with codon 634 mutations, and at 16 for the remaining codons [4, 7].

Conversely, these guidelines do not currently propose a codon-directed therapy of PHPT. However, based on the increased incidence of hyperplasia among those with a codon 634 mutation, performance of a (sub)total parathyroidectomy with autotransplantation could be considered for those with diagnosed PHPT (at the time of thyroidectomy). While for those with a lower risk mutation, the treatment could be similar as for sporadic PHPT (i.e. removal of a single adenoma). Importantly, although this phenotype/genotype correlation is recognised at a population level, there is a range of prevalence within MEN-2A families, suggesting additional influences of, yet unknown, modifying or environmental factors [8, 9].

References

1. Alevizaki M. Management of hyperparathyroidism (PHP) in MEN2 syndromes in Europe. Thyroid Res. 2013;6(Suppl 1):S10.
2. Wells SA, et al. Multiple endocrine neoplasia type 2 and familial medullary thyroid carcinoma: an update. J Clin Endocrinol Metab. 2013;98(8):3149–64.
3. Frank-Raue K, et al. Risk profiles and penetrance estimations in multiple endocrine neoplasia type 2A caused by germline RET mutations located in exon 10. Hum Mutat. 2011;32(1):51–8.
4. Wells SA, et al. Revised American Thyroid Association guidelines for the management of medullary thyroid carcinoma. Thyroid. 2015;25(6):567–610.
5. Schuffenecker I, et al. Risk and penetrance of primary hyperparathyroidism in multiple endocrine neoplasia type 2A families with mutations at codon 634 of the RET proto-oncogene. Groupe D'etude des Tumeurs à Calcitonine. J Clin Endocrinol Metab. 1998;83(2):487–91.
6. Guerin C, et al. Looking beyond the thyroid: advances in the understanding of pheochromocytoma and hyperparathyroidism phenotypes in MEN2 and of non-MEN2 familial forms. Endocr Relat Cancer. 2018;25(2):T15–28.
7. Machens A, et al. Molecular epidemiology of multiple endocrine neoplasia 2: implications for RET screening in the new millenium. Eur J Endocrinol. 2013;168(3):307–14.
8. Cristina EV, Alberto F. Management of familial hyperparathyroidism syndromes: MEN1, MEN2, MEN4, HPT-jaw tumour, familial isolated hyperparathyroidism, FHH, and neonatal severe hyperparathyroidism. Best Pract Res Clin Endocrinol Metab. 2018;32(6):861–75.
9. Machens A, Dralle H. Advances in risk-oriented surgery for multiple endocrine neoplasia type 2. Endocr Relat Cancer. 2018;25(2):T41–52.

Pregnancy-Associated Hyperparathyroidism Complicated by Seizures

Introduction

Primary hyperparathyroidism which was first reported in 1931 by Hunter and Turnbull is prevalent among 0.1 to 0.4% of the general population [1, 2]. Although 25% of the cases involve women of childbearing age, the reported incidence of hyperparathyroidism in pregnancy is far lower than expected [3]. Indian registry spanning over 15 years shows a prevalence of 2.1% of gestational PHPT, which is higher than the <1% reported among western population [1, 4].

Recent studies reveal that less than a quarter of gestational PHPT (gPHPT) are asymptomatic compared to 80% of nonpregnant women with PHPT. However, a high fetal and neonatal death rate of 20–30% of mothers and pregnancy-related complications in 50–60% remains a challenge in neglected scenarios. This is attributed to endocrine and metabolic changes in pregnancy which obscure the symptoms and signs of PHPT.

Case

An otherwise healthy 31-year-old woman, gravida 1, para 0 at 38 weeks of gestation, presented with pain in abdomen and one episode of generalized tonic-clonic seizure (GTCS). The patient underwent LSCS with the delivery of live-born baby which subsequently succumbed to unknown causes within 12 h.

In the postpartum period, the patient had multiple seizure episodes which increased in increasing frequency and was resistant to multiple anti-epileptic medications. The patient's general condition deteriorated, and she developed an altered sensorium. The patient was sedated, intubated and kept on ventilator support. She had no history suggestive of pre-eclampsia. She did not have any other comorbidities and was not on any medications or substance abuse. There was no significant family history. She was found to have hypertension that was difficult to stabilize.

Anand Mishra is the lead author of this chapter.

A. Agarwal et al., *Case Studies in Thyroid and Parathyroid Tumors*,
https://doi.org/10.1007/978-981-99-0938-4_36

Laboratory analysis showed markedly elevated serum ionized calcium, hypophosphatemia, elevated parathyroid hormone (PTH) level of 744.2 pg/mL, and Vitamin D deficiency. Urinary calcium levels were within normal limits. Renal function and cerebrospinal fluid analysis were unremarkable. High-resolution ultrasonography of the neck showed a 22 × 12 mm lesion in the region of the right inferior thyroid pole.

The hypercalcemic state was managed by forced saline diuresis and Zoledronic acid. Subsequently, with normalization of serum calcium levels, the patient recovered from the seizure episode without any neurological deficit. She also became normotensive. Clinical examination, CECT, and MRI brain did not reveal any remarkable findings. ^{99}mTc-Sestamibi scan confirmed a focal, persistent, and intense uptake inferior to Rt lobe of thyroid which was concordant with USG. She underwent focused parathyroidectomy and is doing well.

Discussion

A single parathyroid adenoma is the commonest cause encountered in gPHPT. However, other causes of hypercalcemia are tertiary hyperparathyroidism, humoral hypercalcemia of malignancy, granulomatous disorders, medications, miscellaneous causes-immobilization, etc. [5].

Genetic mutations are encountered in about 10% of gPHPT below 40 years and include multiple endocrine neoplasia (MEN 1, MEN 2A, MEN 4), hyperparathyroidism-jaw tumor syndrome (HPT-JT), and familial isolated hyperparathyroidism (FIHP) [6]. Familial hypocalciuric hypercalcemia (FHH), diagnosed by calcium-creatinine-clearance ratio, is an important differential diagnosis of PHPT. The sensitivity and specificity calcium-creatinine-clearance ratio is reduced (80% and 88% respectively) due to hypercalciuria [7].

Physiological Changes Obscuring Gestational PHPT

Physiological changes in pregnancy prevent the depletion of maternal calcium stores while meeting the fetal requirement for its skeletal development. Levels of 1, 25 Vit D increases as pregnancy advances, leading to increased absorption of calcium from intestines and retention of calcium by the kidneys. Levels of PTH and calcitonin remain unchanged. Contrary to the previous concept of physiological secondary hyperparathyroidism in pregnancy due to falling total serum calcium levels, the recent 2-site "intact" assays and "bio-intact" PTH assays have shown fall in PTH levels at the first trimester followed by return to normal levels during the second and third trimesters. However, in contrast to western studies of women consuming calcium-replete diet, a higher serum PTH has been seen in Asian women consuming calcium-deplete diet and phytate-rich diet [8].

PTH, 1,25(OH)Vit D, calcitonin does not cross the placenta, while 25-hydroxyvitamin D3 (25-OHVitD) traverses' placenta and is converted to its active form by placental 1-O-hydroxylases. About 300 gm/day of calcium is transported via the placenta and reaches a peak in the third trimester. Total serum calcium decreases during pregnancy due to decrease in serum albumin, due to increase in intravascular fluid volume and decrease in glomerular filtration rate (GFR). However, the ionized calcium levels remain unchanged throughout pregnancy. Phosphorus and magnesium levels remain in the lower limit of normal. Parathyroid hormone-related protein (PTHrP) secreted by placenta or fetal parathyroid, protect mother's bones from demineralization and enhances placental calcium transport. The major source of calcium for the fetus is from shunting of maternal intestinal calcium across placenta [8].

Fetal parathyroids commence secreting PTH by tenth week, however, its levels remain low. Secretion of fetal PTH is further influenced by maternal calcium levels. Maternal hypercalcemia can suppress the function of fetal PTH levels, vice versa, maternal hypocalcemia can cause secondary hyperparathyroidism in neonates. During parturition, placental source of calcium ceases causing fall in the total and ionic fetal calcium levels by 0.5 mmol/L, with the lowest levels at 24–48 hours. Calcium levels subsequently increase to normal levels by one week [3].

The fetal demand of calcium during pregnancy is met by active transport via placenta with maternal to fetal gradient of 1:1.4. However, this gradient is eliminated in gPHPT leading to marked suppression of fetal PTH secretion [9]. Postpartum, the sudden interruption of maternal calcium supply results in dreaded neonatal hypocalcemia and tetany, while the mother has the risk of suffering from complications of hypercalcemic crisis [10].

Hypercalcemic crisis is an endocrine emergency characterized by albumin-corrected serum calcium levels of >14 mg/dL (>3.5 mmol/L) associated with multiorgan dysfunction. Various complication of hypercalcemic status can be encountered but hypercalcemia causing generalized tonic-clonic seizures is not commonly reported.

Several underlying pathophysiological mechanisms have been proposed for this rare complication. Chen et al. hypothesized that hypercalcemia causes reversible cerebral vasospasm (actin-myosin coupling induced vascular contraction) resulting in reduced cerebral perfusion which manifests as focal or generalized seizure. Vasospasm may also lead to endothelial damage resulting in endothelin I-induced renin-angiotensin system activation causing hypertension-induced cerebral damage and subsequent epilepsy [11].

Other possible mechanisms include hypertensive encephalopathy secondary to increased vascular resistance, hypokalemia or hypomagnesemia. Undiagnosed hyperparathyroidism leads to chronic hypercalcemia and metabolic alkalosis, which causes hypokalemia. Hypokalemia is a well-known risk factor for developing seizures [12]. Excess calcium has also been reported to cause microthrombus formation leading to petechial hemorrhage, where EEG analysis shows "diffuse electrical slowing with focal paroxysmal regional slowing" [13]. The rate of rise in calcium levels and the duration of hypercalcemia have profound neurological impact. Rapid rise to moderate hypercalcemia (12–13.9 mg/dL) produces more neurological dysfunction than chronic severe hypercalcemia (≥14 mg/dL).

Clinical Features

Physiological symptoms of pregnancy like nausea, vomiting, weakness, epigastric pain, polyuria, polydipsia, constipation, depression, confusion often obscure the diagnosis of PHPT. Nonspecific complaints (depression, constipation, fatigue) are seen with calcium levels of <12 mg/dL. Patients with moderate hypercalcemia present with nausea, anorexia, dehydration, polyuria, polydipsia, and muscle weakness. Severe forms of hypercalcemia/hypercalcemic crisis present as altered mental status with lethargy, stupor, and coma [14].

Maternal complications in gestational PHPT can occur in up to 67% of all cases. Most common complications include renal calculi (24–36%), radiographic evidence of bone disease (13–19%), pancreatitis (7–13%), pre-eclampsia (25%), HELLP syndrome, and hyperemesis gravidarum (rarely), recurrent miscarriages (3.5-fold higher) [15, 16].

Fetal complications have been observed in up to 80% of mothers with untreated PHPT, with 27–31% culminating in death. Postpartum hypocalcemia leading to neonatal tetany is observed in 15–50%. Other complications include intrauterine growth restriction, fetal demise, low birth weight, and preterm delivery. Neonatal hypoparathyroidism due to hypercalcemia may extend from few months to permanent hypoparathyroidism due to the teratogenic effect of hypercalcemia on third and fourth branchial clefts during its development [15].

Diagnosis

Serum calcium concentration of more than 10.1 mg/dL (2.52 mmol/L) or 8.8 mg/dL (2.2 mmol/L) at the second or third trimester should alert the clinician to investigate for hyperparathyroidism. However, it lacks specificity and may be elevated in patients with deranged renal function, and in those with elevated PTH-like peptide, also seen in pregnancy. Assays measuring N-terminal fragment of PTH (biological active) are more specific and highly sensitive.

Radiation exposure due to ^{99}mTc Sestamibi and computed tomography should be avoided in pregnancy to prevent fetal anomalies and subsequent risk of malignancy. One study had considered low-dose sestamibi scan safe during pregnancy reaching a dose of <5 mGy" which is unlikely to cause fetal harm" as stated by ACOG [17]. USG and MRI can be safely performed to localize the offending glands during pregnancy.

Management

The management of gPHPT is individualized based on the period of gestation at diagnosis, severity of symptoms, and associated complications. Limited options are available for management in view of fetal safety concerns.

Mild hypercalcemia in PHPT is usually treated conservatively first by discontinuing any offending medications (calcium supplements, thiazide diuretics, lithium…) followed by adequate correction of dehydration by intravenous fluid administration. Some reports have suggested using frusemide (pregnancy category C), which reduces calcium levels by inhibiting bone resorption through anti-osteoclastic activity and by increasing renal excretion of calcium. Calcitonin though plagued by tachyphylaxis does not cross the placenta and hence can be used in refractory hypercalcemia during pregnancy with caution where benefits outweigh the risks. Cinacalcet (Pregnancy category C) increases sensitivity of CaSR receptors to extracellular calcium leading to reduced secretion of PTH from the parathyroids. It crosses the placenta disrupting the placental calcium homeostasis. Long-term safety profile of the drug in pregnancy has not been established. Bisphosphonates should not administered during pregnancy as it crosses the placenta and has adverse effects on the developing fetus by preventing bone absorption by inhibiting the activity of osteoclasts [15]. Similarly RANK ligand inhibitors, Denosumab (a monoclonal antibody) prevent osteoclast-medicated bone resorption. It also crosses the placenta causing adverse skeletal outcomes in fetus, and hence avoided in pregnancy [18].

Patients with controlled calcium levels by medication are given the option of conservative management throughout the course of pregnancy or surgical intervention preferably in the second trimester. The patient should be informed about exacerbation of hypercalcemia and resultant complications in the later stages of pregnancy and the postpartum period. Patients opting for conservative management are advised "serial fetal anatomical survey" [15].

Surgical excision of the diseased gland/s forms the mainstay of cure in PHPT during pregnancy. Although surgery can be contemplated at any stage, the second trimester is the safest period. Surgery in the first trimester is associated with high risk of miscarriage (10.5%) [17]. Successful parathyroidectomy in the third trimester of pregnancy has also been described [15].

Preoperative localization is of paramount importance in the management of PHPT. In the absence of radiographically identifiable disease, the perplexed surgeon is left with the limited intraoperative adjuncts such as IOPTH (serial intraoperative parathyroid hormone assay), interoperative ultrasonography, and frozen section. Successful excision not only reduces the complications of hypercalcemia, but also eliminates the risk of unidentified parathyroid carcinoma (1%).

Conclusion

Primary hyperthyroidism poses significant morbidity to both the mother and fetus. Corrected calcium levels and serum ionic calcium serves to screen patients with asymptomatic disease.

Conservative expectant management is a valid option in those with mild hypercalcemia. Medical options are limited and their safety profile during pregnancy remains elusive for many agents. Surgery may be a feasible option in select cases and preoperative localization improves cure rates. High index of suspicion and multidisciplinary team approach is essential for optimal outcome.

References

1. Komarowska H, Bromińska B, Luftmann B, Ruchała M. Primary hyperparathyroidism in pregnancy - a review of literature. Ginekol Pol. 2017;88(5):270–5.
2. Felger EA, Kandil E. Primary hyperparathyroidism. Otolaryngol Clin N Am. 2010;43(2):417–32.
3. Quintana EV, Vázquez DE. Hyperparathyroidism and pregnancy. Am Surg. 2010;76(6):648–9.
4. Pal R, Bhadada SK, Gupta N, Behera A, Aggarwal N, Aggarwal A, et al. Primary hyperparathyroidism in pregnancy: observations from the Indian PHPT registry. J Endocrinol Investig. 2021;44(7):1425–35.
5. Ahmad S, Kuraganti G, Steenkamp D. Hypercalcemic crisis: a clinical review. Am J Med. 2015;128(3):239–45.
6. Marini F, Cianferotti L, Giusti F, Brandi ML. Molecular genetics in primary hyperparathyroidism: the role of genetic tests in differential diagnosis, disease prevention strategy, and therapeutic planning. A 2017 update. Clin Cases Miner Bone Metab. 2017;14(1):60–70.
7. Jones AR, Hare MJL, Brown J, Yang J, Meyer C, Milat F, et al. Familial Hypocalciuric Hypercalcemia in Pregnancy: Diagnostic Pitfalls. JBMR Plus. 2020;4(6):1–5.
8. Kovacs CS. Calcium and bone metabolism disorders during pregnancy and lactation. Endocrinol Metab Clin N Am. 2011;40(4):795–826.
9. Kohlmeier L, Marcus R. Calcium disorders of pregnancy. Endocrinol Metab Clin N Am. 1995;24(1):15–39.
10. Pieringer H, Hatzl-Griesenhofer M, Shebl O, Wiesinger-Eidenberger G, Maschek W, Biesenbach G. Hypocalcemic tetany in the newborn as a manifestation of unrecognized maternal primary hyperparathyroidism. Wien Klin Wochenschr. 2007;119(3–4):129–31.
11. Chen TH, Huang CC, Chang YY, Chen YF, Chen WH, Lai SL. Vasoconstriction as the etiology of hypercalcemia-induced seizures. Epilepsia. 2004;45(5):551–4.
12. Nakasone Y, Uchino S, Sato Y, Yamauchi K, Aizawa T. Seizure and profound hypokalemia: unusual presentation of primary hyperparathyroidism. Eur J Case Reports Intern Med. 2015;2(3):7–9.
13. Cherry TAD, Kauffman RP, Myles TD. Primary hyperparathyroidism, hypercalcemic crisis and subsequent seizures occurring during pregnancy: a case report. J Matern Neonatal Med. 2002;12(5):349–52.
14. Health JPC, Cho HJ. A case of primary hyperparathyroidism-induced myoclonic seizure during the third trimester of pregnancy. J Pregnancy Child Heal. 2014;01(01):1–3.
15. Diaz-Soto G, Linglart A, Sénat MV, Kamenicky P, Chanson P. Primary hyperparathyroidism in pregnancy. Endocrine. 2013;44(3):591–7.
16. Norman J, Politz D, Politz L. Hyperparathyroidism during pregnancy and the effect of rising calcium on pregnancy loss: a call for earlier intervention. Clin Endocrinol. 2009;71(1):104–9.
17. DiMarco AN, Meeran K, Christakis I, Sodhi V, Nelson-Piercy C, Tolley NS, et al. Seventeen cases of primary hyperparathyroidism in pregnancy: a call for management guidelines. J Endocr Soc. 2019;3(5):1009–21.
18. Rodrigo N, Learoyd D, Glastras SJ. Complexities surrounding the diagnosis and management of hypercalcaemia in pregnancy. Endocrinol Diabetes Metab Case Rep. 2021;2021(1):20-0163.

HPT-JT Syndrome

Case
A 30-year-old female, with a history of swelling over the lower jaw for 8 months, loosening of teeth of the lower jaw for 7 months and bony and large joint pain in the past 5 months, was found to have hypercalcemia and hyperparathyroidism on evaluation. Bone mineral density revealed osteoporosis of forearm (T score: −3.2), hip (T score: −2.9), and vertebrae (T score: −4.6). MIBI scintigraphy revealed a large focally increased area of radiotracer concentration in the region of the lower pole of the left thyroid lobe; USG of the neck did not pick up any typical lesions in parathyroid. Ultrasound of the abdomen was normal. She underwent a bilateral neck exploration and cystic 1.5 × 1.5 cm left inferior parathyroid lesion was excised which was reported as parathyroid adenoma on HPE. Jaw tumor was excised by Oro Maxillofacial surgeons in the second sitting and the patient continues to do well at 2 years follow-up. Genetic tests were not carried out due to financial constraints.

Discussion

Jaw tumors or odontogenic tumors are growths that develop in the jawbone or soft tissues of the mouth and face. They are usually benign, but vary greatly in size and may be locally invasive causing tooth loss and facial disfigurement [1].

Differential diagnosis of jaw tumors includes: ameloblastoma, giant cell granuloma, dentigerous cysts, cementoblastomas, aneurysmal bone cysts, ossifying fibromas, etc.

Ossifying fibromas or cemento-ossifying fibroma are encapsulated, slow growing, often benign neoplasms composed of varying amounts of bone or cementum-like tissue in fibrous tissue stroma. It commonly affects females in their third and

Anand Mishra is the lead author of this chapter.

A. Agarwal et al., *Case Studies in Thyroid and Parathyroid Tumors*,
https://doi.org/10.1007/978-981-99-0938-4_37

fourth decades of life (M:F – 5:1). The mandible adjoining the molars and premolars is affected more often than the maxilla [2].

To begin with, early lesions appear radiolucent, well-defined, rounded, or oval expansile lesions with a shard border which becomes radio opaque over time [3]. The surrounding thin fibrous capsule makes the periphery appear radiolucent. These lesions typically occur in the medullary part of the bone and grow to cause equal outward expansion in all directions [4]. This expansion displaces the adjoining mandibular canal inferiorly and results in resorption or displacement of the root of involved teeth.

On histopathology, the tumor shows hypercellular fibroblastic stroma with calcifications in variable amounts [5]. The nuclei are hyperchromatic but atypia is present. The calcifications often seen in a characteristic quilted pattern arise because of osteoid or bones or cementum-like tissue in varied proportions. Multiple ossifying fibromas may be associated with hyperparathyroidism-jaw tumor syndrome.

Jaw Tumor Hyperparathyroidism Syndrome

Familial hyperparathyroidism(FHP) comprises various syndromes like multiple endocrine neoplasia type 1, type 2A and type 4, familial hypocalciuric hypercalcemia, hyperparathyroidism-jaw tumor syndrome (HPT-JT), and familial isolated hyperparathyroidism which are distinct from each other clinically and responsible genetic aberration [6]. FHP should be suspected in any young patient presenting with HPT.

HPT-JT shows autosomal dominant inheritance with incomplete penetrance (70%) presenting with parathyroid lesions, ossifying fibromas, and renal/uterine neoplasms [7]. The underlying genetic mutation affects the cell division cycle 73 (CDC73) tumor suppressor gene located on Chromosome 1q31.2 which codes for parafibromin [8]. Parafibromin promotes cell cycle arrest and regulates the expression of various genes and chromatin structure (via RNA polymerase-II associated factor 1 complex) [9]. Three-quarters of all HPT-JT patients have germline mutations in the coding region whereas others may have abnormalities in promoter regions, gene deletions, or epigenetic modifications.

PHPT is the commonest clinical manifestation of his syndrome and commonly a single adenoma is encountered which is often cystic [10]. The hypercalcemia in HPT-JT manifests earlier (mean 27 years) and is more severe compared to other familial syndromes. Malignant transformation is common (up to 15%) and should be suspected in any individual presenting with severe hypercalcemia due to a single lesion and PTH elevated more than 3 folds [11].

Women commonly have menorrhagia and multiple miscarriages. Uterine involvement is seen in almost half of the patients with HPT-JT syndrome [12]. Many patients also undergo hysterectomy at an early age.

Jaw tumors (ossifying fibromas), despite the nomenclature, are seen in only 30% to 50% of individuals [10]. Renal involvement commonly manifesting as unilateral or bilateral renal cysts is seen in 1 of every 5 patients. Renal hamartomas, Wilms' tumor, mixed epithelium-stromal tumor, and papillary renal carcinoma are other associations [10].

Neoplasms of pancreas, testes, thyroid (Hurtle cell), colon, pituitary, bile ducts and chronic lymphocytic leukemia are even rarer associations of this rare syndrome [13].

Management

HPT JT syndrome should be suspected in any young individual presenting with hypercalcemia secondary to a cystic parathyroid lesion, parathyroid carcinoma, ossifying jaw fibroma, and uterine or renal lesions. Documenting a CDC73 germline mutation confirms the diagnosis of this syndrome. Parathyroid lesions are best dealt by surgery if feasible. Focussed parathyroidectomy suffices in most. Should a carcinoma be suspected, a enbloc resection is performed and offers the best chance of cure [14]. Despite best efforts, hyperparathyroidism is likely to recur in 25%. Cinacalcet is a valid and effective option for patients who are poor surgical candidates [10].

Jaw tumors depending upon their size, location, and symptoms may benefit by surgery but are plagued by recurrence [15]. The management of gynecological manifestations and renal anomalies is individualized on a case to case to basis. Attaining normocalcemia is advocated in those contemplating pregnancy before conception to reduce fetal and maternal complications. Occasionally a hysterectomy may be required.

Patients are best kept on lifelong follow as recurrence is common. Surveillance is best carried out by

1. Serum Calcium, PTH and Vit D – Annually.
2. USG Neck if indicated.
3. Panoramic X-ray of Jaws – 5 yearly.
4. Ultrasound/MRI/CT (Renal) 5-yearly.
5. Pelvic Ultrasound in women.

Conclusion

HPT-JT syndrome though rare is a challenge for the treating team. A high index of suspicion, multi-disciplinary involvement, and follow up is necessary for optimal outcome.

References

1. Koenig LJ, Tamimi DF, Petrikowski CGPS. Diagnostic imaging: oral and maxillofacial. 2nd ed. Philadelphia, PA: Elsevier; 2017.

2. Kleihues P, Eds CWK. World Health Organization classification of Tumours. In: Pathology and Genetics of Tumours of the Lung, Pleura, Thymus and Heart; 2014. p. 85–90.
3. du Preez H, Adams A, Richards P, Whitley S. Hyperparathyroidism jaw tumour syndrome: a pictoral review. Insights Imaging. 2016;7(6):793.
4. Liu Y, You M, Wang H, Yang Z, Miao J, Shimizutani K, et al. Ossifying fibromas of the jaw bone: 20 cases. Dentomaxillofacial Radiol. 2010;39(1):57–63.
5. El-Mofty SK. Fibro-osseous lesions of the craniofacial skeleton: an update. Head Neck Pathol. 2014;8(4):432.
6. Weaver TD, Shakir MKM, Hoang TD. Hyperparathyroidism-jaw tumor syndrome. Case Rep Oncol. 2021;14(1):29–33.
7. Mehta A, Patel D, Rosenberg A, Boufraqech M, Ellis RJ, Nilubol N, et al. Hyperparathyroidism-jaw tumor syndrome: results of surgical management. Surgery. 2014;156(6):1315.
8. Carpten JD, Robbins CM, Villablanca A, Forsberg L, Presciuttini S, Bailey-Wilsons J, et al. HRPT2, encoding parafibromin, is mutated in hyperparathyroidism-jaw tumor syndrome. Nat Genet. 2002;32(4):676–80.
9. Yart A, Gstaiger M, Wirbelauer C, Pecnik M, Anastasiou D, Hess D, et al. The HRPT2 tumor suppressor gene product parafibromin associates with human PAF1 and RNA polymerase II. Mol Cell Biol. 2005;25(12):5052–60.
10. Torresan F, Iacobone M. Clinical features, treatment, and surveillance of hyperparathyroidism-jaw tumor syndrome: an up-to-date and review of the literature. Int J Endocrinol. 2019:2019.
11. Van Der Tuin K, Tops CMJ, Adank MA, Cobben JM, Hamdy NAT, Jongmans MC, et al. CDC73-related disorders: clinical manifestations and case detection in primary hyperparathyroidism. J Clin Endocrinol Metab. 2017;102(12):4534–40.
12. Bradley KJ, Hobbs MR, Buley ID, Carpten JD, Cavaco BM, Fares JE, et al. Uterine tumours are a phenotypic manifestation of the hyperparathyroidism-jaw tumour syndrome. J Intern Med. 2005;257(1):18–26.
13. Barnett M, Ahmed F, Mihai R, Rattan A, Humayun MA. The unforeseen diagnosis: hyperparathyroidism-jaw tumour syndrome case report and review of the literature. Case Rep Endocrinol. 2021;2021:5551203.
14. Iacobone M, Ruffolo C, Lumachi F, Favia G. Results of iterative surgery for persistent and recurrent parathyroid carcinoma. Langenbeck's Arch Surg. 2005;390(5):385–90.
15. Iacobone M, Carnailee B, Palazzo FF, Vriens M. Hereditary hyperparathyroidism- a consensus report of European Society of Endocrine Surgeon (ESES). Langenbeck's Arch Surg. 2015;400(8):867–86.

Part IV

PHPT: Pathological Enigma

Atypical Parathyroid Adenoma

Case

A 52-year-old gentleman presented with a history of intractable vomiting for which he was evaluated and found to have hiatus hernia with raised ALP, evaluated further and was found to have elevated serum calcium and PTH. On evaluation with high-resolution USG neck and MIBI scan, there was a concordant lesion in the right inferior parathyroid gland. After optimization and adequate hydration, he was taken up for focused parathyroidectomy. However, intraoperatively in view of the adenoma being adherent to thyroid and nodular hard surface with suspicious features of parathyroid carcinoma (Fig. 1), he underwent en bloc removal of the parathyroid gland along with ipsilateral hemithyroidectomy. Gross ex vivo weight of the specimen (Parathyroid + Right hemithyroidectomy) was 18.6 g (Fig. 2). The histopathology was reported as atypical parathyroid adenoma. The detailed report was as follows: Sections from parathyroid show a tumor disposed diffusely in nests, trabeculae and diffuse pattern with interspersed broad fibrous bands. Tumor cells show mild pleomorphism, coarse chromatin, conspicuous nucleoli in some and moderate amount of cytoplasm (Fig. 3). Focal capsular and vascular invasion are seen. Occasional mitotic figures are also noted. On follow-up he is still eucalcemic after 8 years of surgery.

Amit Agarwal is the lead author of this chapter.

A. Agarwal et al., *Case Studies in Thyroid and Parathyroid Tumors*,
https://doi.org/10.1007/978-981-99-0938-4_38

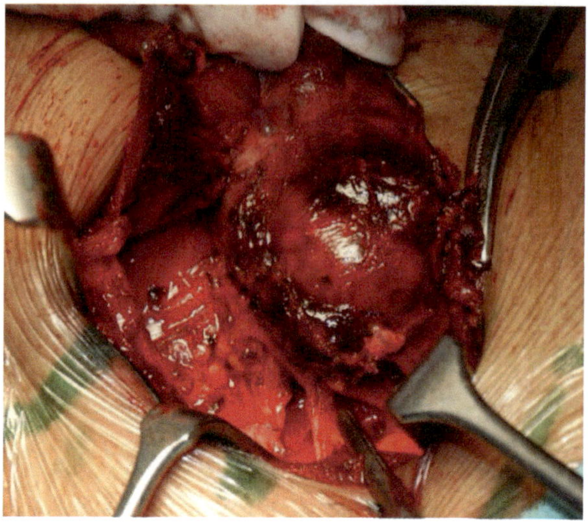

Fig. 1 Intra-operative picture showing the hard, nodular parathyroid

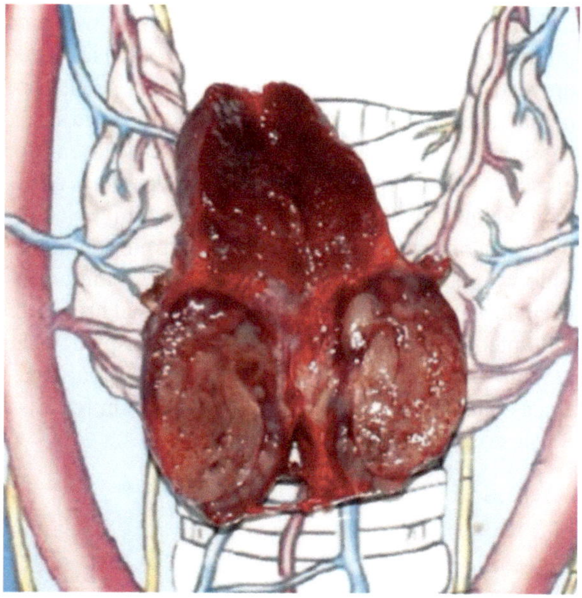

Fig. 2 Specimen picture showing the bisected parathyroid adenoma densely adherent to the thyroid lobe

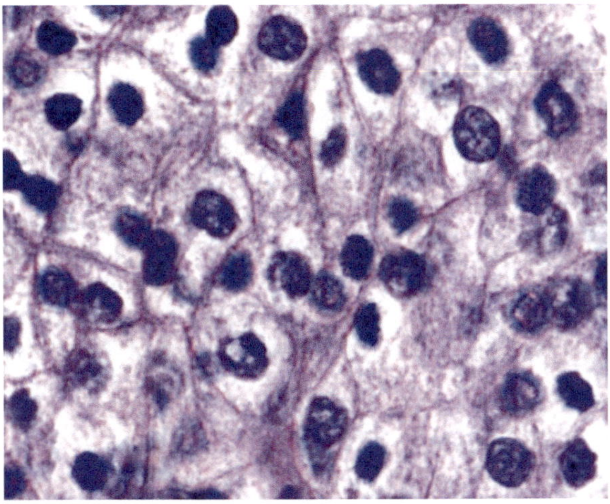

Fig. 3 Microphotograph showing nuclear atypica in atypical parathyroid adenoma

Discussion

Atypical parathyroid adenoma or parathyroid neoplasm of uncertain malignant potential is a rare histopathologic entity. In most consecutive series of patients undergoing surgery for PHPT, the incidence of atypical parathyroid adenoma ranged from 0.5 to 4.4% [1]. An incidence as high as 14% has been reported in the Asian countries [2]. Atypical parathyroid adenomas represent a group of intermediate form of parathyroid neoplasms of uncertain malignant potential which show some atypical histological features (i.e., solid growth pattern, fibrous bands and cellular atypia), which represent a challenge for the differential diagnosis with parathyroid carcinomas. However, the macroscopic appearance at surgery is of limited help since in both cases the parathyroid lesions may appear firm and adherent to the adjacent structures, features that may guide the surgeon to perform a more radical surgical approach suspecting parathyroid carcinoma. In some cases, the initial diagnosis of atypical adenoma needs to be revised to carcinoma because of the occurrence of local or distant metastasis during the follow-up. The reverse, even less frequently, may also occur when the initial diagnosis of parathyroid carcinoma not confirmed by an expert endocrine pathologist [3]17). Common features seen in atypical adenoma include cellular pleomorphism (30%), nuclear atypia (24%), tumor necrosis without unequivocal signs of capsular or vascular invasion. The presence of mitosis should certainly lead to further investigation toward the elimination of malignancy.. Genetic alterations, exclusive CDC73 somatic mutations are very rare in atypical parathyroid adenomas, suggesting a minor pathogenic role, if any, in these neoplasms [4–8]. Immunohistochemical markers have been sought to help identifying atypical parathyroid adenoma carrying the risk of malignant behavior. The proliferation marker Ki-67 is mainly overexpressed in malignant tumors and appears of limited diagnostic value to distinguish atypical adenomas from carcinomas. A significant heterogeneity of the loss of parafibromin staining ranging from 0 to 50% has been observed in atypical parathyroid adenomas. Role of adenomatous polyposis coli (APC) as a tool for help differentiating parathyroid neoplasms is of limited value because of the overlap in the loss of APC expression between benign and malignant lesions; Galectin-3 overexpression (range 32–100%) was found at a rate similar to that observed in parathyroid carcinoma, indicating that this marker, when used alone, does not help to differentiate these two categories of parathyroid neoplasms. PGP9.5 overexpression in atypical parathyroid adenomas ranges between 22 and 35%, whereas in carcinomas between 35 and 71%. PGP9.5 overexpression may be the strongest predictor for recurrent hypercalcemia after the first operation either in atypical adenomas or carcinoma.

References

1. Christofer Juhlin C, Nilsson I-L, Johansson K, Haglund F, Villablanca A, Höög A. Catharina Larsson Parafibromin and APC as Screening Markers for Malignant Potential in Atypical Parathyroid Adenomas. Endocr Pathol. 2010;21:166–77.
2. Agarwal A, Pradhan R, Kumari N, Krishnani N, Shukla P, Gupta SK, Chand G, Mishra A, Agarwal G, Verma AK, Mishra SK. Molecular characteristics of large parathyroid adenomas. World J Surg. 2016;40(3):607–14.
3. Kumari N, Chaudhary N, Pradhan R, Agarwal A, Krishnani N. Role of histological criteria and immunohistochemical markers in predicting risk of malignancy in parathyroid neoplasms. Endocr Pathol. 2016;27:87–96.
4. Tan MH, Morrison C, Wang P, et al. Loss of parafibromin immunoreactivity is a distinguishing feature of parathyroid carcinoma. Clin Cancer Res. 2004;10(6629–6637):8.
5. Gill AJ, Clarkson A, Gimm O, et al. Loss of nuclear expression of parafibromin distinguishes parathyroid carcinomas and hyperparathyroidism-jaw tumor (HPT-JT) syndrome-related adenomas from sporadic parathyroid adenomas and hyperplasias. Am J Surg Pathol. 2006;30:1140–9.
6. Carpten JD, Robbins CM, Villablanca A, et al. HRPT2, encoding parafibromin, is mutated in hyperparathyroidism-jaw tumor syndrome. Nat Genet. 2002;32:676–80.
7. Howell VM, Haven CJ, Kahnoski K, et al. HRPT2 mutations are associated with malignancy in sporadic parathyroid tumours. J Med Genet. 2003;40:657–63.
8. Juhlin C, Larsson C, Yakoleva T, Leibiger I, Leibiger B, Alimov A, Weber G, Hoog A, Villablanca A. Loss of parafibromin expression in a subset of parathyroid adenomas. Endocr Relat Cancer. 2006;13:509–23.

Parathyroid Carcinoma

Case

A 75-year-old male presented to the emergency department with generalized, progressive weakness for about 2 months with frequent falls. His past medical history included two strokes with a right-sided hemiparesis. Due to the severity of his functional decline, he was admitted for further investigations, none of which showed any acute deviations responsible for the patient's symptoms. He also underwent screening laboratory tests; and these showed a very high adjusted calcium of 3.19 mmol/L, with a parathyroid hormone (PTH) of 89.3 pmol/L. His vitamin D was only 9.6 μg/L.

The patient's neck was examined, a palpable mass was appreciated. His calcium:creatinine clearance ratio was 0.0417, excluding familial hypocalciuric hypercalcemia (FHH). With the diagnosis of primary hyperparathyroidism (PHPT) made, the patient was started on IV fluids, vitamin D replacement, and to start IV Zoledronic acid once the vitamin D levels had improved, to prevent the occurrence of refractory hypocalcemia. He subsequently underwent dual localization studies. His Technetium 99 m Sestamibi (MIBI) revealed a MIBI-avid focus at the upper pole of the right thyroid lobe is in keeping with a parathyroid lesion (Fig. 1a). His ultrasound scan (US) confirmed this as a structure measuring 2.2 in largest diameter was noted, posterior to the upper pole of the right thyroid lobe.

The patient was subsequently referred to the endocrine surgery team for the performance of early parathyroidectomy. This decision was due to the suspicion of this being a parathyroid cancer, based on the very high levels of calcium (>3.00 mmol/L) and PTH (> three times the upper limit); as well as on the appearance of the lesion on US, with its overall size and irregular margins (Fig. 1b).

About 1 week after his diagnosis, he underwent a right superior parathyroidectomy with en-bloc right hemithyroidectomy for a hard, nodular, and infiltrative right superior parathyroid gland, measuring 4 cm in the largest diameter (Fig. 2a, b). There were no abnormal lymph nodes.

Rajeev Parameswaran is the lead author of this chapter.

A. Agarwal et al., *Case Studies in Thyroid and Parathyroid Tumors*,
https://doi.org/10.1007/978-981-99-0938-4_39

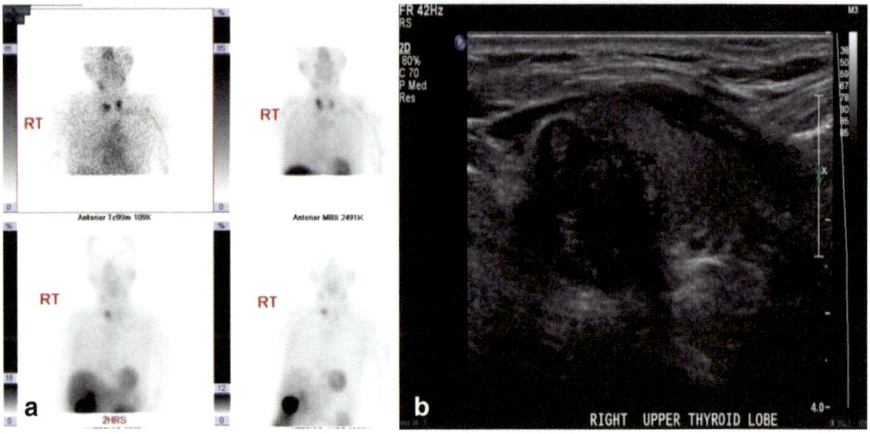

Fig 1 (**a**, **b**) Preoperative Sestamibi and US images of the patient

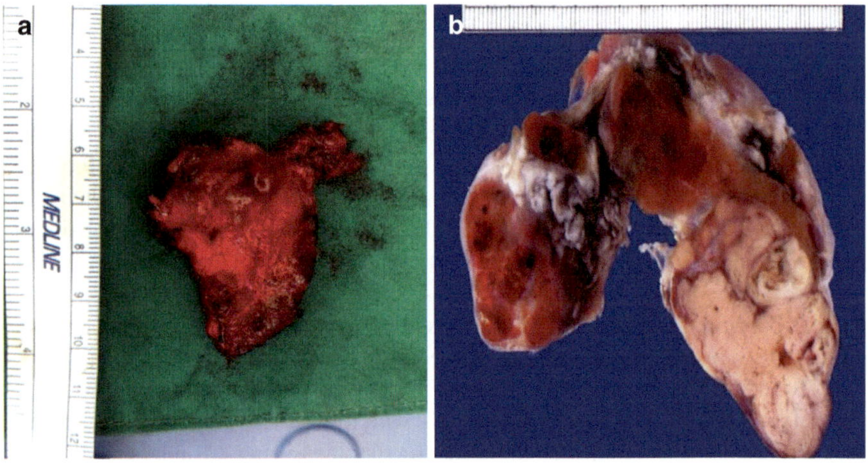

Fig. 2 (**a**, **b**) En-bloc excised specimen and the gross histology of the parathyroid cancer

Histology confirmed the suspicion of malignancy, as the parathyroid tumor was found to be arranged in closely packed trabeculae and nests, separated by delicate vascular septa. These lobules were separated by thick, densely fibrous septa. Capsular invasion and extracapsular lymphovascular invasion were also identified, while perineurial invasion was not. Moreover, there was focal tumor invasion into the adjacent thyroid and perithyroidal soft tissue.

The patient recovered well from the operation. He had no issues regarding his scar or voice. He was discharged to a community care facility on postoperative day 11 on ongoing vitamin D supplements. His PTH levels had dropped initially (nadir 0.5 pmol/L) but became stable at normal levels soon. His calcium levels followed a similar pattern. Moreover, it was noticed that he had become much more alert and less drowsy compared to before his operation. He has been under follow-up for well over 3 years and has not shown signs of recurrent disease, either biochemically or on serial imaging.

Discussion

Parathyroid carcinoma (PC), first described in 1933, [1] is a rare, malignant, neoplasm originating from parathyroid parenchymal cells, which accounts for less than 1% of cases of primary hyperparathyroidism [2]. Conversely to primary hyperparathyroidism, which is more common among females, the incidence for parathyroid cancer is equal among men and women. Moreover, the average age at presentation has been noted to be approximately a decade younger than for patients with a benign disease; with younger patients generally with disease associated with familial syndromes. Conditions predisposed to parathyroid cancer are highlighted in Table 1.

The overall diagnosis of PC has proven to be challenging, due to the lack of distinct clinical and histopathological features. There are several clinical features increasing the suspicion of PC, such as PTH-levels increased more than three times the upper limit of normal and an adjusted calcium of more than 3.00 mmol/L. [3] Moreover, the presence of a palpable neck mass has also been reported [4]. Suspicious features on imaging include signs of infiltration or calcification, while there is usually uniglandular disease [5]. Schantz and Castleman in 1973 established a set of criteria for the pathological diagnosis of this malignancy based on their analysis of 70 parathyroid cancers [6]. Table 2 highlights the histological

Table 1 Factors predisposing to parathyroid cancer

Hereditary hyperparathyroid-jaw tumor syndrome (HPT-JT)
Multiple endocrine neoplasia syndromes (MEN-1 and MEN-2A)
History of irradiation of the head and neck
Familial isolated primary hyperparathyroidism (PHPT)
Parathyroid adenoma or hyperplastic parathyroid gland
Prolonged secondary hyperparathyroidism
End-stage renal disease

Table 2 Histological features of parathyroid carcinoma

Most definitive features
• Capsular invasion with growth into adjacent tissues • Vascular invasion (vessels in capsule or surrounding tissue) • Perineural invasion
Non-definitive features that may be seen in malignancy
• Band-forming fibrosis • Solid growth pattern • Coagulative necrosis[a] • Mitotic activity >5 figures per 50 high power fields[a] • Macronucleoli[a]

[a] When seen together, this triad of features is associated with malignant behavior

features that are associated with a higher risk of malignant behavior. Moreover, the loss of parafibromin expression is also often observed [7].

As there is a paucity of prospective data, the gold standard surgical approach for patients with PC has not been fully established for either the preferred initial surgical approach or regarding indications for the performance of a second-stage surgery [8]. However, in general – if there is suspicion of a PC – performance of an en-bloc resection of the affected parathyroid gland with the surrounding thyroid lobe is recommended, as this has shown to result in improved local control and is possibly also associated with better long-term outcomes [8, 9]. One of the challenging scenarios encountered in clinical practice is when histologic examination of an adenoma suggests the possibility of parathyroid cancer following a simple parathyroidectomy. If the features are suggestive of an aggressive disease with vascular and capsular invasion, early reoperation with excision of adjacent structures may be considered [10]. However, in the absence of any invasive features, monitoring of serum calcium and PTH is sufficient.

Parathyroid cancer is a radioresistant cancer and EBRT has no effect on the treatment of local recurrence or metastatic disease. The role of chemotherapy in the management of parathyroid carcinoma is limited. Generally, chemotherapy is not effective and the results published from the case series have been disappointing [11, 12]. Long-term follow-up for patients is necessary, as disease recurrence is very common (reported rates: 25–100%), sometimes occurring as late as 20 years after initial diagnosis [13].

References

1. Sainton P. Degenerence maligne d'un adenome parathyroidien eosinophile au cours d'une maladie de Recklinghausen. Ann Anat Pathol. 1933;10:813–8.
2. Marcocci C, et al. Parathyroid carcinoma. J Bone Miner Res. 2008;23(12):1869.
3. Schulte KM, Talat N. Diagnosis and management of parathyroid cancer. Nat Rev Endocrinol. 2012;8(10):612–22.
4. Wynne AG, et al. Parathyroid carcinoma: clinical and pathologic features in 43 patients. Medicine (Baltimore). 1992;71(4):197–205.
5. Sidhu PS, et al. Ultrasound features of malignancy in the preoperative diagnosis of parathyroid cancer: a retrospective analysis of parathyroid tumours larger than 15 mm. Eur Radiol. 2011;21(9):1865–73.
6. Schantz A, Castleman B, Parathyroid carcinoma. A study of 70 cases. Cancer. 1973;31(3):600–5.
7. Erickson LA, Mete O. Immunohistochemistry in diagnostic parathyroid pathology. Endocr Pathol. 2018;29(2):113–29.
8. Pelizzo M, et al. Parathyroid carcinoma. Therapeutic strategies derived from 20 years of experience. Minerva Endocrinol. 2001;26(1):23–9.
9. Busaidy NL, et al. Parathyroid carcinoma: a 22-year experience. Head Neck. 2004;26(8):716–26.
10. Shane E. Clinical review 122: parathyroid carcinoma. J Clin Endocrinol Metab. 2001;86(2):485–93.
11. Lumachi F, Basso SM, Basso U. Parathyroid cancer: etiology, clinical presentation and treatment. Anticancer Res. 2006;26(6C):4803–7.
12. Obara T, et al. Surgical and medical management of patients with pulmonary metastasis from parathyroid carcinoma. Surgery. 1993;114(6):1040–8. Discussion 1048–9.
13. McClenaghan F, Qureshi YA. Parathyroid cancer. Gland Surg. 2015;4(4):329.

Part V

PHPT: Postoperative Issues

Post Parathyroidectomy Thyrotoxicosis

Case
A 23-year-old girl presented to orthopedic emergency with fracture sustained on trivial trauma. She was evaluated and found to have a subtrochanteric femur fracture (Fig. 1) which was managed by closed reduction and internal fixation with long proximal femoral nail along with biopsy.

In view of pathological fracture, a MDP bone scan was ordered which was suggestive of a superscan indicative of underlying metabolic bone disease.

Hence the patient was evaluated with serum calcium and iPTH levels, which were found to be high, therefore the patient was subsequently referred to the endocrinology department. On biochemical evaluation her calcium was 15.2 mg/dL (N-8.8–10.6 mg/dL), phosphorus 2.1 and iPTH was 766 pg/mL with ALP of 687 U/L (Normal 50-140 U/L). The patient had normal vitamin D and serum creatinine levels. Hence a diagnosis of primary hyperparathyroidism with hypercalcemic crisis was made. Subsequently, imaging studies were performed. High-frequency ultrasound showed a hypoechoic solid lesion measuring 3.6 × 1.1 × 1 cm at the inferior aspect of the left thyroid lobe extending from the upper lobe to the lower lobe with peripheral vascularity. Sestamibi scan was s/o left superior parathyroid adenoma. In view of discordant imaging results and due to the large size of the lesion, unilateral exploration with a standard thyroid incision was planned.

At operation, a superior enlarged parathyroid was identified, measuring approximately 4 × 2 × 1 cm (Fig. 2) and was found adhered all along to the left thyroid lobe extending up to the inferior pole but could be separated with fine dissection. The inferior parathyroid gland was found to be normal and was preserved. IOPTH showed drop of more than 50% according to Miami's criteria.

On postoperative day one, the patient developed symptomatic hypocalcemia and was managed with calcium infusion (at the rate of 2 mg/kg) along with oral calcium

---

Roma Pradhan is the lead author of this chapter.

A. Agarwal et al., *Case Studies in Thyroid and Parathyroid Tumors*,
https://doi.org/10.1007/978-981-99-0938-4_40

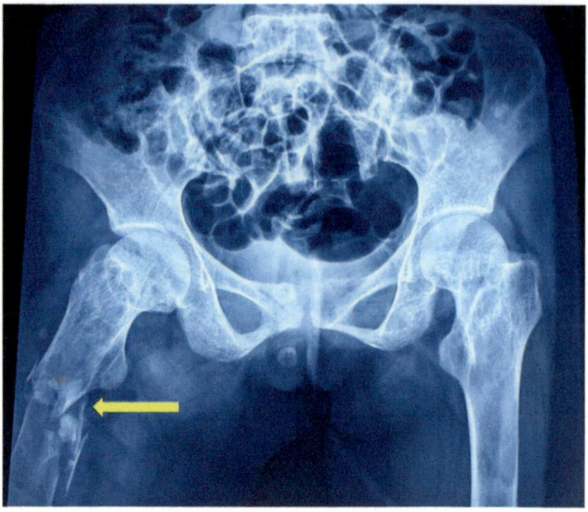

Fig. 1 Subtrochanteric fracture (yellow arrow)

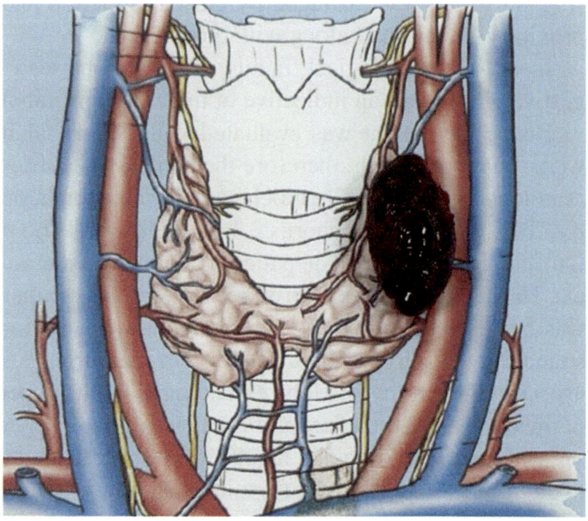

Fig. 2 Specimen measuring 4 × 2 × 1 cm

and active vitamin d supplements. The infusion could only be tapered and stopped over 5 days as she continued to have hypocalcemia despite gradual escalation of oral supplements (max dose-3 g per day). After 12 h of stopping infusion patient had febrile episodes and was managed by antipyretics. On sixth postoperative day, the patient developed unexplained restlessness and agitation with constant tossing over bed as well as having difficulty in breathing. She was found to be having tachycardia (pulse rate: 140-150 beats/min) but saturation levels were maintained. Keeping the possibility of hypocalcemia due to hungry bone syndrome, we gave her injectable calcium but she continued to have these symptoms despite normal calcium levels. With the possibilities like septicemia, pulmonary embolism (as the patient was bedridden because of fracture), relevant investigations were sent but her blood cultures were sterile with normal leucocyte count and she had a normal chest x-ray. We also thought of thyrotoxicosis and thyroid function tests were sent which were found to be suggestive of thyrotoxicosis (normal TSH 2.7 and elevated FT4 Levels—27.94 pmol/L). Meanwhile, she responded well to beta-blockers (propranolol at a dosage of 20 mg BD) and after her symptoms settled she was discharged on 11TH POD.

Discussion

Thyrotoxicosis is an unrecognized and unknown complication following parathyroidectomy. It is thought to be due to release of thyroid hormones due to excessive manipulation of the thyroid gland and is hence labeled as palpation thyroiditis. The rate of postoperative hyperthyroidism after parathyroid surgery is around 20% [1] though the majority of them are asymptomatic hence not detected postoperatively unless routine thyroid tests are performed in the postoperative period. In the study by Rudoskfy et al. [2] maximum levels of fT4 and fT3 were reached on postoperative days 1–3, and the TSH nadir was reached by day 5. By day 40, there was spontaneous resolution of clinical symptoms and biochemical normalization in all cases with no significant long-term sequelae reported. Few of the patients develop severe thyrotoxic symptoms which can often be confused with post-parathyroidectomy hypocalcemia, septicemia, or pulmonary embolism in PHPT patients with severe bone disease and fractures. Therefore, it is important to suspect a possibility of post-parathyroidectomy thyrotoxicosis whenever the patient develops unexplained adrenergic symptoms following parathyroidectomy in order to manage these patients and also to avoid other extensive evaluation.

Although there are many case repost of post-parathyroidectomy thyrotoxicosis following surgery for secondary hyperparathyroidism [2–4] which involved bilateral neck exploration and extensive manipulation of the thyroid gland. However, very few case reports have been published documenting post-parathyroidectomy thyrotoxicosis following surgery for primary hyperparathyroidism [5]. In our case of primary hyperparathyroidism, the superior gland was extending up to the inferior pole and was adhered to thyroid. In such circumstances we usually do en-bloc excision due to clinical suspicion of carcinoma, therefore thyrotoxicosis is not manifested. In our case we made effort to dissect parathyroid and hence there was excessive manipulation of gland which manifested as thyrotoxicosis in the postoperative period.

Awareness of this complication holds importance for parathyroid surgeons to avoid extensive evaluation postoperatively if the patient develops adrenergic symptoms. Patients should also be counseled of such a complication in the same way we explain about post-parathyroidectomy hypocalcemia. This complication assumes more significance in elderly patients and those with underlying heart problems, hence careful watch needs to be maintained in the postoperative period.

Our case highlights the importance of recognizing the possibility of transient palpatory thyroiditis in post-parathyroidectomy scenario even after a unilateral exploration for a parathyroid adenoma and perhaps recommend routine thyroid hormone evaluation following parathyroidectomy.

References

1. Walfish PG, Caplan D, Rosen IB. Postparathyroidectomy transient thyrotoxicosis. J Clin Endo Metab. 1992;75:224–7.
2. Rudofsky G, Tsioga M, Leowardi C, Kopf S, Grafe A, Mawroth PP, Isermann B. Transient hyperthyroidism after surgery for secondary hyperparathyroidism: a common problem. Eur J Med Res. 2011;16:375–80.
3. Stang MT, Yim JH, Challinor SM, Bahl S, Carty SE. Hyperpa rathyroidism after parathyroid exploration. Surgery. 2005;138:1058–65.
4. Espiritu R, Dean D. Parathyroidectomy induced thyroiditis. Endocr Pract. 2010;16:656–9.
5. Calle RA, Cohen KL. Transient thyroiditis due to surgical trauma. Am J Med. 1993;95:546–8.

Hungry Bone Syndrome: Still a Challenge in the Post-Operative Management of Primary Hyperparathyroidism

Case

A 24-year-old unmarried female student presented with pain in lower jaw for which she had a tooth extraction. However, she continued to have swelling & protrusion of lower jaw (left side) and underwent resection of the lower jaw swelling. Three years later she developed generalized weakness, pain in both thighs, difficulty in walking and also gave a history of reduction in her height. She sustained right femur fracture (Fig. 1) after trivial trauma (fall from standing bike) and was treated by nailing. Subsequently, she sustained fracture of left forearm from trivial trauma which was managed with POP cast. On examination she was found to have short stature with malar prominence, pectus excavatum (Fig. 2), kyphosis (Fig. 3) and genu varum. Neck examination showed about 4 × 4 cm smooth surfaced, nontender, firm swelling in right lower neck moving with deglutition. Her biochemistry was as follows:

Date	May 2014	2016
Calcium	12.59	12.0
Phosphorus	2.6	2.1
ALP	2674	1849
PTH	3691	3067
Vitamin D	11.95	3.64

MIBI and USG Neck 3.5 × 2.9 × 5.0 cm mass lesion near right inferior pole of thyroid. She underwent unilateral neck exploration with En- bloc Right inferior parathyroidectomy and hemithyroidectomy (due to dense adhesions) with

Amit Agarwal is the lead author of this chapter.

A. Agarwal et al., *Case Studies in Thyroid and Parathyroid Tumors*,
https://doi.org/10.1007/978-981-99-0938-4_41

intraoperative parathyroid hormone (IOPTH) monitoring. IOPTH values (pg/mL): Pre-incision—2500, Pre-excision—541, Post-excision (5 min)—270, Post-excision (10 min)—183, post-excision (15 min)—160. Specimen weighed 32.6 gm. Post-operative Course: POD1—Ca leve—9.8 mg/DL with no signs & symptoms of hypocalcemia. POD2; T-sign positive in less than a minute. Started on Calcium infusion at 1.5 mg/kg/h. Despite calcium levels being in the normal range, T-sign persisted to be positive. In view of hypomagnesaemia Magnesium infusion at 2 meq/kg/h was started along with oral Phosphorus -500 mg BD. T-Sign and C-sign continued to be persistently positive though her PTH was within normal range: 4.01 pmol/L. The patient was finally discharged with oral calcium (2 g/day) and vitamin D supplements (Rocaltrol 1.5 µg/day) on POD 21

Date	Calcium	Phosphorus	Magnesium	Sodium	Potassium
POD1	11.0/2.16		0.8		
POD2	9.7/1.7				
POD3	9.4/1.6	1.46			
POD4	9.5	2.0	1.5	140	4.1
POD5	9.2	1.9	1.5	141	4.0
POD6	8.2	2.7	1.6[a]	145	4.2
POD7	6.8[b]	2.98	1.8	134	3.8
POD8	6.5/0.7	2.29	1.5	133	4.0
POD9	6.4/0.8	2.44	1.3		
POD9	8.0	2.45	1.5		
POD10	7.7	2.24	1.5	142	3.8
POD11	7.8/1.07	1.72	1.4	138	3.9
POD12					

[a] Magnesium infusion stopped
[b] Calcium infusion raised to 2 mg/kg/h

Date	Calcium	Phosphorus	Magnesium	Sodium	Potassium
POD13	9.0/1.0	1.27	1.0	139	4.6
POD14	9.3/1.2	1.4	1.00	139	4.2

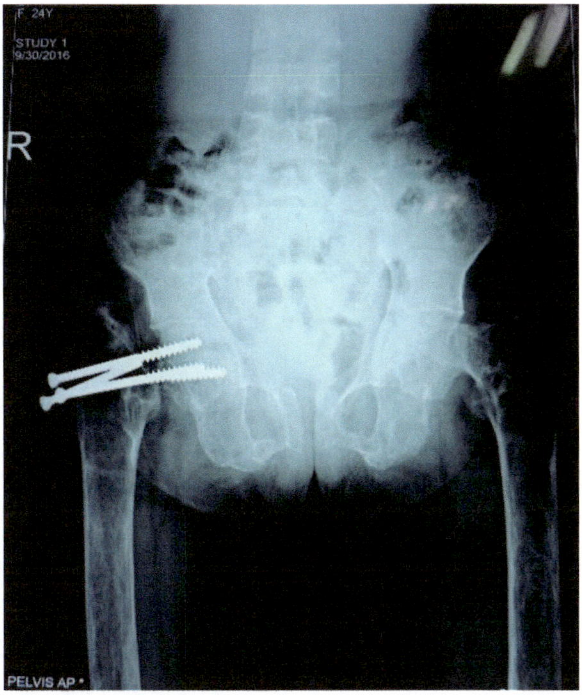

Fig. 1 severely osteoporotic femur with nailing done for fracture neck femur

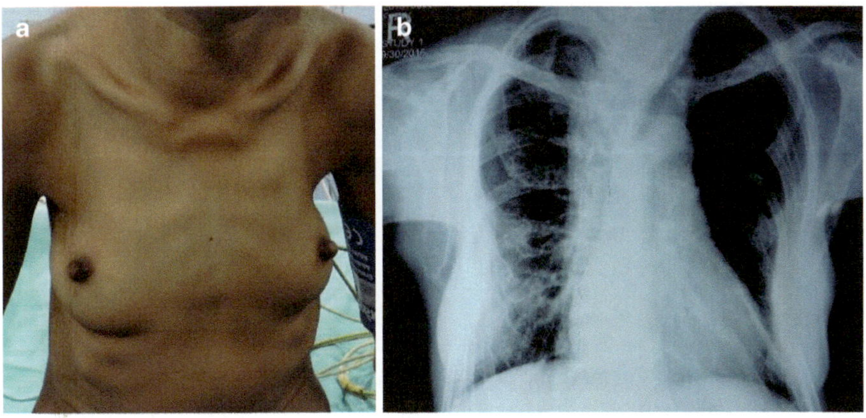

Fig. 2 (**a**, **b**) Clinical picture and X-ray chest showing pectus excavatum

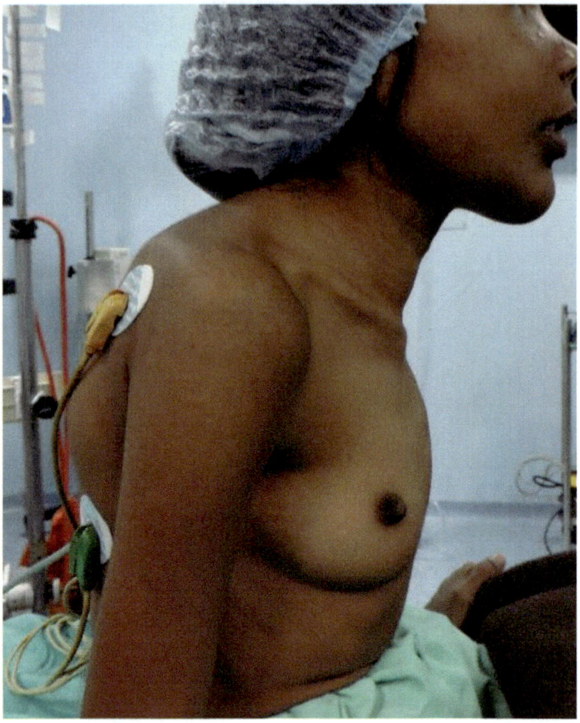

Fig. 3 Patient with kyphosis

Date	Calcium	Phosphorus	Magnesium	Sodium	Potassium
POD15	8.9/1.1	1.32	1.1		
POD16	7.5	1.58	1.0		
POD17	7.6/1.0	1.8	1.3		
POD18	7.3	2.47	1.3	135	3.7
POD19	8.4	2.0	1.1	137	2.0
POD20	7.4/1.07	2.0	1.6		
POD21	7.8	1.2	1.79	5.3	

Discussion

The differential diagnosis of HBS includes: permanent hypoparathyroidism, transient hypoparathyroidism and un-masking of vitamin D deficiency. The term "hungry bone syndrome" (HBS) has been coined to define the rapid, profound and prolonged (longer than fourth day post-operatively) hypocalcemia, which follows parathyroidectomy for severe hyperparathyroidism, with normal or elevated PTH levels along with hypophosphatemia and hypomagnesemia [1]. Pathophysiology of HBS involves bone remodeling which is a process of bone resorption lasting for about 2 weeks followed by a reversal phase of 2–3 weeks duration, before new bone is formed, which lasts about 3 months. In those patients with pre-operative high rates of bone turnover, successful parathyroidectomy curbs osteoclastic resorption. In addition, hypophosphatemia and hypomagnesemia in HBS is probably due to an increase in bone uptake that facilitates matrix remineralization. Clinical manifestations of HBS include severe hypocalcemia (serum calcium concentration <2.1 mmol/L), associated with neuromuscular irritability, clinically manifested by carpopedal spasms, perioral paresthesiae, tingling extremities, Chvostek sign and Trousseau sign [2]. Patients can also develop generalized convulsions, which can lead to pathological fractures, and ultimately if remaining uncorrected to coma and even death. Congestive heart failure, which is reversible after normalization of serum calcium concentration, has also been reported. Biochemical changes associated with HBS include a rapid decrease in serum PTH levels to a mean of 1.7 ± 0.4 pmol/L, reduced serum calcium levels to 12.1 mmol/L within the first 3–4 days but decrease further after the fourth post-operative day in patients with HBS, serum phosphate levels decrease post-operatively and remain so for the duration of the syndrome; Hypomagnesaemia is frequently encountered, serum alkaline phosphatase levels increase significantly post-operatively and remain elevated sometimes for up to 9 months after surgery. HBS after parathyroidectomy develops post-operatively in up to 13% of patients with PHPT [3]. Recent case series from Asia reported much higher prevalence rates of 24–87% [4]. Risk factors for the development of HBS include older age at the time of surgery, higher preoperative levels of serum calcium, two-fold increased levels of PTH (> 45 pmol/L has 90% chance of developing HBS), and elevated alkaline phosphatase, radiological bone disease before surgery, presence of Osteitis fibrosa cystica, increased volume and weight of resected parathyroid glands. Management of HBS is aimed, in the short term, primarily at replenishing the depleted skeletal calcium stores. The reported amount of calcium supplementation required to treat the severe hypocalcemia varies between 6 and 12 g/day [5]. Initially, calcium is supplemented intravenously, but treatment with oral preparations should be initiated as early as possible; adequate doses of active metabolites of vitamin D (calcitriol) or alfacalcidol (2–4 mg/day). Replenishment of magnesium stores as required either given intravenously as magnesium chloride or sulfate or orally as magnesium sulfate. When calcium-containing solutions are given intravenously, administration into large veins or via a central venous catheter is recommended to minimize the risk of local irritation or tissue necrosis by accidental extravasation in surrounding tissues. Electrocardiographic monitoring is recommended as dysrhythmias may occur in case of too rapid correction of the hypocalcemia. In prescribing oral calcium preparations, it is important to realize that different calcium preparations contain different amounts of elemental calcium. Of the available oral preparations: calcium carbonate has the highest percentage of elemental calcium (40%), followed by citrate salts (20%). calcium lactate (13%), calcium gluconate (9%) and calcium glubionate (6.6%), although they do not contain sufficient elemental calcium per tablet and compliance may be affected by the large number of tablets required to be taken orally to achieve the same calcium level. It should be kept in mind that refractory hypocalcemia does not resolve until the magnesium deficiency has been corrected. A randomized study showed that daily high-dose vitamin D supplementation of 2800 IU for 6 months preoperatively and 6 months postoperatively is a safe way to improve vitamin D status in PHPT patients, without increasing plasma or urinary calcium [6]. Boyle et al. [7] showed that preoperative treatment of severe hyperparathyroidism with 1,25(OH)2D (calcitriol) at a dose of 2 mg/day for 1–10 weeks significantly decreased preoperative alkaline phosphatase levels. Preoperative treatment with bisphosphonates is controversial because short-term preoperative bisphosphonate treatment may exacerbate postoperative hypocalcemia by reducing bone resorption, without allowing time for a coupled decrease in bone formation. Duration of HBS has been defined as the time needed for bone remineralization and normalization of bone turnover markers, as well as the time required for normalization of serum calcium following successful parathyroidectomy. In addition, improvement or normalization of bone mineral density (BMD) is considered to be a criterion for resolution of HBS, and several studies adopting this notion have reported that HBS may last from 4.5 to 16 months.

References

1. Witteveen JE, van Thiel S, Romijn JA, Hamdy NAT. Hungry bone syndrome: still a challenge in the post-operative management of primary hyperparathyroidism: a systematic review of the literature. Eur J Endocrinol. 2013;168:R45–53.
2. Kuzucu A, Soysal O, Savli H. Giant mediastinal parathyroid adenoma presenting with a hyperparathyroid crisis and leading to postoperative hungry bone syndrome. Eur J Surg. 2002;168:747–9.
3. Brasier AR, Nussbaum SR. Hungry bone syndrome: clinical and biochemical predictors of its occurrence after parathyroid surgery. Am J Med. 1988;84:654–60.
4. Bhansali A, Masoodi SR, Reddy KS, Behera A, das Radotra B, Mittal BR, Katariya RN & Dash RJ. Primary hyperparathyroidism in North India: a description of 52 cases. Ann Saudi Med. 2005;25:29–35.
5. Demirci H, Suyani E, Karakoc A, Toruner FB, Yetkin I, Ayvaz G, Taneri F, Cakir N, Arslan M. A longstanding hungry bone syndrome. Endocrinologist. 2007;17:10–2.
6. Rolighed L, Rejnmark L, Sikjaer T, et al. Vitamin D treatment in primary hyperparathyroidism: a randomized placebo controlled trial. J Clin Endocrinol Metab. 2014;99(3):1072–80.
7. Boyle IT, Fogelman I, Boyce B, Thomson JE, Beastall GH, McIntosh WB, McLennan I. 1a-Hydroxyvitamin D3 in primary hyperparathyroidism. Clin Endocrinol. 1977;7(Suppl):215s–22s.

Persistent Hyperparathyroidism After Parathyroidectomy for Primary Hyperparathyroidism. Are We Missing the Obvious?

Case

A 65-year-old Chinese female is referred to the Endocrinologist for the management of recurrent hyperparathyroidism. She had a recent dual energy X-ray absorptiometry (DXA) scan that showed osteoporosis (lowest T-score at NOF: −2.9). She has not been started on any anti-osteoporosis medications. She also has hypertension which is well controlled on monotherapy with a calcium channel blocker—amlodipine.

She denies any gastrointestinal or neurological symptoms. She has not had previous kidney stones. She does not have any pituitary, thyroid, or pancreatic problems. Her family history is unavailable as she is adopted.

On physical examination, there are no obvious abnormalities detected.

She had been diagnosed with primary hyperparathyroidism 5 years ago when a health screening biochemical assessment had revealed mildly raised serum adjusted for albumin calcium levels of 2.8 mmol/L (Normal Range (NR): 2.1–2.6) with a simultaneous intact parathyroid hormone (iPTH) level of 9.3 pmol/L (NR: 0.9–6.2). Her serum phosphate level was 0.80 mmol/L (NR: 0.77–1.38). Her renal function was normal, and a fractional excretion of calcium (FeCa) was calculated to be 0.014. The rest of her biochemistry results are listed in Table 1.

She subsequently had an ultrasound scan (USS) and nuclear imaging with technetium 99 m-sestamibi scanning. The scan did not show increased tracer uptake (Fig. 1). The concurrent USS also did not show any lesion. It was deemed that she would benefit from surgery, and she underwent a bilateral exploration parathyroidectomy. A right-sided superior enlarged gland (2 × 3 mm) was identified and removed. Post-operatively, her serum calcium and iPTH levels remained elevated ranging between 2.68 to 2.8 mmol/L and 7.2 to 9 pmol/L respectively. The possibility of familial hypocalciuric hypercalcemia was considered. A genetic analysis was

Rajeev Parmeshwaran is the lead author of this chapter.

A. Agarwal et al., *Case Studies in Thyroid and Parathyroid Tumors*,
https://doi.org/10.1007/978-981-99-0938-4_42

Table 1 Biochemistry at presentation

Biochemistry	Result	Reference range
Serum calcium	2.58	2.1–2.6 mmol/L
Serum albumin	29	37–51 mg/L
Serum adjusted calcium	2.8	
Serum phosphate	0.8	0.77–1.38 mmol/L
Serum intact parathyroid hormone	9.3	0.9–6.2 mmol/L
Serum creatinine	83	Micromole/L
Serum alkaline phosphatase (ALP)	45	39–99 U/L
25hydroxy vitamin D	30	Ng/mL
24 h urine calcium	1.4	Mmol/day
24 h urine creatinine	2.65	Mmol/day
Fractional excretion of calcium (FeCa)	0.014	

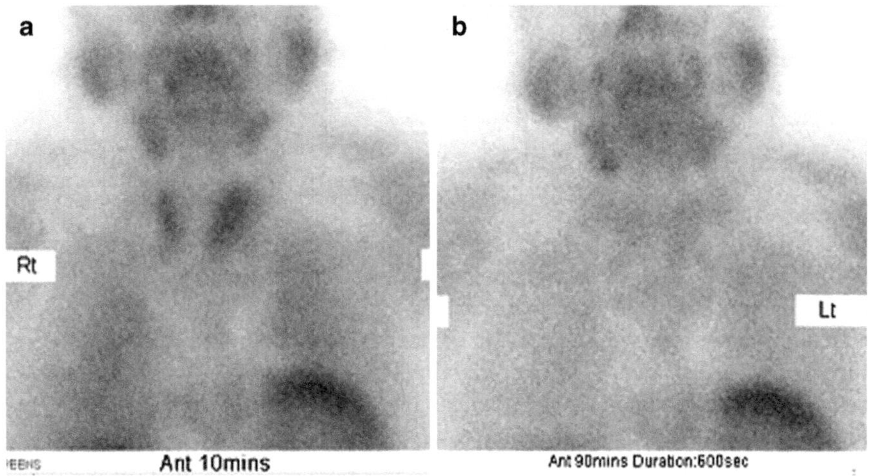

Fig. 1 Technetium-99 m sestamibi scan showing no increased uptake in parathyroid glands

conducted, and a heterozygous mutation (NM_000388, c.644A > G, p.Asp215Gly in exon 4) for the pathogenetic calcium sensing receptor variant was identified.

Discussion

Primary hyperparathyroidism (PHPT) is a biochemical diagnosis, based on an elevated serum calcium level in combination with a normal or raised iPTH level. It is characterized by hypersecretion of parathyroid hormone, independent of serum calcium levels. Parathyroid hormone acts on the kidney, gut, and bone. Hyperparathyroidism increases renal absorption of calcium, increases bone turn over and increases activated vitamin D. This leads to bone loss, nephrolithiasis and nephrocalcinosis, declining renal function and a range of neurocognitive, gastrointestinal and musculoskeletal complaints, though most PHPT today is asymptomatic [1]. The most common causes of PHPT include parathyroid adenomas and parathyroid hyperplasia. Multiglandular disease is typically seen in familial PHPT syndromes [2]. Syndromic forms of PHPT comprise <10% of cases [2]. Parathyroidectomy is recommended for symptomatic or asymptomatic patients who suffer from complications of the hypercalcemia [3]. When performed in patients with PHPT, it is usually curative, with a decrease in complications post-operatively [4].

Post-operatively, serum-adjusted calcium or PTH may remain elevated or may progressively increase either independently or concurrently. Recurrent PHPT is a new finding of hypercalcemia in association with elevated PTH, after a period of 6 months of documented normocalcemia in a successfully operated patient [5]. The prevalence is between 2.5 and 9.8% [6–8]. Persistent PHPT on the other hand is defined as hypercalcemia and elevated PTH within 6 months following surgery [5]. These definitions consider calcium levels. Isolated elevation of PTH levels with normocalcemia does not represent this condition [5].

Up to one-third of patients present with elevated PTH concentrations after successful surgery for sporadic PHPT [9]. Though the obvious concern is that this may be an early marker of autonomous parathyroid secretion, [9] this finding has not been shown to be consistently associated with recurrent PHPT. It is therefore not recommended for routine PTH checks in normocalcemic individuals post-parathyroidectomy [10]. The differentials for a persistently elevated PTH in the context of eucalcemia are vast. It could be due to unrecognized vitamin D deficiency, hungry bone syndrome, impaired renal function, inadequate calcium intake and some have reported a peripheral insensitivity to parathyroid hormone with an altered set point. A higher PTH level pre-operatively and an older age at presentation has been associated with the phenomenon (Table 2) [9, 10]. Other more uncommon causes include gastrointestinal disorders associated with calcium malabsorption, medications (e.g. diuretics, lithium, anti-resorptives) [10].

The first step in evaluating post-operative abnormal biochemistry is therefore to check serum-adjusted calcium and PTH levels. If there is eucalcemia concurrently with raised PTH, the differentials in Table 2 should be considered. If persistent or recurrent hyperparathyroidism is present (i.e. raised serum-adjusted calcium and PTH levels), one must reconsider the underlying diagnosis. Previous records need to be reviewed as well as a careful review of family history, biochemistry (at diagnosis, intra-operatively and post-operatively) and radiological and pathological records. Familial conditions such as familial hypocalciuric hypercalcemia should be considered at this point. Other conditions to consider are listed in Table 2.

Table 2 Causes of raised intact parathyroid hormone levels post-parathyroidectomy

Hypocalcemia/normocalcemia	Hypercalcemia
Vitamin D deficiency	Inadequate pre-operative localization
Impaired renal function	Ectopic lesions
Hungry bone syndrome	Familial conditions such as FHH (familial hypocalciuric hypercalcemia)
Inadequate calcium intake	
Peripheral insensitivity to parathyroid hormone	

Familial hypocalciuric hypercalcemia (FHH) is an autosomal dominant disease with high degree of penetrance. In the most common type – Type 1 FHH (FHH1), a loss-of-function mutation of the calcium-sensing receptor gene ([11, 12] occurs. Type 2 FHH (FHH2) results from inactivation in the germline of the G protein α11 subunit encoded by GNA11 [13, 14]. Lastly, type 3 FHH (FHH3) occurs due to a germline loss-of-function mutation in adaptor-related protein complex 2 subunit sigma 1 (AP2S1) [13, 14]. In FHH, a lifelong non-progressive elevation in calcium and magnesium with a normal or mildly raised parathyroid hormone level occurs ([1, 15, 16]. Hypercalcemia is typically asymptomatic and rarely has clinically significant consequences [11]. Rare cases of accompanying chondrocalcinosis and acute pancreatitis have been reported [17, 18]. The prevalence is difficult to estimate since many affected individuals remain asymptomatic and go undetected [11]. It has been reported that of those patients who underwent failed neck exploration for PHPT, 9–23% of them ultimately have FHH [15, 16, 19]. FHH has a biochemical phenotype that is quite similar to primary hyperparathyroidism, but the unique feature of this disease is that there is low or inappropriately normal urinary calcium excretion [11]. It is important to differentiate the two diagnoses as FHH does not require surgical intervention. Analytical variations may exist and therefore, biochemistry should be repeated two to three times especially if the clinical findings are not compelling [16]. Hypocalciuria is explained by abnormalities of the calcium-sensing receptor in the proximal renal tubule [15]. 24-h urine calcium and creatinine are usually collected to help calculate the calcium/creatinine clearance ratio in the initial workup of hypercalcemia.

The difficulty with using the calcium/creatinine clearance ratio alone as the diagnostic threshold is that there is no consensus regarding a cut-off value for the ratio. It is important to bear in mind that the ratio has not been validated for diagnosing FHH in patients with renal impairment, vitamin D deficiency or in pregnancy [10]. Some studies have considered a cut-off of <0.01 to be specific [19, 20]. With the recent availability of genetic screening, some have suggested this as an alternative route to diagnosis, but there could be novel genes that are not tested for on the panel. To increase the diagnostic sensitivity (~98%), some have proposed adopting a 2-step diagnostic procedure with calcium/creatinine clearance ratio of 0.02 or less and testing for mutations in the CASR gene [16] as diagnostic of FHH Type 1- the commonest form. When genetic testing is unavailable, clinicians need to use all biochemical and patient data to guide accurate diagnosis [11]. Radiology is typically unrevealing. On imaging, there have been reports of benign parathyroid adenomas described in FHH [20–23]. Majority of cases of FHH do not need treatment and morbidity is often as a result of inappropriate surgical intervention [11].

In conclusion, there are many reasons for persistently elevated PTH levels after parathyroidectomy. FHH needs to be considered as a differential diagnosis especially if the hypercalcemia is mild. Taking a good family history can give insight into the diagnosis. Inappropriately low urinary calcium excretion is a clue that FHH may be the explanation and subsequent genetic testing should be considered, especially in cases with positive family history [11]. The condition has important implications for management of a patient and potentially his or her entire family [11]. Identification of FHH pre-operatively avoids unnecessary surgery and its attendant complications.

References

1. Islam AK. Advances in diagnosis and management of primary hyperparathyroidism. Ther Adv Chronic Dis. 2021;12:1–20. https://doi.org/10.1177/20406223211015965Therapeut.
2. Bilezikian JP, Cusano NE, Khan AA, Liu JM, Marcocci C, Bandeira F, et al. Primary hyperparathyroidism. Nat Rev Dis Primers. 2016;2(1):1174. https://doi.org/10.1038/nrdp.2016.33.
3. Bilezikian JP, Brandi ML, Eastell R, Silverberg SJ, Udelsman R, Marcocci C, et al. Guidelines for the management of asymptomatic primary hyperparathyroidism: summary statement from the fourth international workshop. J Clin Endocrinol Metabol. 2014;99(10):3561–9. https://doi.org/10.1210/jc.2014-1413.
4. Udelsman R, Lin Z, Donovan P. The superiority of minimally invasive parathyroidectomy based on 1650 consecutive patients with primary hyperparathyroidism. Ann Surg. 2011;253(3):585–91. https://doi.org/10.1097/SLA.0b013e318208fed9.
5. Udelsman R. Approach to the patient with persistent or recurrent primary hyperparathyroidism. J Clin Endocrinol Metabol. 2011;96(10):2950–8. https://doi.org/10.1210/jc.2011-1010.
6. Nordenstrom E, Westerdahl J, Bergenfelz A. Long-term follow-up of patients with elevated PTH levels following successful exploration for primary hyperparathyroidism. World J Surg. 2004;28(6):570–5. https://doi.org/10.1007/s00268-004-7124-y.
7. Ryder CY, Jarocki A, McNeely MM, Currey E, Miller BS, Cohen MS, et al. Early biochemical response to parathyroidectomy for primary hyperparathyroidism and its predictive value for recurrent hypercalcemia and recurrent primary hyperparathyroidism. Surgery. 2021;169(1):120–5. https://doi.org/10.1016/j.surg.2020.05.049.
8. Solorzano CC, Mendez W, Lew JI, Rodgers SE, Montano R, Carneiro-Pla DM, et al. Long-term outcome of patients with elevated parathyroid hormone after success parathyroidectomy for sporadic primary hyperparathyroidism. Arch Surg. 2008;7(14):659–63.
9. Oltmann SC, Maalouf NM, Holt S. Significance of elevated parathyroid hormone after Parathyroidectomy for primary hyperparathyroidism. Endocr Pract. 2011;17(Suppl 2):57–62. https://doi.org/10.4158/EP10324.RA.
10. Bollerslev J, Rejnmark L, Zahn A, Heck A, Appelman-Dijkstra NM, Cardoso L, et al. European expert consensus on practical management of specific aspects of parathyroid disorders in adults and in pregnancy: recommendations of the ESE educational program of parathyroid disorders (PARAT 2021). Eur J Endocrinol. 2022;186(2):R33–63. https://doi.org/10.1530/EJE-21-1044.
11. Lee JY, Shoback DM. Familial hypocalciuric hypercalcemia and related disorders. Best Pract Res Clin Endocrinol Metab. 2018;32(5):609–19. https://doi.org/10.1016/j.beem.2018.05.004.
12. Pollak MR, Brown EM, Chou YH, Hebert SC, Marx SJ, Steinmann B, et al. Mutations in the human Ca(2+)-sensing receptor gene cause familial hypocalciuric hypercalcemia and neonatal severe hyperparathyroidism. Cell. 1993;75:1297–303.
13. Nesbit MA, Hannan FM, Howles SA, Reed AAC, Cranston T, Thakker CE, et al. Mutations in AP2S1 cause familial hypocalciuric hypercalcemia type 3. Nat Genet. 2013a;45(1):93–7. https://doi.org/10.1038/ng.2492.
14. Nesbit MA, Hannan FM, Howles SA, Babinsky VN, Head RA, Cranston T, et al. Mutations affecting G-protein subunit α 11 in hypercalcemia and hypocalcemia. N Engl J Med. 2013b;368(26):2476–86. https://doi.org/10.1056/NEJMoa1300253.
15. Heath DA. Familial Hypocalciuric Hypercalcemia. Rev Endocr Metab Disord. 2000;1:291–6.
16. Christensena SE, Nissenb PH, Vestergaarda P, Mosekilde L. Familial hypocalciuric hypercalcemia: a review. Curr Opin Endocrinol Diabetes Obes. 2011;18:359–70. https://doi.org/10.1097/MED.0b013e32834c3c7c.
17. Pearce SH, Wooding C, Davies M, Tollefsen SE, Whyte MP, Thakker RV, et al. Calcium-sensing receptor mutations in familial hypocalciuric hypercalcaemia with recurrent pancreatitis. Clin Endocrinol. 1996;45(6):675–80.
18. Volpe A, Guerriero A, Marchetta A, Caramaschi P, Furlani L. Familial hypocalciuric hypercalcemia revealed by chondrocalcinosis. Joint Bone Spine. 2009;76(6):708–10. https://doi.org/10.1016/j.jbspin.2009.02.001.

19. Marx SJ, Stock JL, Attie MF, Downs RW Jr, Gardner DG, Brown EM, et al. Familial hypocalciuric hypercalcemia: recognition among patients referred after unsuccessful parathyroid exploration. Ann Intern Med. 1980;92(3):351–6.
20. Marx SJ. Familial hypocalciuric hypercalcemia as an atypical form of primary hyperparathyroidism. J Bone Miner Res. 2018;33(1):27–31. https://doi.org/10.1002/jbmr.3339.
21. Brachet C, Boros E, Tenoutasse S, Lissens W, Andry G, Martin P, et al. Association of parathyroid adenoma and familial hypocalciuric hypercalcaemia in a teenager. Eur J Endocrinol. 2009;161(1):207–10. https://doi.org/10.1530/EJE-09-0257.
22. Forde HE, Hill AD, Smith D. Parathyroid adenoma in a patient with FHH. BMJ Case Rep. 2014;2014:30–60. https://doi.org/10.1136/bcr-2014-.
23. Marstrand SD, Tofteng CL, Jarløv A, Borgwardt L, Schwarz P. Concomitant familial hypocalciuric hypercalcemia and single parathyroid adenoma: a case report. J Med Case Rep. 2021;15(1):168. https://doi.org/10.1186/s13256-021-03051-6.

Part VI

Benign Thyroid Diseases

Recurrence in a Pyramidal Lobe

Case

This 32-year-old lady presented with a recurrent goiter. She had a total thyroidectomy 8 years prior to the presentation and the recurrence was in the pyramidal lobe (Fig. 1a, b). It was confirmed as thyroid tissue by Isotope scan (Fig. 2).

This required surgery as it was cosmetically unacceptable. There is a small risk of malignancy developing in the remnant.

The difficulty was doing it through a low cervical incision of the previous thyroidectomy. This emphasizes the importance of removing the embryological remnants during total thyroidectomy [1–3].

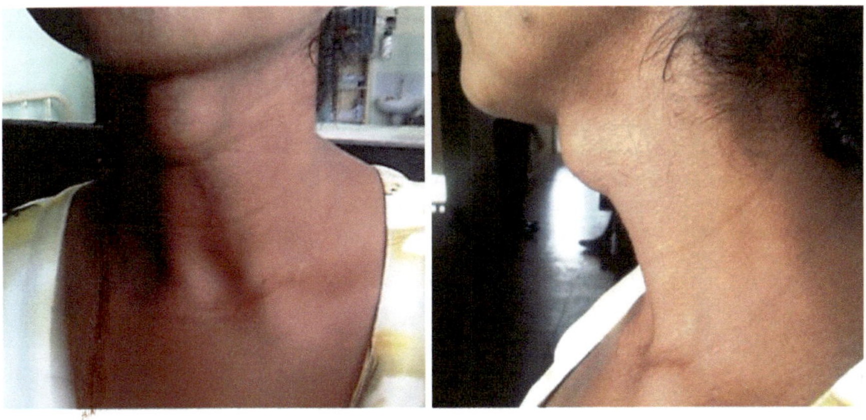

Fig 1 (**a**) Clinical picture of the patient with anterior neck swelling (pyramidal lobe recurrence). (**b**) lateral view

Ranil Fernando is the lead author of this chapter.

A. Agarwal et al., *Case Studies in Thyroid and Parathyroid Tumors*,
https://doi.org/10.1007/978-981-99-0938-4_43

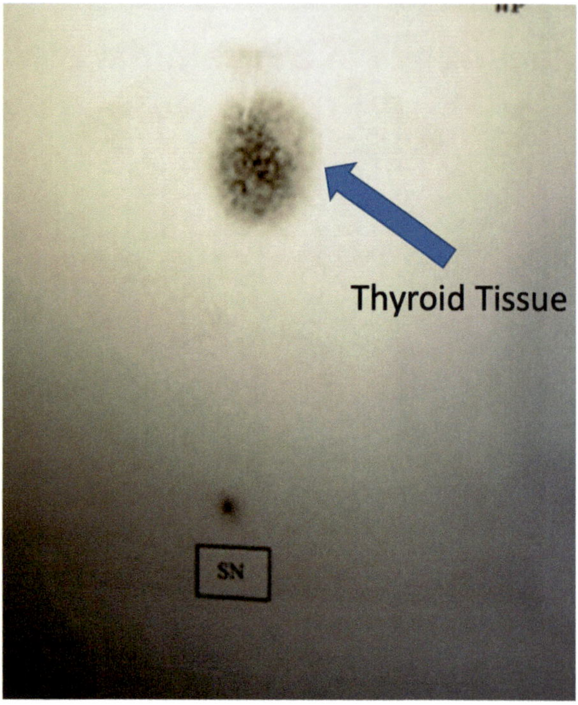

Fig 2 Thyroid tissue (arrow) on isotope scan

References

1. Snook KL, Stalberg PLH, Sidhu SB, Sywak MS, Edhouse P, Delbridge L. Recurrence after total thyroidectomy for benign multinodular goiter. World J Surg. 2007;31(3):593–8. https://doi.org/10.1007/s00268-006-0135-0.
2. Fernando R, Rajapaksha A, Ranasinghe N, Gunawardana D. Embryological remnants of the thyroid gland and their significance in thyroidectomy. World J Endocr Surg. 2014;6(3):110–2.
3. Fernando R. Recurrent goiters. World J Endoc Surg. 2019;11(1):15.

Goitre and Dermoid

Case

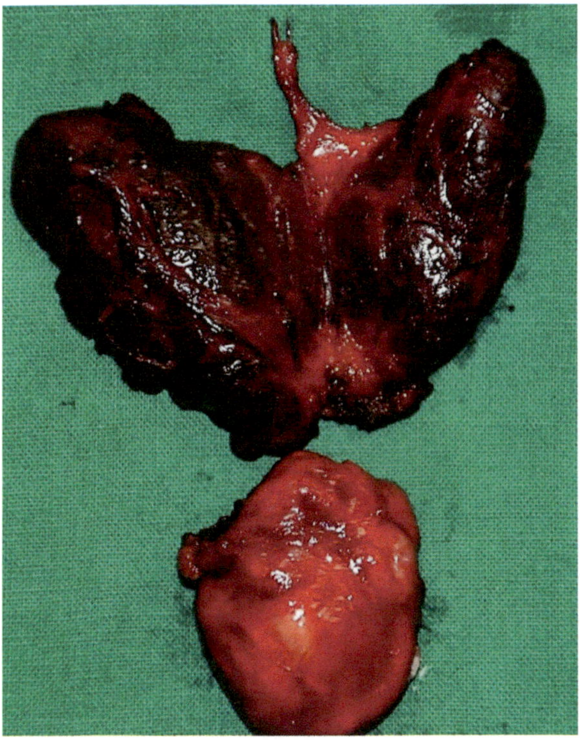

Ranil Fernando is the lead author of this chapter.

A. Agarwal et al., *Case Studies in Thyroid and Parathyroid Tumors*,
https://doi.org/10.1007/978-981-99-0938-4_44

A 56-year-old female presented with multinodular (MNG) goiter of 10 years duration with compressive symptom. She was assessed to have a euthyroid Grade 2 MNG.

At surgery a MNG and a retrosternal dermoid cyst (confirmed histologically) were found and removed. The dermoid cyst may have contributed to the compressive features. This is again an uncommon cause of compression.

Dermoid cysts are the most common teratomatous lesions. They occur in the head and neck region as well as other regions. The occurrence of a dermoid masquerading as a thyroid nodule is very rare [1].

Reference

1. Diercks GR, Iannuzzi RA, McCowen K, Sadow PM. Dermoid cyst of the lateral neck associated with the thyroid gland: a case report and review of the literature. Endocr Pathol. 2013;24(1):45–8. https://doi.org/10.1007/s12022-013-9234-2.

Hemi Agenesis of Thyroid

Case

A 34-year-old female presented with a large thyroid nodule of the right lobe of thyroid causing compressive features. On assessment, it was a euthyroid solitary nodule of the right lobe with a significant deviation of the trachea. The US scan could not visualize the left lobe clearly.

Due to the significant compressive features, she underwent surgery.

At surgery, it was clear that she had hemi agenesis of the left lobe with gross nodular enlargement of the right lobe (Fig. 1).

R hemi thyroidectomy was undertaken and the patient was put on replacement thyroxine therapy. The family was screened and close follow up arranged.

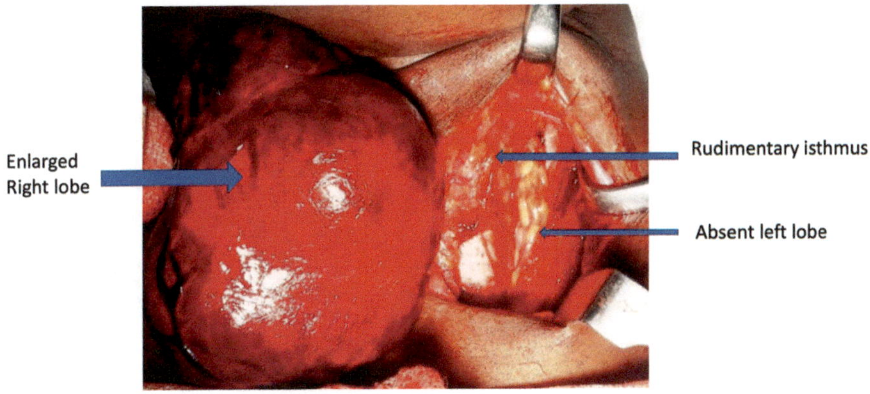

Fig. 1 Picture shows enlarged right lobe with rudimentary isthmus and absent left lobe

---

Ranil Fernando is the lead author of this chapter.

A. Agarwal et al., *Case Studies in Thyroid and Parathyroid Tumors*,
https://doi.org/10.1007/978-981-99-0938-4_45

Thyroid hemiagenesis (THA) is a rare congenital disorder [1]. The significance of it remains undefined, but it is stated that patients with THA have a tendency to develop additional thyroid and nonthyroidal pathologies [2]. Hence they need close follow-up.

References

1. Szczepanek-Parulska E, Zybek-Kocik A, Wartofsky L, Ruchała M. Thyroid hemiagenesis: incidence, clinical significance, and genetic background. J Clin Endocrinol Metab. 2017;102(9):3124–37. https://doi.org/10.1210/jc.2017-00784.
2. Trueba SS, Augé J, Mattei G, Etchevers H, Martinovic J, Czernichow P, Vekemans M, Polak M, Attié-Bitach T. PAX8, TITF1, and FOXE1 gene expression patterns during human development: new insights into human thyroid development and thyroid dysgenesis-associated malformations. J Clin Endocrinol Metab. 2005;90(1):455–62.

Autonomously Functioning Thyroid Nodule

Case

A 36-year-old female had been investigated and treated for a left-sided thyroid nodule for 2 years in another institution. She had been having compressive symptoms such as orthopnoea for 1 year before her presentation to our institution.

She was referred for consideration of surgery for a solitary nodule of the left lobe. Investigations including an Isotope Scan (Fig. 1) confirmed that it was an autonomously functioning thyroid nodule (AFTN).

She underwent left hemi thyroidectomy (Fig. 2). The right lobe was normal at surgery. She remains euthyroid without any treatment.

Fig. 1 Isotope scan showing left AFTN (arrow)

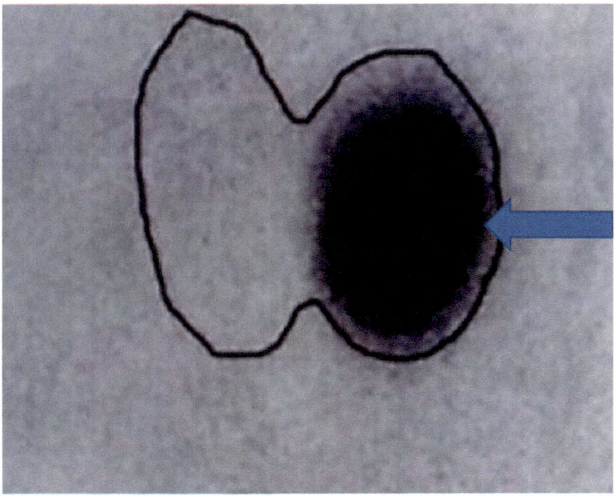

Ranil Fernando is the lead author of this chapter.

A. Agarwal et al., *Case Studies in Thyroid and Parathyroid Tumors*,
https://doi.org/10.1007/978-981-99-0938-4_46

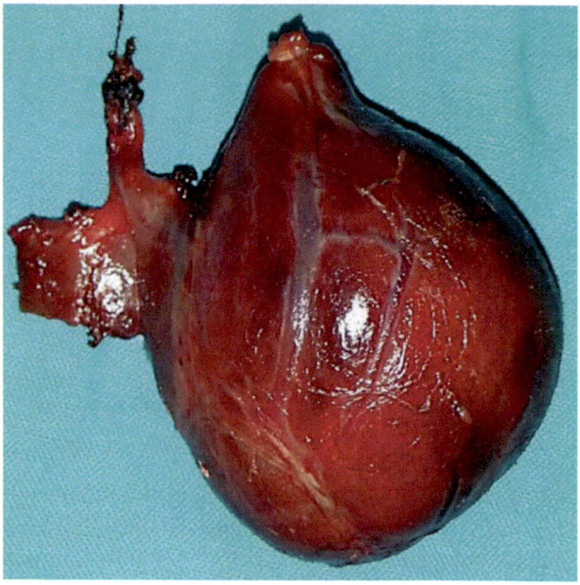

Fig. 2 Left Hemithyroidectomy specimen

The reported incidence of AFTN is about 1% on the investigation of thyroid nodules. Only about 10–30% become hyperfunctioning. Due to the rarity and lack of understanding of its characteristic clinical behavior, AFTNs are often overlooked and undertreated [1].

Reference

1. Pinto D, Fernando R. Autonomously functioning thyroid nodule: a patient-based review. Sri Lanka J Surg. 2021;39(3):49–54. https://doi.org/10.4038/sljs.v39i3.8857.

Goiter Recurrence

Case

This 40-year-old female underwent a total thyroidectomy 10 years prior to presentation. The histology was not available from the previous surgery. The diagnosis card stated that the patient had undergone a partial thyroidectomy for a nodular goiter. She presented with features of compression (Fig. 1).

The FNAC done prior to revision surgery showed a Beth II lesion. She underwent revision total thyroidectomy. The operative specimen is depicted in Fig. 2.

Goiter recurrence is a common problem due to incomplete surgery. This emphasizes the need to undertake proper total thyroidectomy for multinodular goiter otherwise; recurrence is 30–50% [1, 2].

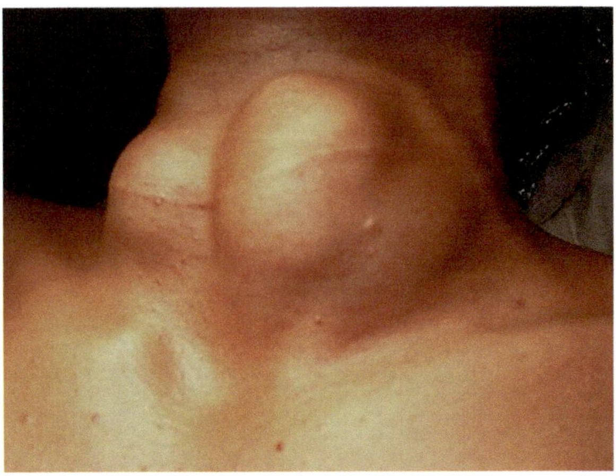

Fig. 1 Presentation, with large recurrence and visible scar

Ranil Fernando is the lead author of this chapter.

A. Agarwal et al., *Case Studies in Thyroid and Parathyroid Tumors*,
https://doi.org/10.1007/978-981-99-0938-4_47

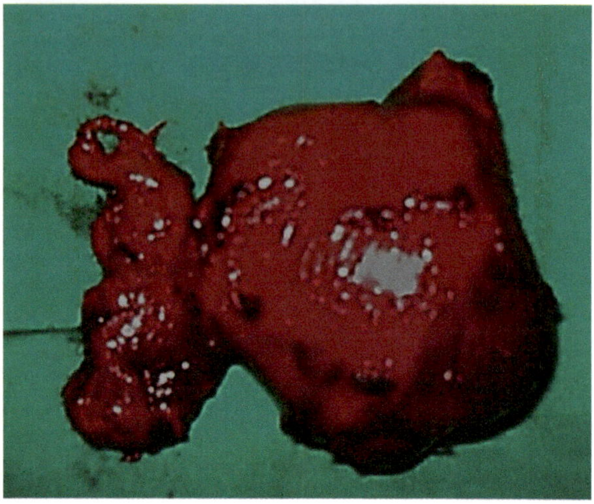

Fig. 2 Total thyroidectomy specimen

References

1. Delbridge L, Guinea AI, Reeve TS. Total thyroidectomy for bilateral benign multinodular goiter. Arch Surg. 1999;134:1389–93.
2. Mishra A, Agarwal A, Agarwal G, Mishra SK. Total thyroidectomy for benign thyroid disorders in an endemic region. World J Surg. 2001;25:307–10.

Retrosternal Component Bigger than Cervical Component of Goiters

In all, 3 patients had large multinodular goiters with features of compression clinically. The retrosternal component was much larger than the goiter in the assessment by imaging (Figs. 1, 2, and 3).

All 3 retrosternal components were delivered through cervical Collar incisions during total thyroidectomy. The **key was that the retrosternal components did not extend much beyond the aortic arch**.

This is a very critical component of the pre-operative assessment. If the retrosternal goiter extends beyond the aortic arch, preparations must be made to undertake sternotomy even though it may not be required always [1, 2].

The other key point is to deliver the retrosternal component slowly and gently. Once the correct plain of the retrosternal component is reached, careful dissection, teasing with gentle traction will deliver it. Harsh pulling or forcing must be NOT done.

Ranil Fernando is the lead author of this chapter.

A. Agarwal et al., *Case Studies in Thyroid and Parathyroid Tumors*,
https://doi.org/10.1007/978-981-99-0938-4_48

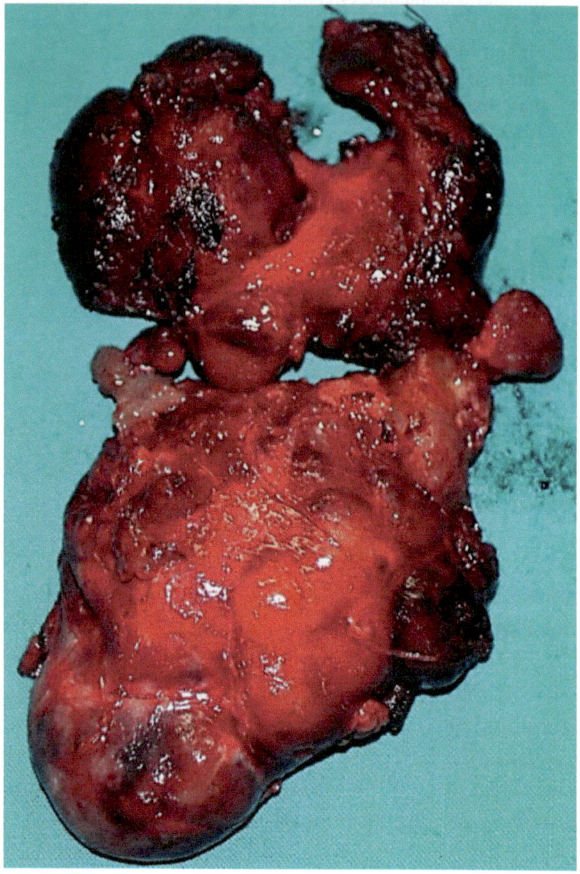

Fig. 1 Patient 1 showing retrosternal thyroid part larger than the normal thyroid

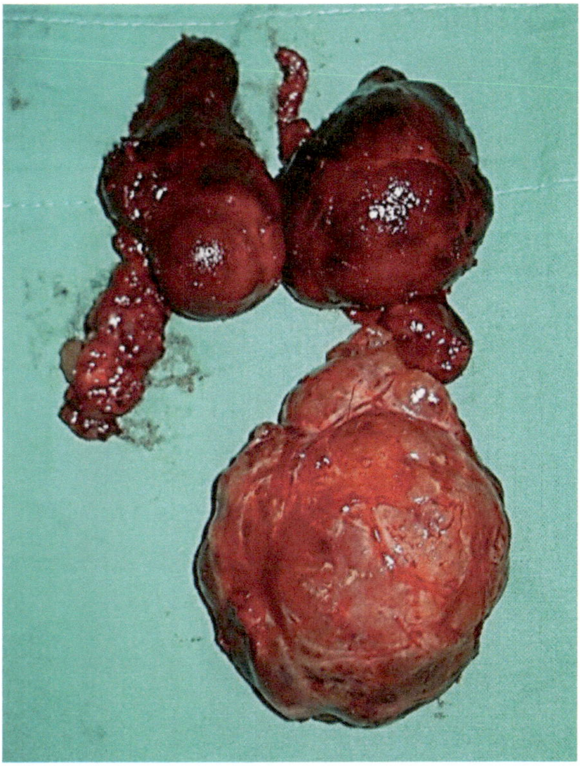

Fig. 2 Patient 2 showing large retrosternal component

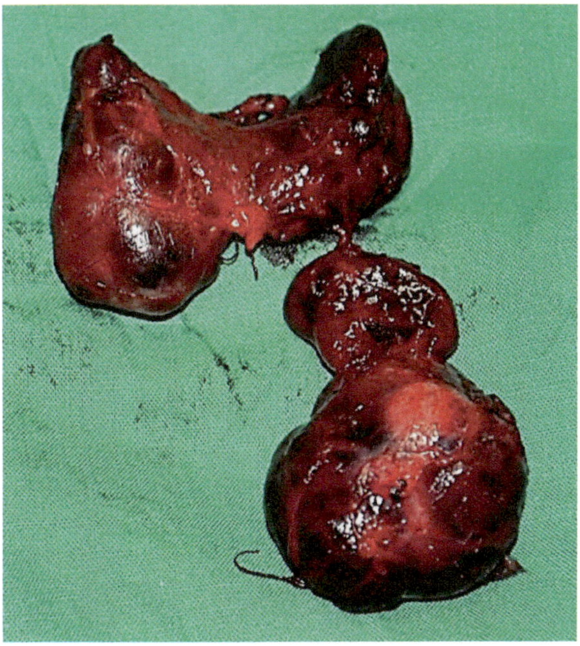

Fig. 3 Patient 3 showing large retrosternal component connected by a thin thyroid tissue

References

1. White ML, Doherty GM, Gauger PG. Evidence-based surgical management of substernal goiter. World J Surg. 2008;32(7):1285–300. https://doi.org/10.1007/s00268-008-9466-3.
2. Rugiu MG, Piemonte M. Surgical approach to retrosternal goitre: do we still need sternotomy? Acta Otorhinolaryngol Ital. 2009;29(6):331–8.

Airway Issues Leading to Difficult Intubation in Goiter

Case
A 54-years-old lady was evaluated for neck swelling which was present for 12 years progressively increasing in size. No history of breathlessness and no dysphagia or change in voice. On examination of neck she had a thyroid swelling of around 10 × 10 cm in front of the neck moving up with deglutition (Fig. 1). No visible veins/pulsations/scars/sinuses. No local rise of temperature/tenderness. Firm in consistency, bosselated surface, regular margin. Retrosternal extension present. No significant palpable cervical LAP. Trachea was central and bilateral carotids were palpable. Investigations: USG neck showed multiple nodules. FNAC was colloid goiter. TFT was normal. On indirect laryngoscopy b\l true vocal cord could not be visualized. CECT neck showed diffusely enlarged thyroid extending superiorly till submandibular region and inferiorly till superior mediastinum on both sides. Rt lobe- 12 × 6.5 × 5.0 cm. X-ray neck showed deviation of trachea along with large retro-tracheal extension (Fig. 2). Anticipating intubation difficulty she was intubated with fiber-optic intubation (Fig. 3). Total thyroidectomy was done and at operation both lobes of thyroid were found to be enlarged with multiple nodules extending from angle of mandible to sterna notch. Following thyroid removal, it was noted that the trachea was collapsed with softened and narrowed tracheal rings. Anticipating post-thyroidectomy tracheomalacia tracheostomy made at the level of second and third tracheal rings. The weight of the specimen was 542.5 gm (Fig. 4). De-cannulation of tracheostomy tube was done on sixth post-operative day and was discharged with normal voice.

Amit Agarwal is the lead author of this chapter.

A. Agarwal et al., *Case Studies in Thyroid and Parathyroid Tumors*,
https://doi.org/10.1007/978-981-99-0938-4_49

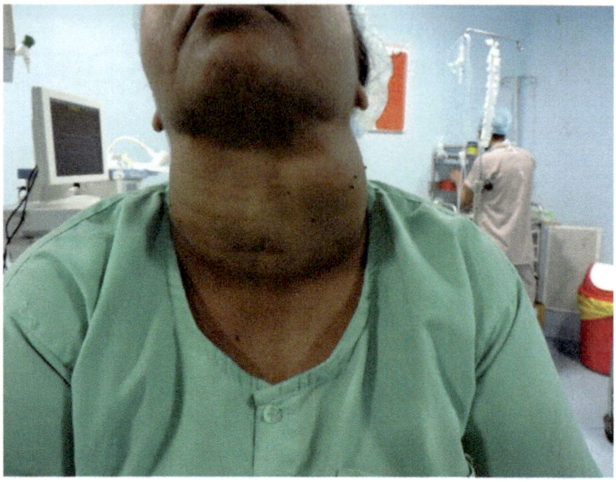

Fig. 1 Patient having large multinodular goiter

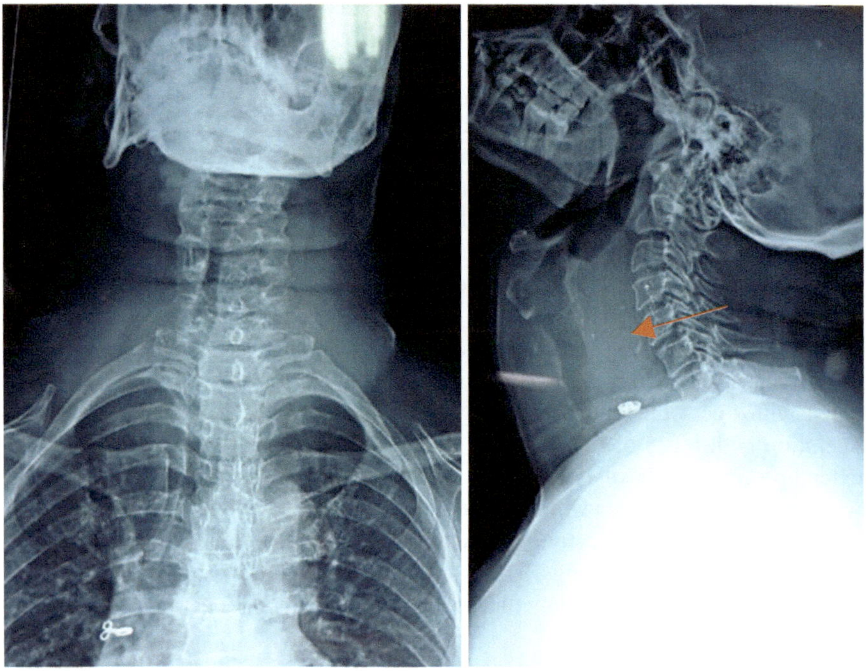

Fig. 2 X-ray neck showing deviation of trachea and a large retro-tracheal component (arrow)

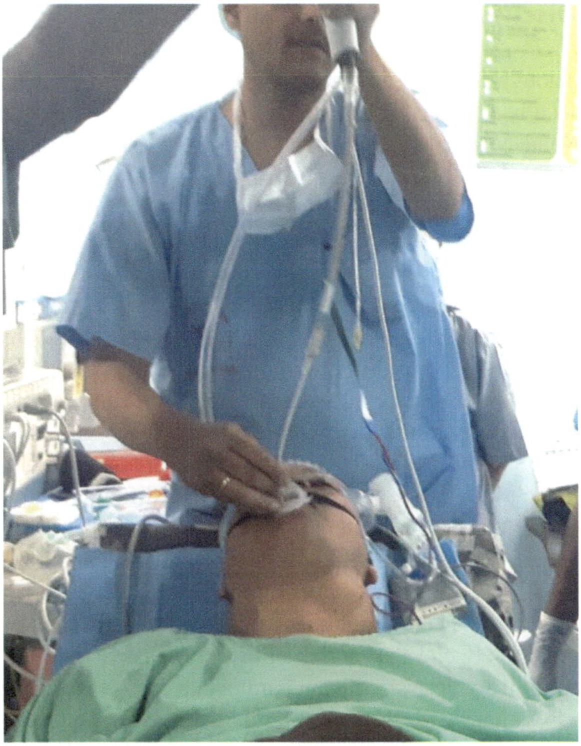

Fig. 3 Fiber-optic intubation in progress

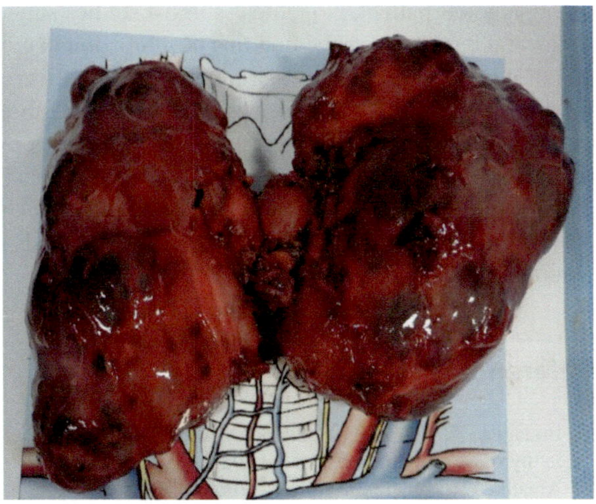

Fig. 4 Total thyroidectomy specimen weighing >500 gm

Discussion

Though difficult intubation (DI) is expected in anaplastic thyroid carcinoma and locally advanced DTC, rate of DI in benign goiter is highly variable in the literature. Some consider thyroid surgery itself as a risk factor for DI, while others do not. Rate of DI in the literature varies from 5% to 11% [1–3]. Most anaesthesiologists follow the IDS (7 criteria scoring system) or the modified IDS scale (8 criteria) to assess the Intubation difficulty. The modified IDS scale includes [3]: number of intubation attempts, number of operators, the use of alternative techniques, Cormack–Lehane grade (no laryngeal manipulation was used to improve this score) and lifting force applied to the laryngoscope, external laryngeal pressure, position of the vocal cords, and the degree of difficulty in passing the endotracheal tube. An easy intubation is defined as a successful single attempt by one operator without the use of any alternative techniques or manipulations under normal conditions and scored as MIDS = 2; A MIDS score > 2 and < 5 is interpreted as a slightly difficult intubation, and a MIDS score >5 is considered as a difficult intubation. The literature is highly variable about the factors that may predict difficult intubation. A meta-analysis [4] suggested that MS ≥ 3, reduced TM distance, and low IG significantly increase the likelihood of difficult intubation in thyroid surgery; while the presence of Tracheal Deviation (TD) (the unique thyroid pathology linked parameter), obesity and males moderately elevate the risk of difficult airway management in this specific clinical setting. So these significant parameters can be used for a more accurate preoperative assessment with the aim to anticipate difficult intubations and to optimize potentially difficult airways in thyroid surgery by selecting the appropriate method of intubation. Again, the literature is divided over the most appropriate method of intubating a goiter patient. Nonetheless, most studies suggest direct laryngoscopy with Trans oral intubation as the first line of intubation in goiter patients [5]. Other methods of intubation include awake intubation with Fiber-optic or video laryngoscopy (including glidedoscopy). Fiber-optic intubation requires a learning curve unlike the videolaryngoscopy. Advantages of video laryngoscopy include shorter intubation time, wider view of airway, no limitation on tracheal tube diameter, and ease in changing the size of the tracheal tube if required while maintaining the airway view [6]. One can also use a combination of these methods in case of failure to intubate by conventional means.

References

1. Bouaggad A, Nejmi SE, Bouderka MA, Abbassi O. Prediction of difficult tracheal intubation in thyroid surgery. Anesth Analg. 2004;99(2):603–6.
2. Amathieu R, Smail N, Catineau J, Poloujadoff MP, Samii K, Adnet F. Difficult intubation in thyroid surgery: myth or reality? Anesth Analg. 2006;103(4):965–8.

3. Tutuncu AC, Erbabacan E, Teksoz S, Ekici B, Koksal G, Altintas F, et al. The assessment of risk factors for difficult intubation in thyroid patients. World J Surg. 2018;42:1748–53.
4. De Cassai A, Boscolo A, Rose K, Carron M, Navalesi P. Predictive parameters of difficult intubation in thyroid surgery: a meta-analysis. Minerva Anestesiol. 2020;86(3):317–26.
5. Loftus PA, Ow TJ, Siegel B, Tassler AB, Smith RV, Schiff BA. Risk factors for perioperative airway difficulty and eval- uation of intubation approaches among patients with benign goiter. Ann Otol Rhinol Laryngol. 2014;123:279–85.
6. Heinz E, Quan T, Nguyen H, Pla R. Intubation of a patient with a large goiter: the advantageous role of videolaryngoscopy. Case Rep Anesthesiol. 2019;2019:1327482.

Benign Goiter Causing Preoperative RLN Palsy

Case

A 66-year-old woman presented to us with a history of anterior neck swelling since childhood and recent onset of change in the character of voice × 2 months. She is a known case of NIDDM fairly controlled on OHA. Examination of the neck revealed nodular swelling in front of the neck measuring 8 × 4.5 cm in the midline; extending in between the medial border of bilateral sternocleidomastoid muscles, superiorly 4 cm from the angle of mandible on either sides, inferiorly extending to below the medial third of the clavicle, moving upwards with deglutition, all borders were well defined except lower border, Pemberton sign negative, trachea was deviated to left and there was no deep cervical lymphadenopathy. CECT showed enlargement of both lobes with multiple nodular lesions showing heterogenous contrast enhancement in both lobes. There was retrosternal extension by 2 cm below the sternal notch. FNAC was colloid goiter with hurthle cell changes. Laryngoscopy showed right vocal cords palsy and x-ray neck showed that trachea was mildly deviated to left with luminal narrowing in AP view. She was taken up for surgery where both RLN were identified and preserved. Right RLN was pulled up and was superior to the tubercle of zuckerkandl. Intraoperative neuromonitoring showed voltage on IONM for right RLN was 80 uv initially but increased to 120 uv at the end of surgery while for the left RLN was 1080 uv at the end of surgery. No tracheomalacia was observed. Grossing—Ex-vivo weight- 200 g Right lobe: 7.5 × 4.5 × 3.5 cm Left lobe- 7 × 3.5 × 2.5 cm and cut section—revealed that both lobes (R > L) contained multiple yellowish colored fleshy nodules of varying sizes along with areas of calcification and hemorrhage. Largest size of the nodule on both the sides was 2 × 2 cm. The histopathology was a multinodular goiter. At follow-up her voice improved and laryngoscopy showed normal VC function (Figs. 1, 2, and 3).

Amit Agarwal is the lead author of this chapter.

A. Agarwal et al., *Case Studies in Thyroid and Parathyroid Tumors*,
https://doi.org/10.1007/978-981-99-0938-4_50

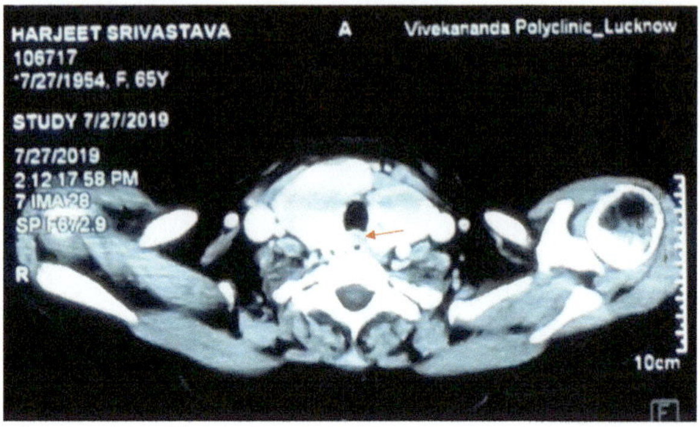

Fig. 1 Cross-sectional imaging showing separation of trachea and esophagus (arrow) by intervening thyroid tissue suggestive of RLN compression in TO-groove

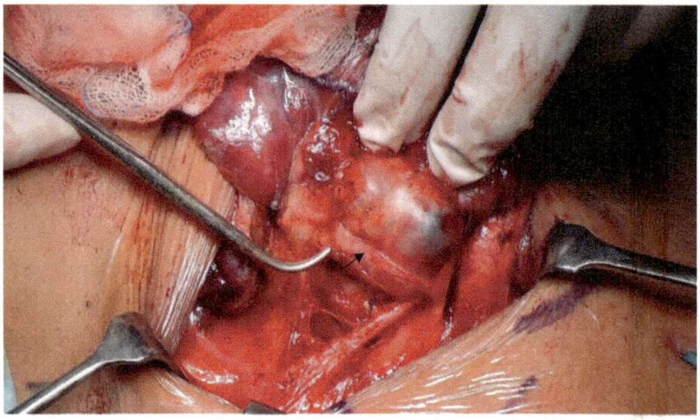

Fig. 2 Intraoperative view of stretching of RLN (black arrow) by the big tubercle of Zuckerkandl (TZ)

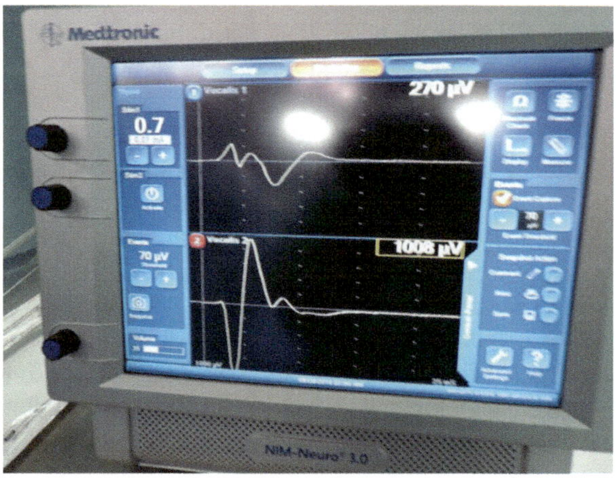

Fig. 3 Neuromonitoring of paralyzed RLN

Discussion

The association of preoperative RLN palsy and thyroid disease is taken as suggestive of locally advanced malignant thyroid disease by invasion of the nerve. However, preoperative RLN palsy may also be due to the benign goiter though the risk of benign thyroid disease causing paralysis of the nerve is extremely rare and has only been reported in isolated case reports and small case series. From the review of the relevant literature, the incidence of preoperative RLNP ranges from 8% to 11% for thyroid malignancy and from 0.7% to 1.0% for benign thyroid diseases in large surgical series [1, 2]. The mechanism of injury in benign goiter is not as clear but compression, stretching, or inflammation have been postulated as possible reasons for palsy. In bilateral benign goiters, it is likely that the RLN is pinched in the trachea-oesophageal groove causing palsy. Further, if there is a large tubercle of Zuckerkandl it may cause compression and stretching of RLN as happened in our patient. In addition, rapid tumor growth predisposes the RLN to injury and hemorrhage into a thyroid cyst [3] or rapid cyst distention due to inflammation could cause sudden compression of the nerve. Clinicians should be aware that up to 50% of patients with RLN palsy may not complain of any symptoms of dysphonia. This may be due to the partial compression or because of slow growth as is seen in benign goiters allowing for compensation of the opposite vocal cord. Patients with RLN palsies and thyroid masses should always be investigated with either CT or MRI scanning from the skull base to the diaphragm to determine the size of the thyroid mass, its characteristics and anatomy, the presence of lymphadenopathy, and possible relationship of the mass with the RLN and upper aero-digestive tract structures. Preoperative radiologic findings usually provide clues about the possible mechanism of RLN palsy. Wang et al [4] have shown that their patients of preoperative RLN palsy had at least two of the following image features: tracheal deviation, tracheoesophageal separation, clavicle extension, and tumor larger than 5 cm in diameter. All of these findings have the potential to cause compression or stretching of the RLN and/or its blood supply. The presence of an RLN palsy at presentation not only represents a diagnostic conundrum, but also a management dilemma. Patients with RLN palsy in benign thyroid disease can experience recovery of the palsy and this has been previously documented [5]. However, the fact that patients may recover highlights the importance of preserving the RLN during definitive surgical management [6]. It is therefore of paramount importance that paralyzed nerves are identified, dissected, and handled in the same way as nerves which are functioning before surgery. A positive electrophysiological response of the RLN during surgery means that there might be residual nerve function in the laryngeal muscles despite overt vocal cord paralysis. Thus, the use of neuromonitoring also allows intraoperative assessment, identification, and dissection of the RLN which may be displaced, as well as assessment of return of function. In conclusion, preoperative RLN palsy does not necessarily indicate malignant disease, careful assessment of cross-sectional imaging should be done and surgeons should not go into surgery with a preconceived notion of nerve resection of the affected nerve given the potential for benign disease and the potential for vocal cord recovery and should utilize the neuromonitoring in such situations.

References

1. Holl-Allen RT. Laryngeal nerve paralysis and benign thyroid disease. Arch Otolaryngol. 1967;85:335–7.
2. Rowe-Jones JM, Rosswick RP, Leighton SE. Benign thyroid disease and vocal cord palsy. Ann R Coll Surg Engl. 1993;75:241–4.
3. Fenton JE, Timon CI, McShane DP. Recurrent laryngeal nerve palsy secondary to benign thyroid disease. J Laryngol Otol. 1994;108:878–80.
4. Wang CC, Wang CP, Tsai TL, et al. The basis of preoperative vocal fold paralysis in a series of patients undergoing thyroid surgery: the preponderance of benign thyroid disease. Thyroid. 2011;21(8):867–72.
5. Chi SY, Lammers B, Boehner H, Pohl P, Goretzki PE. Is it meaningful to preserve a palsied recurrent laryngeal nerve? Thyroid. 2008;18(3):363–6.
6. Chiang FY, Lin JC, Lee KW, Wang LF, Tsai KB, Wu CW, Lu SP, Kuo WR. Thyroid tumors with preoperative recurrent laryngeal nerve palsy: clinicopathologic features and treatment outcome. Surgery. 2006;140:413–7.

Management Issues of Monstrous Goiters

Case 1

A 40-year-old lady presented with anterior neck swelling for 8 years (Fig. 1) with no h/s/o any compressive symptoms or hemoptysis. There was redness and serous discharge at the FNAC site. Non-guided cytology was suggestive of benign. CECT showed 12 × 9.7 × 9.2 cm lesion in the right lobe of the thyroid with multiple areas of calcification (yellow orange) with displacement of hypopharynx, larynx and trachea to the left. Difficult airway intubation as trachea was compressed (Fig. 2 with orange arrow) and deviated was anticipated for this patient so awake fiberoptic intubation was tried after pre-oxygenation with 100% O_2 and nasal spray of xylocard. Superior laryngeal block was not possible due to large thyroid mass. Trachea was deviated and not palpable therefore tracheal block was not given. The procedure was abandoned due to failed awake procedure (vocal cords were not completely visualized). Intubation was again tried after a period of 2 weeks with fiberoptic and lateral position patient and continuous use of xylocard spray with help of epidural catheter (spray as you go technique), the patient could be intubated successfully. Total thyroidectomy with auto implantation of rt. superior gland in rt. scm was done. The tumor was encircling the carotid 270° and was dissected with fine dissection. Bilateral IJV, carotid, and vagus preserved. The tumor involves part of pharyngeal muscles, separated with sharp dissection. Bilateral RLN was preserved. Right carotid was encircled 180°which was separated with sharp dissection (Fig. 3a). The specimen (Fig. 3b) weighed 1.5 kg. Postoperatively the patient was kept on elective ventilation for 18 h and was extubated successfully. The patient was discharged on seventh postoperative day. HPE showed papillary thyroid carcinoma and was planned for RAI treatment.

Roma Pradhan is the lead author of this chapter.

A. Agarwal et al., *Case Studies in Thyroid and Parathyroid Tumors*,
https://doi.org/10.1007/978-981-99-0938-4_51

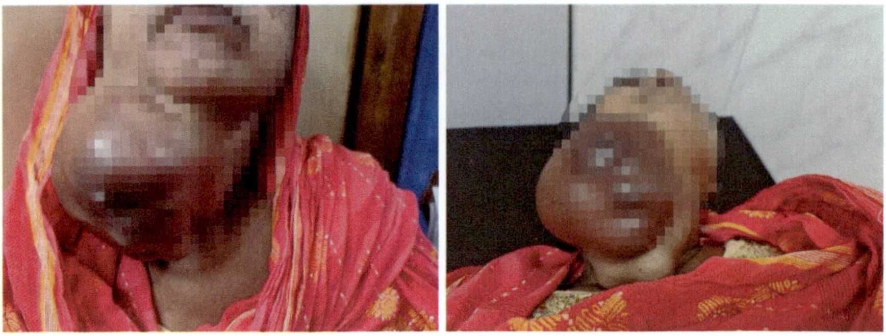

Fig. 1 Clinical picture

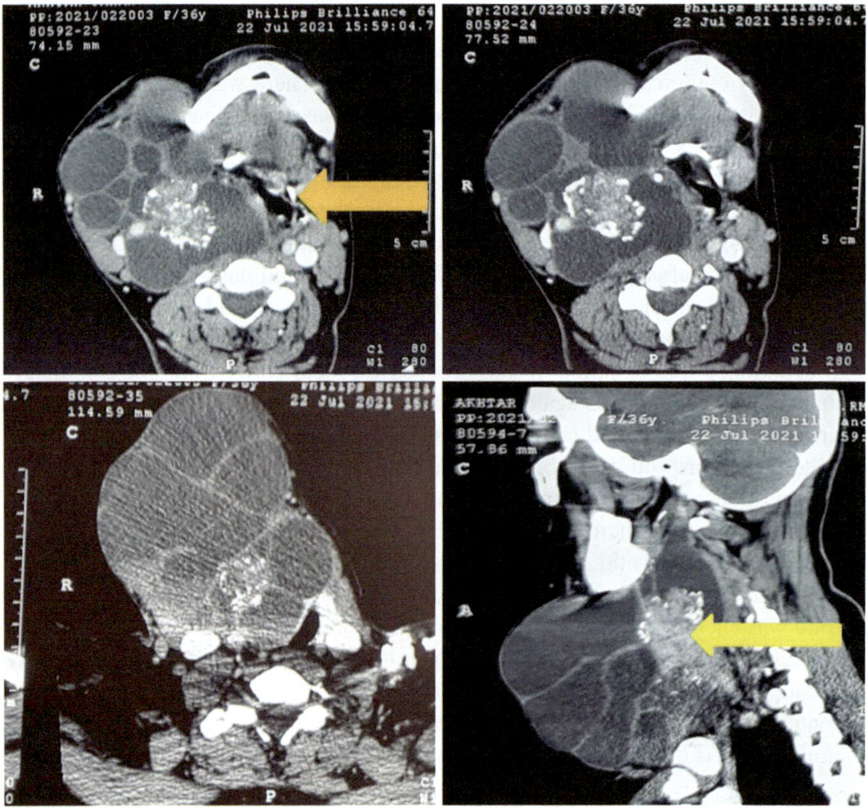

Fig. 2 Orange arrow: deviated and compressed airway, yellow arrow showing suspicious area with calcification

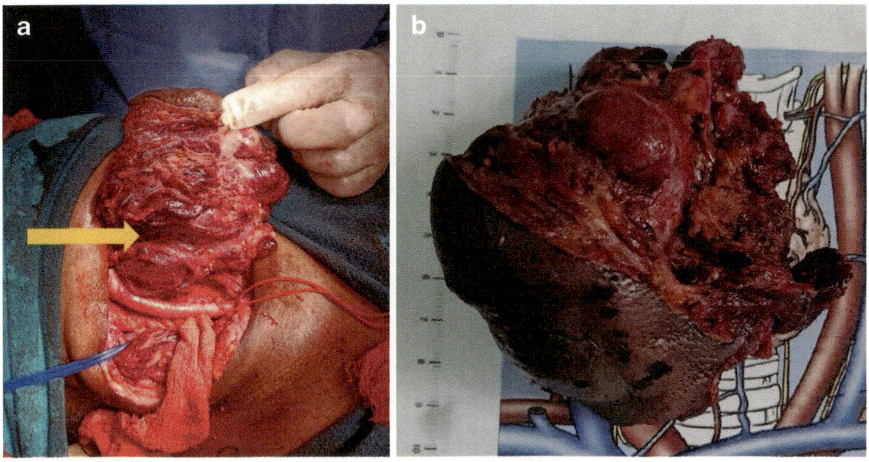

Fig. 3 (**a**) Orange arrow shows the carotid groove after separation of carotid, (**b**) postoperative specimen weighing 1.5 kg

Case 2

A 53-year-old lady presented with anterior neck swelling for 7 years (Fig. 4). The swelling was gradually increasing in size. There was no history suggestive of any compressive symptoms. However patient developed facial nerve palsy because of middle ear infection. The patient was planned first for thyroid surgery after discussion with ENT surgeon for middle ear infection. CECT was done (Fig. 5). Patient was planned for total thyroidectomy with continuous neuromonitoring. Awake intubation was done using fiberoptic. Decrease in voltage (<100 μV) occurred once while delivering the right lobe (Fig. 6 orange arrow), which got reverted. No permanent loss of signal happened on the right side hence we proceeded to the left side. Postoperative specimen weighed 1000 g (Fig. 7). Postoperative recovery was smooth and the patient was discharged on seventh POD.

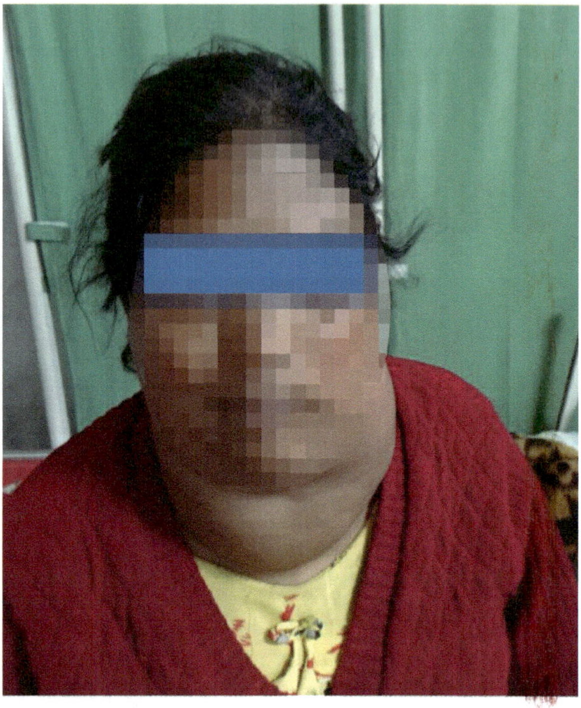

Fig. 4 Clinical picture

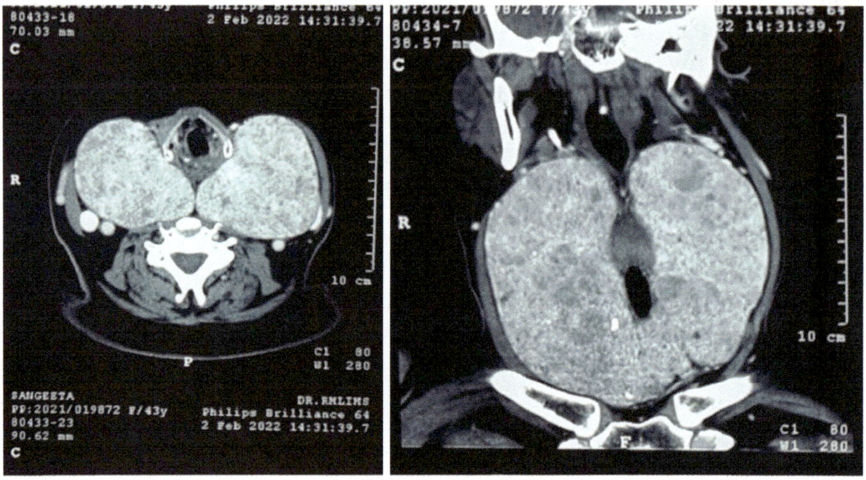

Fig. 5 CECT Neck

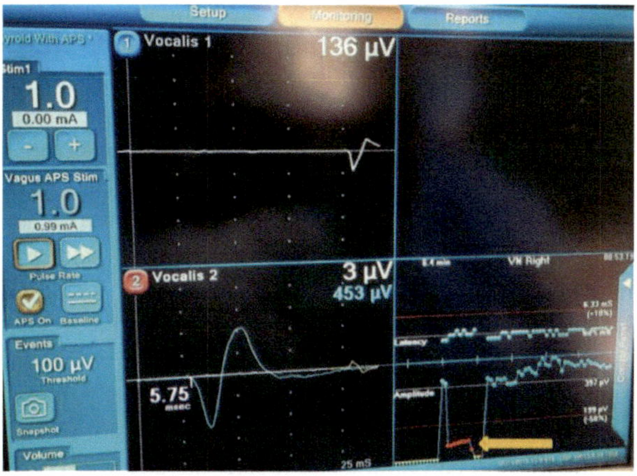

Fig. 6 Continuous neuromonitoring loss of amplitude (orange arrow)

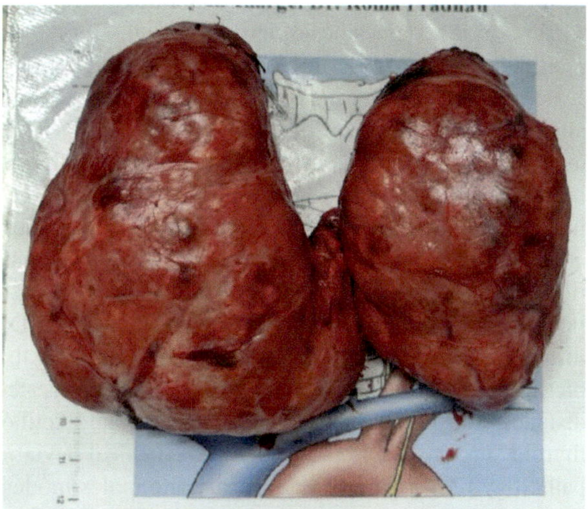

Fig. 7 Specimen weighing 1000 g

Discussion

A huge thyroid tumor is defined as any thyroid tumor with an average weight greater than 500 g, a diameter greater than 100 mm, in which the upper end extends up to the mandibular angle, the lower end extends to the sternum and both sides of the posterior border are normally sternocleidomastoid muscle [1]. Patients with huge thyroid tumor are usually asymptomatic initially and that is the reason for their delay in taking medical help. The most common symptom in patients with obstructive cervical or substernal goiter is exertional dyspnea, which is present in 30–60% of patients [2, 3]. The recommended management of such huge thyroid tumor is surgery especially for those with compressive symptoms. However, it is possible that surgical complications, such as recurrent laryngeal nerve injury, hypocalcemia, and hemorrhage, are higher than in small thyroid goiters because of anatomical changes and difficulty of surgical approach. Hence such patients should be operated in expert endocrine centers where the complication rates are similar as compared to small thyroids. The use of adjuncts like continuous neuromonitoring may help the surgeon to find displaced recurrent laryngeal nerves in huge thyroid or prevent its damage while delivering the thyroid lobe. Difficult intubation is another aspect that needs to be dealt in such cases. Though difficult intubation (DI) is expected in anaplastic thyroid carcinoma and locally advanced DTC, the rate of DI in benign goiter is highly variable in the literature. Some consider thyroid surgery itself as a risk factor for DI, while others do not. The rate of DI in the literature varies from 5% to 11% [4–6]. Most anesthesiologists follow the IDS (7 criteria scoring system) or the modified IDS scale (8 criteria) to assess the intubation difficulty. The modified IDS scale includes [6]: number of intubation attempts, number of operators, the use of alternative techniques, Cormack–Lehane grade (no laryngeal manipulation was used to improve this score) and lifting force applied to the laryngoscope, external laryngeal pressure, position of the vocal cords, and the degree of difficulty in passing the endotracheal tube. An easy intubation is defined as a successful single attempt by one operator without the use of any alternative techniques or manipulations under normal conditions and scored as MIDS = 2; A MIDS score >2 and <5 is interpreted as a slightly difficult intubation, and a MIDS score >5 is considered as a difficult intubation. The literature is highly variable about the factors that may predict difficult intubation. A meta-analysis [7] suggested that MS ≥ 3, reduced TM distance, and low IG significantly increase the likelihood of difficult intubation in thyroid surgery; while the presence of tracheal deviation (TD) (the unique thyroid pathology linked parameter), obesity and males moderately elevate the risk of difficult airway management in this specific clinical setting. So these significant parameters can be used for a more accurate preoperative assessment with the aim to anticipate difficult intubations and to optimize potentially difficult airways in thyroid surgery by selecting the appropriate method of intubation. Again, the literature is divided over the most appropriate method of intubating a goiter patient. Nonetheless, most studies suggest direct laryngoscopy with trans oral intubation as the first line of intubation in goiter patients [8]. Other methods of intubation include awake intubation with fiberoptic or video laryngoscopy (including glidedoscopy). Fiberoptic intubation requires a learning curve unlike the videolaryngoscopy. Advantages of video laryngoscopy include shorter intubation time, wider view of airway, no limitation on tracheal tube diameter, and ease in changing the size of the tracheal tube if required while maintaining the airway view [9]. One can also use a combination of these methods in case of failure to intubate by conventional means.

References

1. Du W, Liu S-T, Li P. Intra—and postoperative complications in 137 cases of giant thyroid gland tumor. Oncol Lett. 2012;4(5):965–9.
2. Katlic MR, Wang CA, Grillo HC. Substernal goiter. Ann Thorac Surg. 1985;39(4):391–9.
3. Banks CA, Ayers CM, Hornig JD. Thyroid disease and compressive symptoms. Laryngoscope. 2012;122(1):13–6.
4. Bouaggad A, Nejmi SE, Bouderka MA, Abbassi O. Prediction of difficult tracheal intubation in thyroid surgery. Anesth Analg. 2004;99(2):603–6.
5. Amathieu R, Smail N, Catineau J, Poloujadoff MP, Samii K, Adnet F. Difficult intubation in thyroid surgery: myth or reality? Anesth Analg. 2006;103(4):965–8.
6. Tutuncu AC, Erbabacan E, Teksoz S, Ekici B, Koksal G, Altintas F, et al. The assessment of risk factors for difficult intubation in thyroid patients. World J Surg. 2018;42:1748–53.
7. De Cassai A, Boscolo A, Rose K, Carron M, Navalesi P. Predictive parameters of difficult intubation in thyroid surgery: a meta-analysis. Minerva Anestesiol. 2020;86(3):317–26.
8. Loftus PA, Ow TJ, Siegel B, Tassler AB, Smith RV, Schiff BA. Risk factors for perioperative airway difficulty and evaluation of intubation approaches among patients with benign goiter. Ann Otol Rhinol Laryngol. 2014;123:279–85.
9. Heinz E, Quan T, Nguyen H, Pla R. Intubation of a patient with a large goiter: the advantageous role of videolaryngoscopy. Case Rep Anesthesiol. 2019;2019:1327482.

Dyshormonogenetic Goiter

Case

A 33-year-old woman presented with swelling in front of the neck since birth. Swelling is progressively increasing in size with rapid progression for 2 years but without compressive symptoms. She was evaluated at age of 5 years and diagnosed to have hypothyroidism and started on Tab Thyroxine 100ug; however, she has been taking her medication irregularly and swelling gradually progressed to present size. Her parents gave a history of psychiatric illness in her for the last 2 years and she was put on Tab Risperidone 2 mg, Fluoxetine 20 mg OD and Tab Olanzapine 1.25 mg HS. She was born of non-consangious marriage and had normal development till age 5. She had an average school performance till fourth standard but later dropped out from school. On examination the patient was conscious, oriented, Pallor present, no icterus, no cyanosis, no clubbing, no lymphadenopathy, mild non-pitting pedal edema. Thyroid-right lobe 25x 18 cm non-tender firm mobile smooth and left lobe 15 x 15 cm, inferior border felt, Pemberton's sign was negative. Systemic examination: CVS – S1 S2 +, No murmur RS – B/L crepitations; abdomen– soft, No organomegaly; CNS – HMF were normal; Field of vision normal; eye movements –normal MOTOR -Normal DTR – biceps ++/++, Triceps ++/++, Knee +/+ Ankle +/+, delayed relaxation present Sensory – Touch, pain, temperature vibration normal. USG thyroid showed multinodular goiter with TIRADS score of 4; guided FNA Showed MNG Bethesda Grade II; TSH-47.3, FT4–3 pmol, TPO-10 IU/L, TRAb-1.13iu/L, Thyroglobulin- 300 ng/ml IDL showed normal cords. I^{131} perchlorate discharge test was negative for organification. The patient's

Amit Agarwal is the lead author of this chapter.

A. Agarwal et al., *Case Studies in Thyroid and Parathyroid Tumors*,
https://doi.org/10.1007/978-981-99-0938-4_52

thyroxine dose was increased to 150ug/day and was planned for surgery after 2 months. Whole genome sequencing was sent to look for genetic causes; however, genetic studies were negative for any mutation of thyroid genes. MRI did not reveal any enlargement of Endolymphatic Sac. BERA studies revealed severe sensory-neural loss in the right ear. On her next visit, 2 months later there was substantial reduction in the size of goiter and her TSH was 10.6. She underwent total thyroidectomy and specimen weighed 545 gm with the right lobe measuring 15 × 10 × 5 cm and the left lobe measuring 10 × 6 × 3 cm. Postoperative period was uneventful and her histopathology was reported as benign multinodular goiter (Figs. 1, 2, and 3).

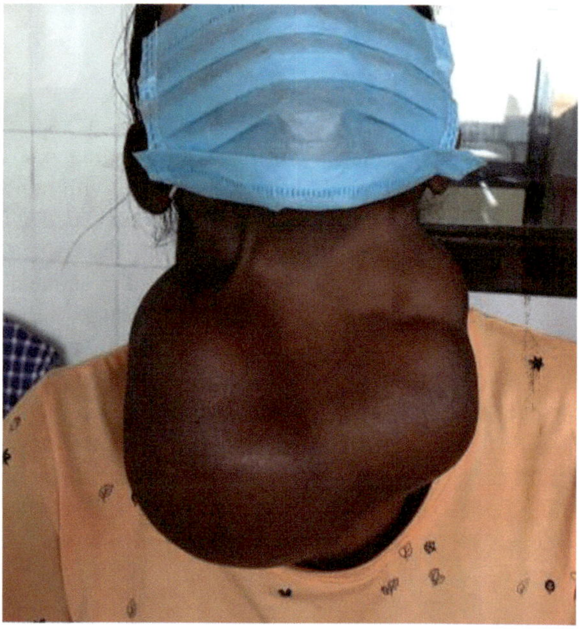

Fig. 1 Patient at presentation

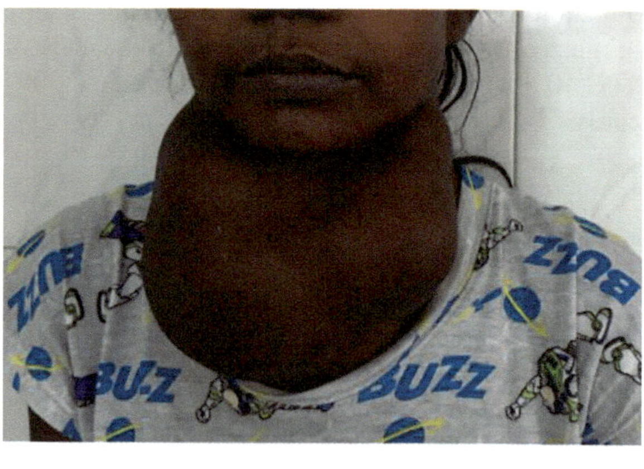

Fig. 2 Reduction in goiter size after thyroxine replacement

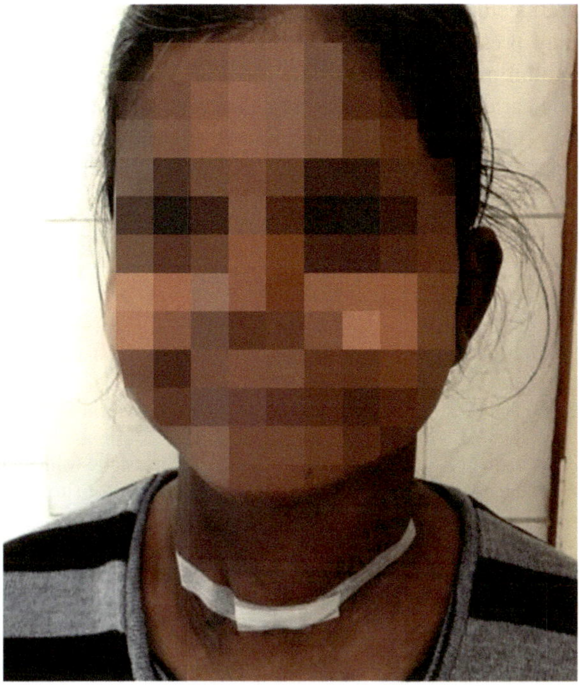

Fig. 3 Smiling patient after thyroidectomy

Discussion

The two most common causes of congenital hypothyroidism are [1, 2]: thyroid dysgenesis (80–85%) and thyroid dyshormonogenesis (15–20%). Dyshormonogenesis may result from genetic defect in any of the 7 key steps resulting in defective hormone synthesis: (1) defect in iodide trapping. (2) defect in transport of iodide into the thyroid colloid, (3) defect in thyroglobulin synthesis, (4) defect in iodide organification, oxidation, and coupling, (5) defect in H_2O_2 generation, (6) defect in synthesis of maturation factors DUOXA1 and A2, (7) defective recovery of iodine leading to loss of iodine in urine. TPO gene abnormality is the most common cause of congenital dyshormonogenetic hypothyroidism followed by TG gene defect. The usual presentation of a TG gene defect is severe hypothyroidism with a goiter being present at birth or shortly thereafter. However, a later presentation with a goiter in childhood is well recognized if diagnosis is delayed or levothyroxine supplementation is started late. Just replacement is not enough because significant goiter reduction occurs only when TSH is suppressed below normal. Another concern is the development of thyroid cancer in the TG deficiency goiter [3, 4]. Hishinuma et al. [4] reported thyroid malignancy in seven of 11 adults with Tg deficiency with surgically removed goiters. Thyroid supplementation appears to have been ineffective in preventing the development of cancer in some of these patients. It must also be remembered that dyshormongenetic goiter is morphologically characterized by architectural and cellular pleomorphism that may mimic thyroid malignancy and may present some difficulties in differential diagnosis. On cytology, DHG may exhibit nuclear atypia in the form of enlarged pleomorphic nuclei with or without nuclear chromatin and these cellular changes can be mistaken for follicular, papillary, medullary, or undifferentiated thyroid carcinoma. Because DHG may exhibit trabecular, solid, insular, and cribriform growth patterns it can be confused with undifferentiated thyroid cancer on histology.

References

1. Grasberger H, Refetoff S. Genetic causes of congenital hypothyroidism due to dyshormonogenesis. Curr Opin Pediatr. 2011;23(4):421–8.
2. Braham E, Rejeb HB, Marghl A, Kilani T, El Mezni F. A rare and particular form of goiter to recognize. Ann Transl Med. 2013;1(2):21.
3. Alzahrani AS, Baitei EY, Zou M, Shi Y. Metastatic follicular thyroid carcinoma arising from congenital goiter as a result of a novel splice donor site mutation in the thyroglobulin gene. J Clin Endocrinol Metab. 2006;91:740–6.
4. Hishinuma A, Fukata S, Kakudo K, Murata Y, Ieiri T. High incidence of thyroid cancer in long-standing goiters with thyroglobulin mutations. Thyroid. 2005;15:1079–84.

Graves' Disease Due to a Large Goiter

Case
A 20-year-old female presented with swelling in front of her neck for 3 years, insidious in onset, non-painful, gradually progressive in size with h/o anxiety, palpitations, exertional dyspnea, proximal muscle weakness, tremors of hands, excessive sweating, heat intolerance, hair fall, and increased appetite. The patient was evaluated and started on antithyroid drugs (carbimazole, 30 mg) by a private practitioner. After 1 year patient stopped the medications on her own when she conceived, but she delivered a stillborn child at 8 months of gestation. Following this swelling again gradually increased in size, and was associated with prominence of eyes with watering of eyes. The patient was then referred to SGPGIMS for further management. On examination there was diffuse enlargement of thyroid lobes, with a palpable thrill near superior pole along with positive eye signs: Nafziger sign, Stelwag sign, Darlymples sign, and with clinical activity score of 1/10. Her T4 was more than 300 (58–161 nmol/L) and T3 was 10 (1.2–2.7 nmol/L). She was re-started on carbimazole in doses of 40 mg, increased to 60 mg and then gradually tapered when referred for surgery. After adequate preparation with collosal iodine, she was taken up for surgery. Total thyroidectomy was performed. Both lobes found to be enlarged, hyper-vascular, with multiple parasitic vessels (more from posterior aspect) with weight of 160 g and measuring: Right lobe -12 × 8 × 4 cm, Left lobe- 10 × 8 × 6 cm. Postoperatively she developed symptomatic hypocalcemia which was managed with intravenous calcium followed by oral supplementation with calcium and active vitamin D for 3 months. Subsequently, she is doing well.

Amit Agarwal is the lead author of this chapter.

A. Agarwal et al., *Case Studies in Thyroid and Parathyroid Tumors*,
https://doi.org/10.1007/978-981-99-0938-4_53

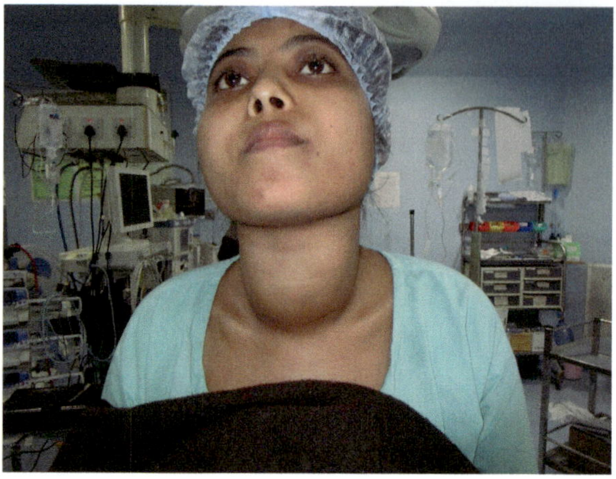

Discussion

Thionamide antithyroid drug therapy, which includes methimazole and propylthiouracil, results in a remission in approximately 40–50% of patients treated for 12–18 months (range, 10–90%). Higher remission rates occur in patients with milder disease and smaller goiters, but for the average patient, laboratory factors do not predict remission. The principal disadvantage of thionamide therapy is adverse effects. The usual starting dose for methimazole is 10–30 mg per day, depending on the severity of the patient's hyperthyroidism. Most patients do not require more than 30–40 mg per day. Higher methimazole doses may be used in more severe thyrotoxicosis (e.g., FT4 >3 times greater than the reference range and large goiters) but are also associated with more adverse effects. Minor adverse effects such as pruritic rash and arthralgias occur in approximately 5% of patients receiving methimazole, and typically begin within the first few weeks of starting therapy. The more severe adverse effects of antithyroid drugs include agranulocytosis, hepatotoxicity, and antineutrophil cytoplasmic antibody–positive vasculitis. Agranulocytosis occurs in approximately 1 in 500 patients, 46 and is both dose-related with methimazole as well as an idiosyncratic reaction. Thus patients with large goiters requiring high doses of methimazole (>60 mg) are prone to develop side effects of anti-thyroid medications and thus are candidates for surgery. Also, it has been shown that a higher thyroidal volume is predictive of lesser remission rates with anti-thyroid medications. Complications of surgery are minimal in the hands of experienced thyroid/endocrine surgeons and thus such patients should be referred to high-volume centers.

Further Reading

Mohlin E, Filipsson Nystrom H, Eliasson M. Long-term prognosis after medical treatment of graves' disease in a northern Swedish population 2000-2010. Eur J Endocrinol. 2014;170:419–27.

Vos XG, Endert E, Zwinderman AH, Tijssen JG, Wiersinga WM. Predicting the risk of recurrence before the start of Antithyroid drug therapy in patients with graves' hyperthyroidism. J Clin Endocrinol Metab. 2016;101:1381–9.

Graves' Disease with Nodule

Case

A 64-year-old lady with a history of anterior neck swelling ×2 years associated with palpitation, sweating, rapid weight loss, and diarrhea. She has been taking antithyroid medication and beta blockers for last 2 years. On examination, she had Lid lag with staring look along with diffuse enlargement of both lobes of thyroid gland with a nodule palpable in both lobes. Ultrasound neck that both thyroid lobes were grossly enlarged but also showed multiple nodules with multiple cystic areas within, largest in right measuring 1.4 × 2.2 cm largest in left lobe measuring 1.5 × 1.8 cm. Her thyroid function tests were suggestive of a diagnosis of GD (TSH:0.005 miu/L (0.4–4), fT4: 16.14 pmol/l (12–22), TRAb: 38.27 IU/L (>1.75 IU/L). Thyroid scan features were suggestive of diffuse toxic goiter. She underwent total thyroidectomy and histopathology was suggestive of primary hyperplasia in resolution and showing multiple nodules in both lobes without any evidence of malignancy.

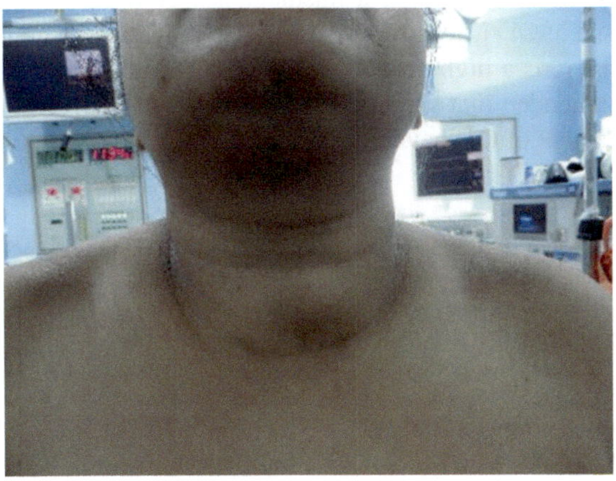

Amit Agarwal is the lead author of this chapter.

A. Agarwal et al., *Case Studies in Thyroid and Parathyroid Tumors*,
https://doi.org/10.1007/978-981-99-0938-4_54

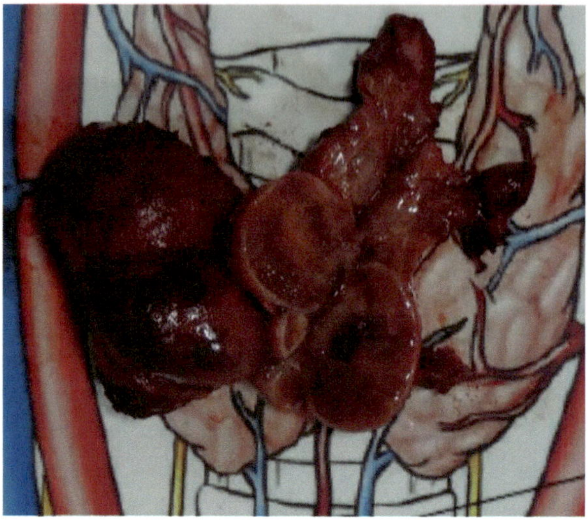

Discussion

The multicentric study by Kraimps et al. [1] found an overall incidence of 3.8% of carcinoma in GD; rate of carcinoma was much higher (15%) if the nodule was present. The incidence of thyroid nodules in patients with GD is reported as 20–35% [2] in the literature. Palpable thyroid nodules to occur in 10–15% of patients with Graves' disease. The use of ultrasonography and scintigraphy as methods of nodule detection is the likely cause of the increased detection rate compared to palpation alone. FNAC from small thyroid nodules is not recommended because of the increased risk of hemorrhage and a misdiagnosis of follicular neoplasm due to hyperplastic tissue of GD [3]. Most malignancies are within the nodule (palpable or otherwise) and there is a high proportion (38%) of papillary micro-carcinoma [4]. Thus, it is recommended that surgery in the form of total thyroidectomy should be advised in any patient of GD having a nodule.

References

1. Kraimps JL, Bovin-Pineau MH, Mathonnet M, De Galan L, Ronceray J, Visset J. Multicentric study of thyroid nodules in patients with graves' disease. Br J Surg. 2000;87:1111–3.
2. Staniforth JUL, Erdirimanne S, Guy D. Eslick thyroid carcinoma in Graves' disease: a meta-analysis. Int J Surg. 2016;27:118–25.
3. Gabriele R, Letizia C, Borghese M, De Toma G, Celi M, Izzo L, Cavallaro A. Thyroid cancer in patients with hyperthyroidism. Horm Res. 2003;60:79e83.
4. Gerenova J, Buysschaert M, de Burbure CY, Daumerie C. Prevalence of thyroid cancer in Graves' disease: a retrospective study of a cohort of 103 patients treated surgically. Eur J Intern Med. 2003;14:321e325.

Graves' Eye Disease

Case

A 35-year-old woman had symptoms of weight loss, diarrhea, heat intolerance, and palpitations along with prominence and protrusion of both eyes. She had a small thyromegaly. She was diagnosed by her general physician as Graves' disease with ophthalmopathy and put on anti-thyroid medications which she received for 15 years before being referred for surgery. When she presented to us, examination of the eyes revealed proptosis, lid lag, lid retraction, absence of forehead wrinkling and convergence was slow and jerky. She underwent total thyroidectomy and in the last 5 years there has been no progression in eye signs and symptoms.

Amit Agarwal is the lead author of this chapter.

A. Agarwal et al., *Case Studies in Thyroid and Parathyroid Tumors*,
https://doi.org/10.1007/978-981-99-0938-4_55

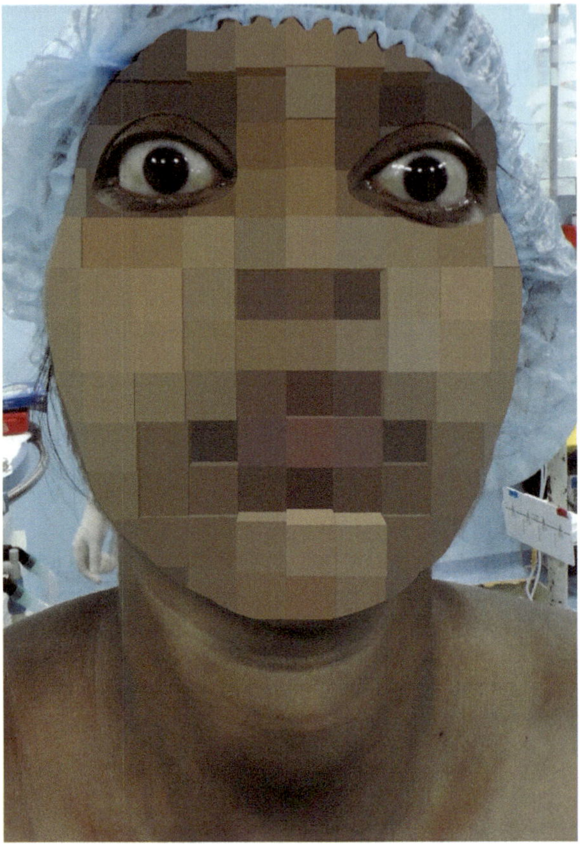

Discussion

The treatment of a patient of GD with eye disease includes the following:

1. Immediate cessation of smoking.
2. Restoration of euthyroidism.
3. Assessment of disease activity.
4. Local protective measures.
5. Specific medications.
6. Rehabilitative eye surgery.

Assessment of Eye disease severity: Several classification schemes have been created to grade the severity of GED [1].

1. The NO SPECS Classification system grades GED-related signs and symptoms by assigning a Global Severity Score.

2. The European Group on Graves Orbitopathy scale is based on 3 categories of disease severity-mild, moderate, or severe.
3. The VISA system to assess GED is based on physical examination findings and patient symptoms.

General guidelines:

- Mild inactive disease: local measures only.
- Mild active disease: observation, selenium or oral glucocorticoids.
- Moderate to severe and active disease: IV glucocorticoids; if still progression then orbital RT, with or without orbital decompression followed by rehabilitative surgery.

Local protective measures: eye lubrication (fresh tear drops or carboxymethylcellulose ointments), sunglasses.

Restoration of euthyroidism: can be achieved through use of either of them: ATD, RAI, or surgery:

Mild active GO: RAI, ATD, or Surgery are equally acceptable therapeutic option. However, RAI may worsen the GO by 3–5 times even in mild disease.

Moderate or severe active GO: RAI is contra-indicated. Either ATD or Surgery are the options. The work by Laurberg et al. [2] has supported the concept that TRAb titres decline fairly soon after thyroidectomy. Recently two important studies have concluded that in such patients where likelihood of remission on ATD is low, the preferred option is surgery [3, 4]. Total or sub-total thyroidectomy have the same response [5].

Specific medications for GO:

1. Selenium: Beneficial effect of selenium is due to its anti-inflammatory and anti-oxidant nature.
2. Glucocorticoids:
   (a) Oral GCs: can be used in mild active disease as stand-alone treatment or as a prophylaxis if RAI is chosen as a therapy in this group of patients.
   (b) IV methylprednisolone in moderate to severe and active GO as a 12-weekly regimen.
3. Orbital RT: can be given along with oral GCs in improving diplopia and GO severity.
4. Cyclosporine: in combination with oral GCs can be used as second-line therapy when there is partial or no response to IV GCs in mod/severe GO.
5. Orbital decompression: In rapidly progressive active disease of at least moderate severity where immunomodulatory therapy has failed, it is sometimes appropriate to consider orbital decompression.
6. Azathioprine: A potential role of azathioprine for preventing long-term GO relapse after steroids are discontinued, has been suggested.

7. Immunomodulatory therapy: Patients have moderate-to-severe disease, which account for only 5% of GO patients can be a potential target for systemic immunotherapy like Rituximab, Tocilizumab, Teprotumumab, Mycophenolate mofetil, Intravenous immunoglobulin, and TNF-alpha inhibitors.

References

1. Kotwal A, Stan M. Current and future treatments for graves' disease and graves' Ophthalmopathy. Horm Metab Res. 2018;50:871–86.
2. Laurberg P, Wallin G, Tallstedt L, Abraham-Nordling M, Lundell G, Torring O. TSH-receptor autoimmunity in graves' disease after therapy with anti-thyroid drugs, surgery, or radioiodine: a 5-year prospective randomized study. Eur J Endocrinol. 2008;158:69–75.
3. Meyer Zu Horste M, Pateronis K, Walz MK, Alesina P, Mann K, Schott M, Esser J, Eckstein AK. The effect of early thyroidectomy on the course of active graves' Orbitopathy (GO): a retrospective case study. Horm Metab Res. 2016;48:433–9.
4. De Bellis A, Conzo G, Cennamo G, Pane E, Bellastella G, Colella C, Iacovo AD, Paglionico VA, Sinisi AA, Wall JR, Bizzarro A, Bellastella A. Time course of Graves' ophthalmopathy after total thyroidectomy alone or followed by radioiodine therapy: a 2-year longitudinal study. Endocrine. 2012;41:320–6.
5. Liu ZW, Masterson L, Fish B, Jani P, Chatterjee K. Thyroid surgery for Graves' disease and Graves' ophthalmopathy. Cochrane Database Syst Rev. 2015;(11):CD010576.

Graves with Vitiligo and Papillary Thyroid Carcinoma

Case

A 30-year-olds gentleman presented with anterior neck swelling for 2 years along with palpitations, sweating, and rapid weight loss. The patient also presented with the development of vitiligo patches for 2 years. Family history: h/o Graves' disease in mother. The patient was on irregular medication when he presented to our outpatient clinic. Clinical examination showed lid lag and prominent eyes with CAS (Clinical activity score) of 0/7. Neck examination showed bilateral diffuse enlargement of thyroid gland along with vitiligo patches (Fig. 1). After clinical diagnosis of Graves' disease biochemical investigations were advised and TSH was found to be low TSH: 0.01miu/L (0.4–4) and high fT4: 10 ng/dL (0.89–1.76 ng/dL). The patient was managed medically with neomercazole for 3 months along with beta blocker. The patient was planned for total thyroidectomy after normalization of FT4 levels. Total thyroidectomy specimen weighed 120 g (Fig. 2) and postoperatively patient was discharged on fourth postoperative day. Histopathology was multifocal PTC with BRAF negative.

Roma Pradhan is the lead author of this chapter.

A. Agarwal et al., *Case Studies in Thyroid and Parathyroid Tumors*,
https://doi.org/10.1007/978-981-99-0938-4_56

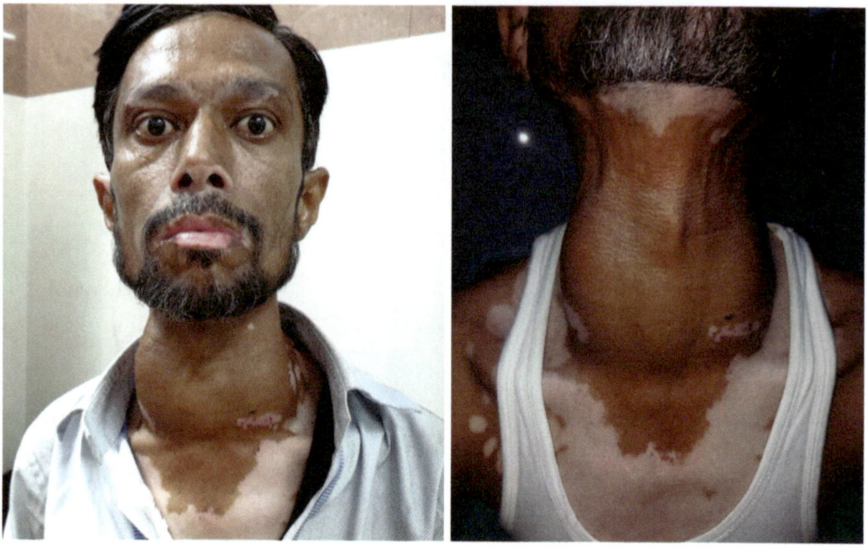

Fig. 1 Clinical picture showing prominent eyes, enlarged thyroid, and vitiligo patches

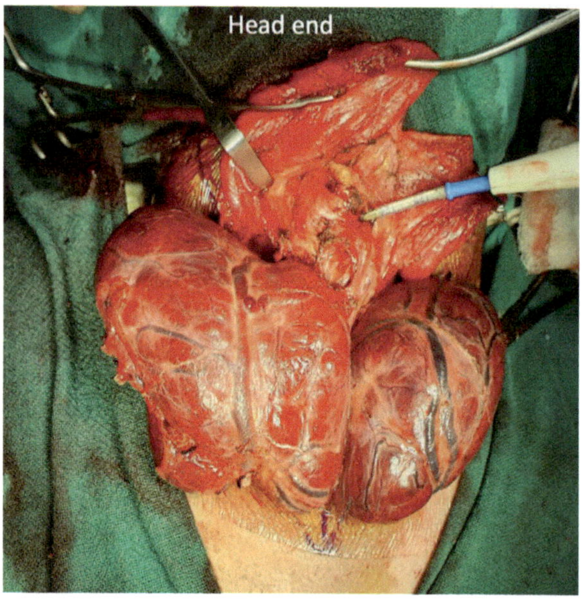

Fig. 2 Total thyroidectomy specimen

Discussion

Graves' disease patients are thought to have an increased risk of thyroid cancer but prevalence varies widely, with rates of up to 21.1% being reported in GD patients [1]. A collective review by Belfiore et al. observed that the malignancy rate of palpable thyroid nodules in GD patients ranged from as low as 2.3% to up to 45.8% [2] while the malignancy rate of palpable nodules occurring in the general population hovered around 5%. The biological behavior of cancers in Graves' disease is controversial and study by Hales et al. did not find any difference between aggressive histology or outcome [3, 4]. However, a study by Ozaki et al. suggested higher incidence of locoregional and distant metastases in thyroid cancer patients with GD [5]. Pellegriti et al. [6] compared long-term outcome and concluded that the cumulative risk for recurrent or progressive distant metastases was approximately threefold higher in Graves' patients than in euthyroid patients. Similar observations were made by other authors too [7].

Vitiligo is characterized by the loss of functional skin and mucosal melanocytes, the estimated prevalence is 0.5–2%. Several studies have suggested vitiligo is associated with a variety of other autoimmune diseases, including thyroid conditions, alopecia areata, type 1 diabetes mellitus, pernicious anemia, and rheumatoid arthritis. Population-based study in Korea [8] enrolled 73,336 vitiligo patients and 146,672 controls. The study found that patients with vitiligo were at increased risks of Graves' disease, Hashimoto thyroiditis, and thyroid cancer compared with the controls.

The systematic review and meta-analysis [9] found that 6 thyroid disorders showed various prevalences in vitiligo. Screening vitiligo patients for thyroid disorders seem plausible, in an effort to detect potential thyroid diseases or to assess the risk of future onset.

References

1. Pazaitou-Panayiotou K, Michalakis K, Paschke R. Thyroid cancer in patients with hyperthyroidism. Horm Metab Res. 2012;44(04):255–62.
2. Belfiore A, Russo D, Vigneri R, Filetti S. Graves' disease, thyroid nodules and thyroid cancer. Clin Endocrinol. 2001;55(6):711–8.
3. Hales IB, Mcelduff A, Crummeretal P. Doesgraves'disease or thyrotoxicosis affect the prognosis of thyroid cancer. J Clin Endocrinol Metabol. 1992;75(3):886–9.
4. Kasuga Y, Sugenoya A, Kobayashi S, Masuda H, Iida F. The outcome of patients with thyroid carcinoma and graves' disease. Surg Today. 1993;23(1):9–12.
5. Ozaki O, Ito K, Kobayashi K, Toshima K, Iwasaki H, Yashiro T. Thyroid carcinoma in graves' disease. World J Surg. 1990;14(3):437–40.
6. Pellegriti G, Belfiore A, Giuffrida D, Lupo L, Vigneri R. Outcome of differentiated thyroid cancer in graves' patients. J Clin Endocrinol Metabol. 1998;83(8):2805–9.
7. Cappelli C, Braga M, DeMartinoetal E. Outcomeofpatients surgically treated for various forms of hyperthyroidism with differentiated thyroid cancer: experience at an endocrine center in Italy. Surg Today. 2006;36(2):125–30.
8. Bae JM, Lee JH, Yun JS, Han B, Han TY. Vitiligo and overt thyroid diseases: a nationwide population-based study in Korea. J Am Acad Dermatol. 2017;76(5):871–8.
9. Yuan J, Sun C, Jiang S, Lu Y, Zhang Y, Gao XH, Wu Y, Chen HD. The prevalence of thyroid disorders in patients with vitiligo: a systematic review and meta-analysis. Front Endocrinol (Lausanne). 2019;9:803.

Toxic MNG

Case

A 36-year-old female presented with a history of swelling over the front of the neck (Fig. 1) for 15 years and associated with weight loss, proximal muscle weakness, palpitations, and hyper-defecation for 5 years. She had been previously diagnosed as Grave's disease, and as per information provided by herself, she was put on anti-thyroid medication followed by 45 mCi of RAI in 3 sittings. However, she failed on RAI therapy and was referred for surgery. Currently on Tab NMZ 10 mg TDS and Inderal 20 mg BD. On examination, both lobes of thyroid enlarged with the right lobe larger than the left. Multiple nodules were palpable both in the right and left lobe. Cervical LN are not palpable. No thrill palpable and no eye signs. On evaluation thyroid function tests were normal, USG Neck showed diffusely enlarged thyroid, IDL: bilateral vocal cords were mobile and thyroid scan showed diffuse toxic goiter with multiple cold nodules. SPECT CT also showed multiple hypodense nodules in both lobes. She was treated by total thyroidectomy. During induction of anesthesia the patient had atrial fibrillations and bradycardia (Fig. 2). Cardiologist's opinion was taken and transcutaneous pacing was done and surgery was completed (Fig. 3).

Amit Agarwal is the lead author of this chapter.

A. Agarwal et al., *Case Studies in Thyroid and Parathyroid Tumors*,
https://doi.org/10.1007/978-981-99-0938-4_57

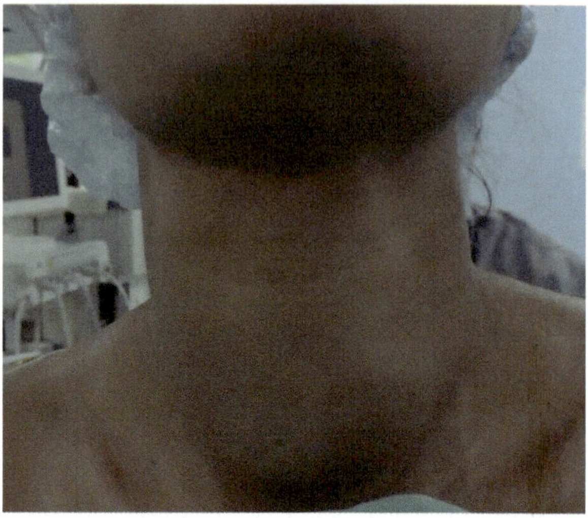

Fig. 1 Clinical picture showing the large neck swelling

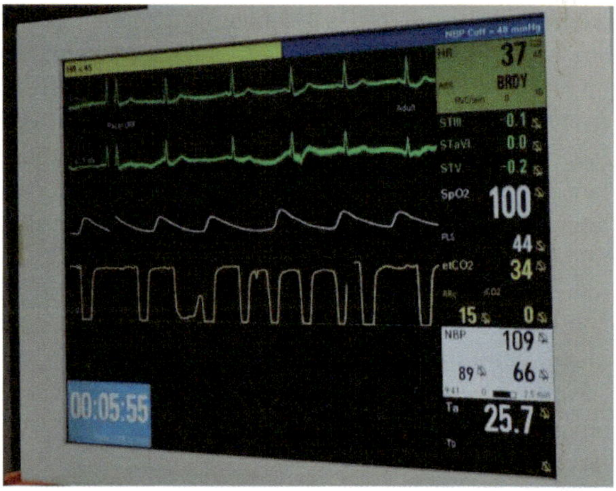

Fig. 2 Patient experienced severe bradycardia requiring pacing for correction

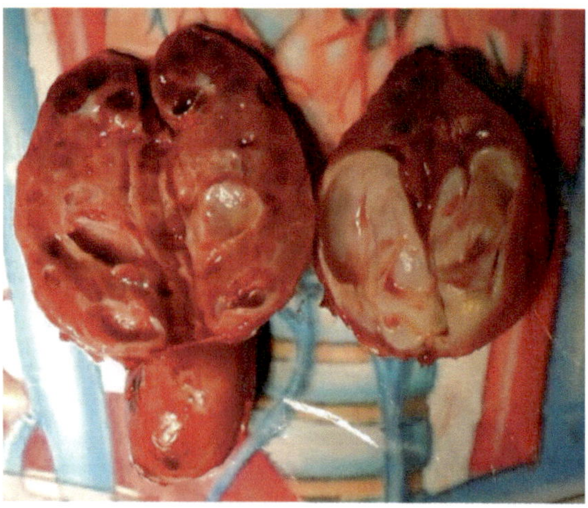

Fig. 3 Specimen showing multiple nodules in both lobes

Discussion

Toxic multinodular goiter develops in the elderly people (>60 years). Thyroid hormone excess associated with thyroid autonomy can have serious cardiovascular consequences such as hypertension, atrial fibrillation, and congestive heart failure, even though the symptoms are often milder than those of Grave's disease [1]. Atrial fibrillation is an important cardiac complication in elderly patients with thyroid autonomy and might not revert even when euthyroidism is restored, if it has been present for a long time and is coexistent with heart disease. Patients aged over 65 years with toxic multinodular goiter and atrial fibrillation are also at an increased risk of stroke. Also, atrial fibrillation is an independent predictor of congestive heart failure in patients with hyperthyroidism. An analysis of rhythm disorders in 219 patients with hyperthyroidism showed an age-dependent distribution of atrial fibrillation, which occurred in 43% of patients with toxic multinodular goiter versus 10% of patients with Grave's disease [2]. The risk of persistent atrial fibrillation is particularly high in patients with toxic multinodular goiter, because of their advanced age at diagnosis, but also because they tend to experience long-term thyroid hormone excess as a result of prolonged subclinical hyperthyroidism. Atrial fibrillation that persists for 4 months or more after the control of hyperthyroidism rarely reverts to sinus rhythm without cardioversion. In patients who do not regain normal rhythm spontaneously within 4 months of normalization of thyroid function, pharmacological or electrical cardioversion should be done [3]. Antiarrhythmic drugs should be used to avoid the recurrence of atrial fibrillation after successful cardioversion. Anticoagulant therapy with warfarin should be administered for at least 3 weeks before cardioversion and should be continued for at least 4 weeks after successful cardioversion to avoid the risk of embolic events [4]. Care should be taken to use a reduced dosage of Warfarin in hyperthyroid patients.

References

1. Doubleday AR, Sippel RS. Hyperthyroidism. Gland Surg. 2020;9(1):124.
2. Agner T, Almdal T, Thorsteinsson B, Agner E. A re-evaluation of atrial fibrillation in thyrotoxicosis. Dan Med Bull. 1984;31:157–9.
3. Biondi B, Kahaly GJ. Cardiovascular involvement in patients with different causes of hyperthyroidism. Nat Rev Endocrinol. 2010;6:431–43.
4. Shimizu T, et al. Hyperthyroidism and the management of atrial fibrillation. Thyroid. 2002;12:489–93.

Histological Surprise of Malignancy in Toxic Goiter

Case

A 55-year-old female was referred to our Endocrine Surgery clinic for discussion of surgical treatment of her toxic multinodular goiter. The patient had presented to her GP, with palpitations and feeling giddy at times. She was diagnosed with atrial fibrillation, for which she was started on a β-blocker. She was then found to have a slightly raised free thyroxine (fT4): 16.3 pmol/L [8.0–16.0] and a suppressed TSH: <0.01 mIU/L [0.45–4.50].

She was subsequently referred to the Endocrine Medicine clinic for further work-up. Neck US scan revealed bilateral, non-suspicious nodules within the thyroid. An isotope scan showed an increased radionuclide uptake in several of the nodules, with a decreased uptake in the surrounding extranodular thyroid tissue, confirming the diagnosis of toxic multinodular goiter.

The patient underwent a total thyroidectomy and was discharged on postoperative day two without any issues regarding her voice, wound, or problems with her calcium home stasis. Histology confirmed the presence of several thyroid adenomas; however, it also revealed an incidental unifocal, papillary thyroid carcinoma (PTC), measuring 15 mm in diameter, and showing signs suspicious for vascular invasion. Based on these findings, her PTC was considered to have an intermediate risk of recurrence, and therefore she was referred for adjuvant radio-iodine treatment.

Discussion

Toxic goiter is one of the most common reasons of hyperthyroidism, and is, in the majority of these patients, comprised of benign follicular neoplasms [1]. The incidence of thyroid cancer in patients presenting with a toxic goiter was initially

Rajeev Parameswaran is the lead author of this chapter.

A. Agarwal et al., *Case Studies in Thyroid and Parathyroid Tumors*,
https://doi.org/10.1007/978-981-99-0938-4_58

thought to be very low (i.e. <5%) [2, 3]; however, more recent studies show the incidence to be slightly higher (i.e. around 20%; compared with 36% among the euthyroid patients in the same cohort) [4]. These data suggest the initial presumed rarity of malignancy in the setting of hyperthyroidism, to be an underestimation of the actual risk [5]. Some of the published series highlighting the incidence of thyroid cancers in TMNG are shown in Table 1.

The 2015 ATA guidelines [13] do currently not recommend cytologic evaluation in the presence of a distinct nodule that is hyperfunctioning. Conversely, those with non-functioning nodules should be considered for cytologic evaluation, based on size and ultrasound features. This difference in approach could be based on the characteristic of thyrotropin (TSH) as a growth factor for thyroid nodules [14]. The hypothesis is that the opposite scenario, thus an increased thyroid hormone coupled with a suppressed TSH, could potentially protect the thyroid tissue from developing into a malignancy [15]. This specific profile is present in patients with toxic nodular goiter, leading some to believe a certain degree of protection against the development of malignancy among these patients in whom there is suppressed extranodular thyroid tissue secondary to the hyperthyroidism [4]. However, robust data to support this statement is unavailable.

Among large series investigating the incidence of incidental thyroid malignancy, PTC was found to be the more common subtype of thyroid cancer (75–95% of cases) than follicular thyroid carcinoma (FTC); [10, 16–18] with the microPTC variant to be more common [19, 20]. While the higher incidence of relatively smaller PTCs could be owed to more meticulous sectioning during histopathological examination, this does not explain the etiology of the development of these incidental thyroid carcinomas. The prevalence of occult PTC found during autopsies has been reported to be as high as 35%, suggesting latent features of this neoplasm [21]. It is generally considered that incidentally found thyroid cancers are frequently determined in early stages, with more favorable histopathological features and better prognosis [20].

Overall, treatment options for patients with a toxic goiter include surgery, radioiodine, or prolonged (probably lifelong) anti-thyroid therapy, generally based on both patient factors as well as and regional availability or preferences. The ATA guidelines advise surgical treatment for patients with very large goiters (>80 g), symptoms or signs of compression/obstruction, the need for rapid return to

Table 1 Published series highlighting the incidence of thyroid cancers in toxic MNG

Study and year	Number of patients	Malignancy rate in TMNG
Smith et al. 2013 [6]	238	18.3%
More et al. 2020 [7]	448	25%
Baser et al. 2019 [8]	364	5%
Slijepcevic et al. 2015 [9]	278	13.7%
Miccoli et al. 2006 [10]	998	8.2%
Phitayakorn et al. 2008 [11]	507	6.2%
Berker et al. 2011 [12]	477	8%

euthyroidism, and the suspicion of thyroid malignancy [13]. The possibly higher incidence of malignancy in this group stresses the importance of yielding patients with a goiter with hyperthyroidism do the appropriate work-up, including cytology, to assess their individual risk of malignancy [5].

If a thyroid cancer is incidentally found during surgery for a toxic goiter, either in the index nodule or in the non-nodular thyroid tissue, adjuvant decision steps should follow the current thyroid cancer guidelines [22].

References

1. Pazaitou-Panayiotou K, Michalakis K, Paschke R. Thyroid cancer in patients with hyperthyroidism. Horm Metab Res. 2012;44(04):255–62.
2. Gelmini R, Franzoni C, Pavesi E, Cabry F, Saviano M. Incidental thyroid carcinoma (ITC): a retrospective study in a series of 737 patients treated for benign disease. Ann Ital Chir. 2010;81(6):421–7.
3. Giles Y, Fatih T, Harika B, Yersu K, Tarik T, Serdar T. The risk factors for malignancy in surgically treated patients for graves' disease, toxic multinodular goiter, and toxic adenoma. Surgery. 2008;144(6):1028–37.
4. Tam AA, Ozdemir D, Alkan A, Yazicioglu O, Yildirim N, Kilicyazgan A, et al. Toxic nodular goiter and thyroid cancer: is hyperthyroidism protective against thyroid cancer? Surgery. 2019;166(3):356–61.
5. Alvarez AL, Mulder M, Handelsman RS, Lew JI, Farra JC. High rates of underlying thyroid cancer in patients undergoing thyroidectomy for hyperthyroidism. J Surg Res. 2020;245:523–8.
6. Smith JJ, Chen X, Schneider DF, Broome JT, Sippel RS, Chen H, et al. Cancer after thyroidectomy: a multi-institutional experience with 1,523 patients. J Am Coll Surg. 2013;216(4):571–7.
7. More Y, Khalil AB, Mustafa H, Gupte M, Al-Abbadi M, Elamin D, et al. Incidental thyroid cancer in patients undergoing surgery for hyperthyroidism. Am J Otolaryngol. 2020;41(2):102187.
8. Baser H, Topaloglu O, Bilginer MC, Ulusoy S, Kılıcarslan A, Ozdemir E, et al. Are cytologic and histopathologic features of hot thyroid nodules different from cold thyroid nodules? Diagn Cytopathol. 2019;47(9):898–903.
9. Slijepcevic N, Zivaljevic V, Marinkovic J, Sipetic S, Diklic A, Paunovic I. Retrospective evaluation of the incidental finding of 403 papillary thyroid microcarcinomas in 2466 patients undergoing thyroid surgery for presumed benign thyroid disease. BMC Cancer. 2015;15(1):1–8.
10. Miccoli P, Minuto MN, Galleri D, D'Agostino J, Basolo F, Antonangeli L, et al. Incidental thyroid carcinoma in a large series of consecutive patients operated on for benign thyroid disease. ANZ J Surg. 2006;76(3):123–6.
11. Phitayakorn R, McHenry CR. Incidental thyroid carcinoma in patients with graves' disease. Am J Surg. 2008;195(3):292–7.
12. Berker D, Isik S, Ozuguz U, Tutuncu YA, Kucukler K, Akbaba G, et al. Prevalence of incidental thyroid cancer and its ultrasonographic features in subcentimeter thyroid nodules of patients with hyperthyroidism. Endocrine. 2010;39(1):13–20.
13. Ross DS, Burch HB, Cooper DS, Greenlee MC, Laurberg P, Maia AL, et al. 2016 American thyroid association guidelines for diagnosis and management of hyperthyroidism and other causes of thyrotoxicosis. Thyroid. 2016;26(10):1343–421.
14. Boelaert K, Horacek J, Holder R, Watkinson J, Sheppard M, Franklyn J. Serum thyrotropin concentration as a novel predictor of malignancy in thyroid nodules investigated by fine-needle aspiration. J Clin Endocrinol Metabol. 2006;91(11):4295–301.
15. Fiore E, Rago T, Provenzale M, Scutari M, Ugolini C, Basolo F, et al. Lower levels of TSH are associated with a lower risk of papillary thyroid cancer in patients with thyroid nodular disease: thyroid autonomy may play a protective role. Endocr Relat Cancer. 2009;16(4):1251–60.

16. Nanjappa N, Kumar A, Swain SK, Aroul TT, Smile SR, Kotasthane D. Incidental thyroid carcinoma. Indian J Otolaryngol Head Neck Surg. 2013;65(1):37–9.
17. Memon W, Khanzada TW, Samad A, Kumar B. Incidence of thyroid carcinoma in multinodular goiters. Rawal Medical J. 2010;35(1):65–7.
18. Pezzolla A, Marzaioli R, Lattarulo S, Docimo G, Conzo G, Ciampolillo A, et al. Incidental carcinoma of the thyroid. Int J Surg. 2014;12:S98–S102.
19. Sakorafas GH, Giotakis J, Stafyla V. Papillary thyroid microcarcinoma: a surgical perspective. Cancer Treat Rev. 2005;31(6):423–38.
20. Evranos B, Polat SB, Cuhaci FN, Baser H, Topaloglu O, Kilicarslan A, et al. A cancer of undetermined significance: incidental thyroid carcinoma. Diagn Cytopathol. 2019;47(5):412–6.
21. Jia Q, Li X, Liu Y, Li L, Kwong JS, Ren K, et al. Incidental thyroid carcinoma in surgery-treated hyperthyroid patients with Graves' disease: a systematic review and meta-analysis of cohort studies. Cancer Manag Res. 2018;10:1201–7.
22. Haugen BR, Alexander EK, Bible KC, Doherty GM, Mandel SJ, Nikiforov YE, et al. 2015 American thyroid association management guidelines for adult patients with thyroid nodules and differentiated thyroid cancer: the American thyroid association guidelines task force on thyroid nodules and differentiated thyroid cancer. Thyroid. 2016;26(1):1–133.

Retrosternal Goiter Delivered by Cervical Route

Case 1

A 60-year-old presented with complaints of swelling in front of neck for 15 years which is progressively increasing in size and associated with voice change from 2 months. She also gave a history of dyspnea on exertion and loss of weight. On examination it was a multinodular goiter with 8 × 8 cm left lobe nodule and 3 × 2 cm right lobe nodule. There were visible veins over neck & upper chest and lower border was not palpable. Trachea was deviated to the right side and there was no significant palpable cervical LAP. Bilateral carotids were palpable but were displaced posteriorly on left and there was a dull note on percussion over sternum. Indirect laryngoscopy showed left vocal cord palsy. USG-guided FNAC showed follicular lesion of undetermined significance—BETHESDA CATEGORY 3. CECT Neck showed left lobe of thyroid is replaced by a mass lesion having large peripheral enhancing solid component and non-enhancing component measuring (5.7 × 5.6 × 15.8 cm) in size long with internal calcification with retrosternal extension (7 cm) up to level of carina (Fig. 1) and two hypodense lesions are seen in the right lobe. Total thyroidectomy was done. Retrosternal portion delivered with sharp and blunt dissection (Fig. 2). Intermittent IONM was done—294 microvolt on the right side & 190 microvolts on the left side. Specimen measured right lobe- 6 × 4 × 2 cm, left lobe—9 × 5 × 4 cm with 8 × 5 × 4 cm nodule at inferior pole extending retro-sternally.

Roma Pradhan is the lead author of this chapter.

A. Agarwal et al., *Case Studies in Thyroid and Parathyroid Tumors*,
https://doi.org/10.1007/978-981-99-0938-4_59

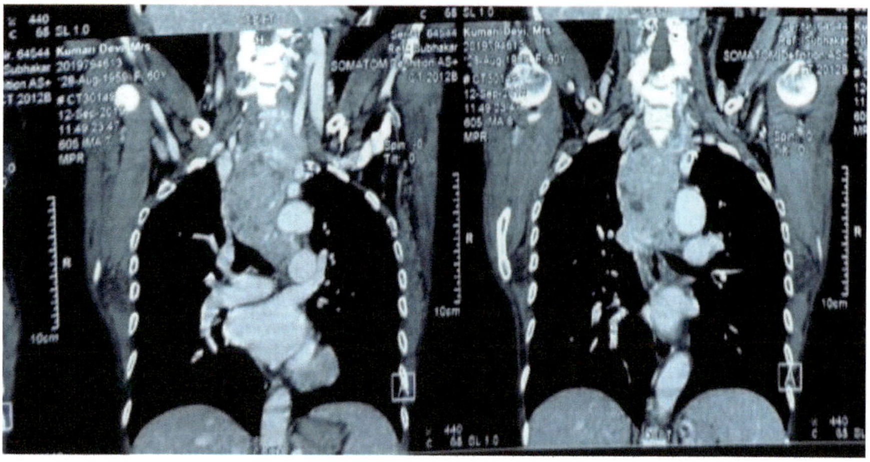

Fig. 1 CECT showing goiter extending retro-sternally up to carina

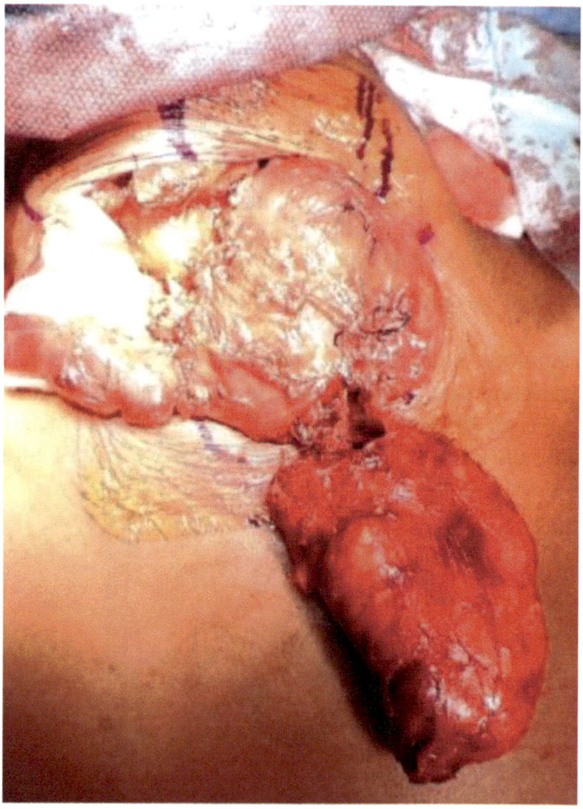

Fig. 2 Intra-operative view of the retro-sternal portion of goiter delivered from the neck without the need for sternotomy

Case 2

A 57-year-old lady presented with anterior neck swelling (Fig. 3) for 6 years. However, she presented to opd due to the appearance of vessels over anterior chest wall and discomfort in breathing on raising arm. Neck examination showed multinodular goiter with dilated veins over chest wall with pembertons sign positive. Bilateral carotids were palpable, however it was possible to get below the swelling. Due to suspicion of extension of tumor posteriorly in mediastinum CECT was advised. CECT (Fig. 4) showed enlarged thyroid gland with the right lobe extending into the mediastinum up to lower paratracheal region and closely abutting arch of azygos vein posteriorly, while the left lobe is extending up to the prevascular region of mediastinum. As the tumor was above the level of T4 vertebra, plan was delivery

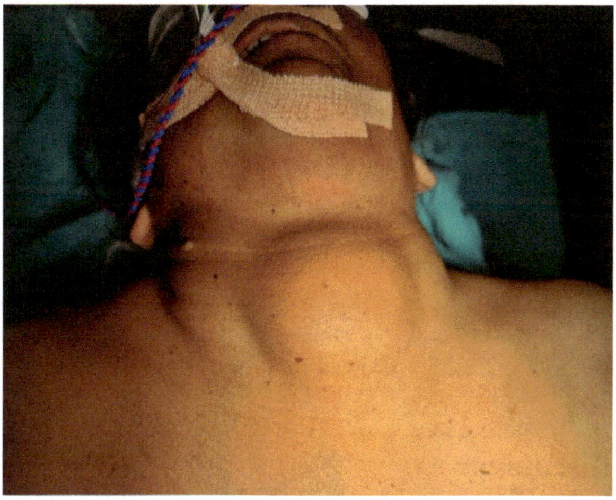

Fig. 3 Clinical picture (Patient intubated with neuromonitoring tube)

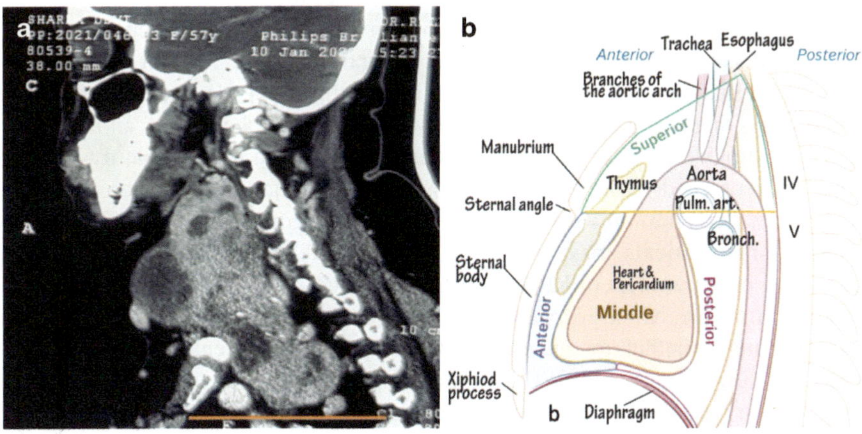

Fig. 4 (**a**) CT sagittal section of a patient with orange line drawn at level of sternal angle, (**b**) Image showing various divisions with corresponding yellow line at sternal angle

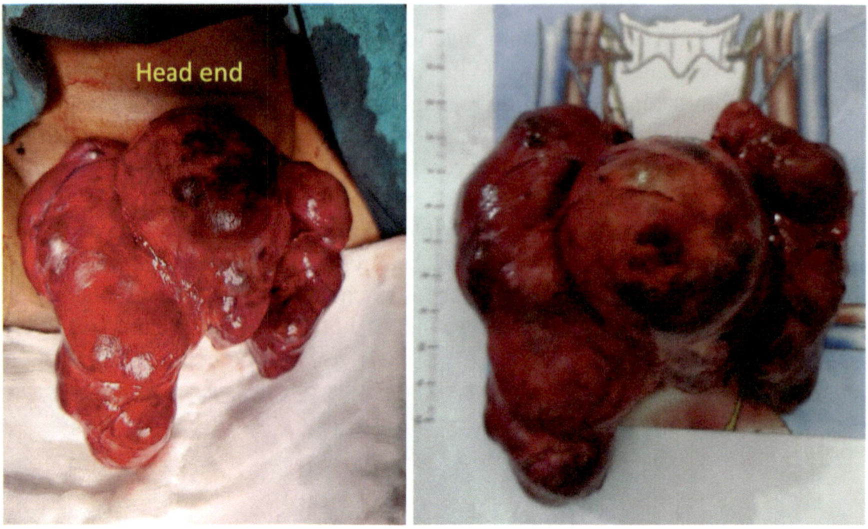

Fig. 5 Post-operative specimen weighing 500 g

of the tumor by cervical incision. Total thyroidectomy was planned with cionm. Specimen weighed 500 g (Fig. 5). Post-operative recovery was smooth. The patient developed clinical hypocalcemia and was managed with oral calcium and vitamin D. Histopathology showed multinodular goiter.

Discussion

Commonly accepted definitions are: All goiters with a lower pole lying below the thoracic inlet, those goiters in which at least 50% of the thyroid mass is below the thoracic inlet, those goiters whose lower border radiographically reaches the transverse process of the fourth thoracic vertebrae and those with a major intrathoracic component that required reaching into the mediastinum [1]. Six to forty percentage are asymptomatic and incidentally discovered on plain chest films and 20–30% have no palpable cervical goiter [2]. Patients may give a history that dyspnea or cough is worsened by some positions such as lying flat or rolling on one side. Sometimes the symptoms resulting from substernal goiters mimic those of bronchial asthma. Patients may also have pre-operative RLN palsy resulting from stretching or entrapment of RLN. At times hoarseness may be present in spite of a functioning nerve, hence every attempt should be made to preserve the nerve. It has been debated whether to operate upon asymptomatic patients harboring retrosternal goiter. Patients with RSG may develop acute airway obstruction. A delay in diagnosis or treatment changed the grading of the retrosternal mass - from grade I (those extending nearly to the arch of the aorta) to grade II (those extending to the arch of the aorta or beyond). Alfonso et al. [3] recommended early surgery when radiographic signs of tracheal deviation became evident. The authors observed tracheal or esophageal compression in 90 (33%) of 273 consecutive patients with benign goiter. Newman et al. [4] reported that out of a group of 120 patients with airway compression secondary to goiters, 30 (25%) patients presented with acute airway distress requiring either intubation or semi-emergent surgery. The authors also made a strong case for surgical decompression even if the patient was asymptomatic, because 50% compression of their trachea may not cause symptoms but further compression can be catastrophic. Also, postoperative morbidity is more common in patients undergoing substernal goiter resection and morbidity rates for substernal goiter resection range from 4% to 12% in the literature and include: recurrent laryngeal nerve injury, hypoparathyroidism, and airway complications such as neck hematoma and prolonged intubation. A study by Khan et al. [5] demonstrated that a trans-thoracic approach is associated with increased rates of several critical postoperative morbidities, and the data indicate the potential of increased overall mortality. Thus all retrosternal goiters whether asymptomatic should be treated with early surgery rather than having it run the risk of acute airway distress. A review study by McKenzie et al. [6] describes the risk factors for sternal split to include: history of goiter with retrosternal extension beyond 160 months, increased thyroid tissue density, posterior Mediastinal location, and subcarinal extension. It is often not just the size that predicts need for sternotomy but the shape of retrosternal portion of goiter; iceberg, hourglass, and dumb-bell shape or discontinuity of the gland that is important. Thyroid tissue density has been described as the strongest predictor of need for sternotomy. CT can predict the need for sternotomy by documenting the extent, shape and density of the retrosternal portion [7, 8]. Sternotomy, either partial or total split, is required only in 2–8% of cases. Thus, in conclusion, early surgical removal of asymptomatic RSG by an experienced endocrine or thyroid surgeon is to be done with a surgical team familiar with sternotomy at stand-by.

References

1. Lin Y-s, Wu H-Y, Lee C-W, Hsu C-C, Chao T-C, Yu M-C. Surgical management of substernal goitres at a tertiary referral centre: a retrospective cohort study of 2,104 patients. Int J Surg. 2016;27:46–52.
2. Wax MK, Briant TDR. Management of substernal goitre. J Otolaryngol. 1992;21:165–70.
3. Alfonso A, Christoudias G, Amaruddin Q, Herbsman H, Gardner B. Tracheal or oesophageal compression due to benign thyroid disease. Am J Surg. 1981;142:350–4.
4. Newman E, Shaha AR. Substernal goitre. J Surg Oncol. 1995;60:207–12.
5. Khan MN, Goljo E, Owen R, Park RCW, Yao M, Miles BA. Retrosternal Goiter: 30-day morbidity and mortality in the Transcervical and transthoracic approaches. Otolaryngol Head Neck Surg. 2016;155(4):568–74.
6. McKenzie GA, Rook W. Is it possible to predict the need for sternotomy in patients undergoing thyroidectomy with retrosternal extension? Interact Cardiovasc Thorac Surg. 2014;19:139–43.
7. Sarı S, Erbil Y, Ersoz F, Sarıcam G, Salmasloglu A, Issever H, Ozarmagan S. Predictive value of thyroid tissue density in determining the patients on whom sternotomy should be performed. J Surg Res. 2012;174(2):312–8.
8. Shen WT, Kebebew E, Duh QY, Clark OH. Predictors of airway complications after thyroidectomy for substernal goiter. Arch Surg. 2004;139:656–9.

Retrosternal Goiter Treated by Partial Sternotomy

Case

A 40-year-old lady presented with a history of anterior neck swelling for 20 years with a history of breathlessness on lying down but no complaints of dysphagia or change in the character of voice. On examination, she had a diffuse goiter 4 cm × 3 cm whose lower border was not palpable. X-ray chest revealed mediastinal widening. Hence with suspicion of retrosternal extension CECT was done. CECT thorax showed a large well-defined lobulated heterogeneously enhancing mass measuring 8.2 × 4.8 × 11.8 cm involving the right lobe and isthmus of thyroid (Fig. 1) and extending inferiorly into the mediastinum up to the level of T4/5 intervertebral disc with retrosternal extension of approximately 4.7 cm; lesion is seen extending across the midline and displacing left carotid vessels left laterally (Fig. 2). In view of extension of retrosternal portion beyond aortic arch, partial sternotomy was planned. At operation right lobe of thyroid was found to be enlarged and crossing midline to the left extending below the Brachiocephalic vein for about 6 cm (Fig. 3a). The specimen weighed 225 g and measured: RL-10 cm × 6 cm × 5 cm; LL-2 cm × 1 cm × 1 cm. HPE: multi-nodular goiter. Post operative picture of the patient seen in Fig. 3b.

Amit Agarwal is the lead author of this chapter.

A. Agarwal et al., *Case Studies in Thyroid and Parathyroid Tumors*,
https://doi.org/10.1007/978-981-99-0938-4_60

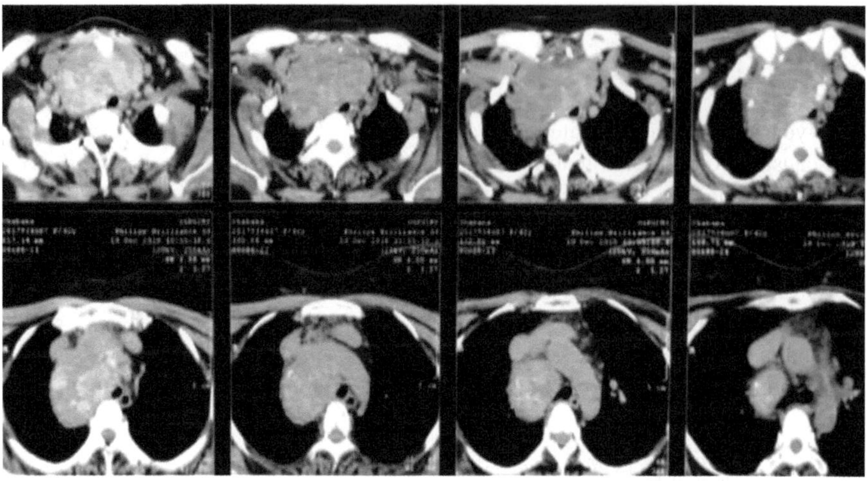

Fig. 1 Non-contrast CT neck and upper thorax axial sections showing a large isodense mass lesion with internal foci of calcification epicentered in lower neck with extension into superior mediastinum abutting the mediastinal great vessels and trachea and right bronchus

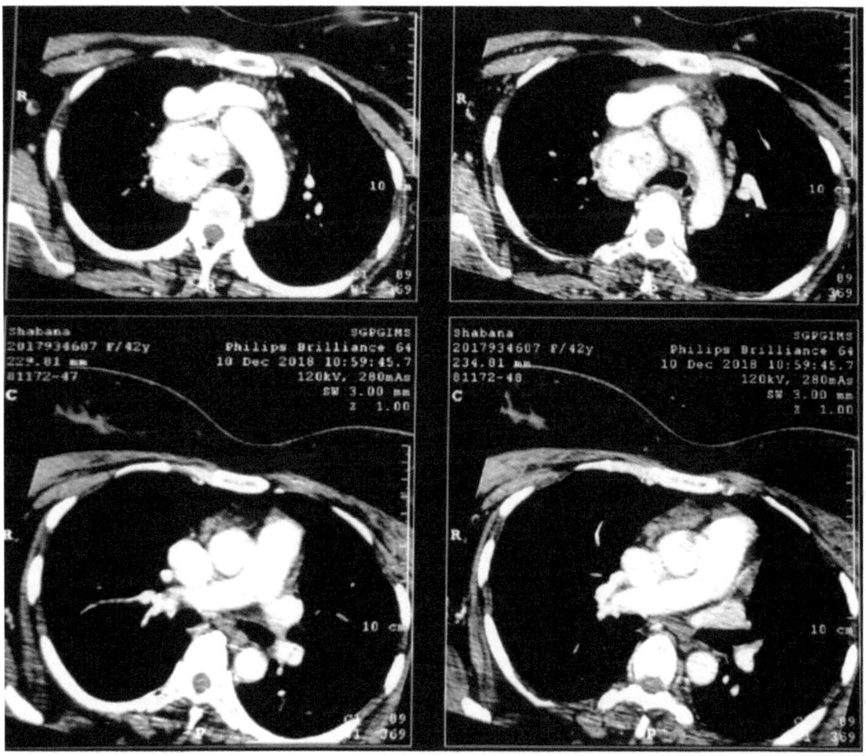

Fig. 2 Contrast-enhanced ct thorax in axial sections showing lower most extent of the mass lesion in mediastinum as avidly enhancing lesion with central necrosis abutting arch of aorta, svc and reaching up to the level of carina

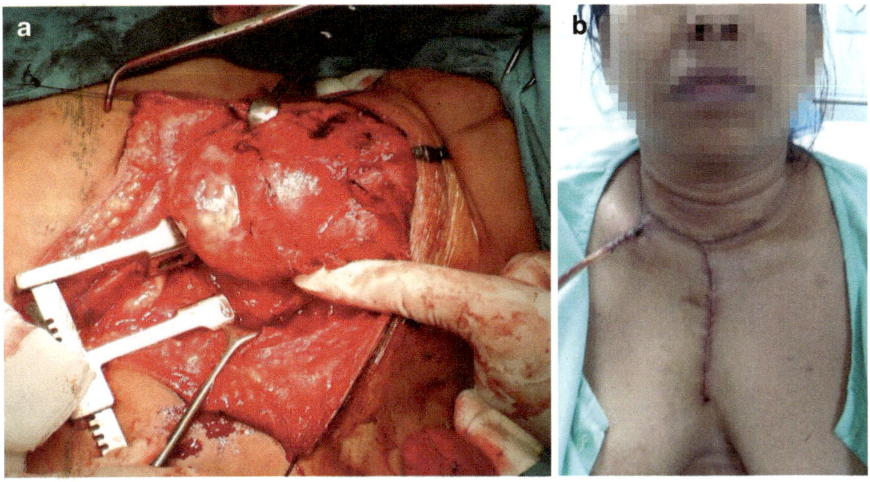

Fig. 3 (**a**) Intra-operative view after manubriotomy. (**b**) Post-operative wound closure

Discussion

Surgery remains the most effective treatment for symptomatic patients of retrosternal goiter, with most retrosternal goiters safely removed through a cervical incision. The cervical approach can be utilized in the majority of cases [1]; however, it may increase the inherent risks of surgery due to poor access in cases which extend beyond aortic arch. For these cases where the cervical approach is not adequate, 'intrathoracic' approaches have been employed, including manubriotomy, full sternotomy, and lateral thoracotomy. In the classification proposed by Huins et al. [2] retrosternal goiters reaching beyond aortic arch can safely be removed via a manubriotomy, thus avoiding the full sternotomy and its morbidity. Manubriotomy is especially useful for cases which extend below the aortic arch and up to the pericardium. Manubriotomy, or full sternotomy, have many advantages over lateral thoracotomy. They have been proven in cardiac surgery to employ an incision that can be performed quickly, reliably and with very low morbidity, providing excellent mediastinal exposure to allow delivery of the retrosternal portion of the gland. Moreover, it can be performed without having to reposition the patient. The use of a lateral thoracotomy would seem unnecessary since an RSG is essentially a midline structure and hence should be easily approached via a midline incision. However, full sternotomy may increase the hospital stay and has potential for leading to increased morbidity.

References

1. Monchik JM, Marerazzi G. The necessity for a thoracic approach in thyroid surgery. Arch Surg. 2000;135(4):467e71. [discussion, 471e2].
2. Huins CT, Georgalas C, Mehrzad H, Tolley NS. A new classification system for retrosternal goitre based on a systematic review of its complications and management. Int J Surg. 2008;6:71–6.

Retrosternal Goiter Treated by Tracheal Stenting

Case

An 80-year-old frail lady presented to us with a history of progressively increasing breathlessness for 3 months and stridor ×7 days. She had been evaluated under Cardiology for rest pain and evaluated on lines of Acute Coronary Syndrome/ NSEMI, Angiography was normal but the patient was found to have a substernal mass with external compression over trachea. On examination there was a 3 × 3 cm nodule palpable in the region of the left lobe of thyroid gland without cervical LAP. CT Neck and Thorax showed both lobes of thyroid had multiple heterogeneously enhancing nodules with coarse calcification and severe luminal narrowing of trachea (Fig 1) and deviation towards the right side with mediastinal extension up to D3. The patient presented with unacceptable surgical risk (Fig 2) and was referred to a pulmonologist for the possibility of tracheal stenting. They performed rigid bronchoscopy which revealed >70% tracheal narrowing due to external compression and narrowing extended from 2.8 cm distal to the vocal cord. Stenting Y-Shaped Silicon stent No. 18 was put without any procedure-related complication (Fig 3). There was a significant improvement in stridor. At follow-up of 6 months the patient is well without any episode of stridor or airway compromise.

Amit Agarwal is the lead author of this chapter.

A. Agarwal et al., *Case Studies in Thyroid and Parathyroid Tumors*,
https://doi.org/10.1007/978-981-99-0938-4_61

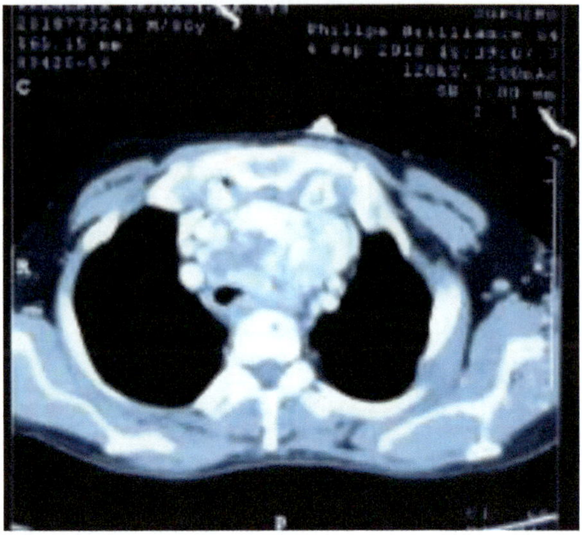

Fig. 1 CECT thorax showing massive retrosternal goiter with severe tracheal stenosis

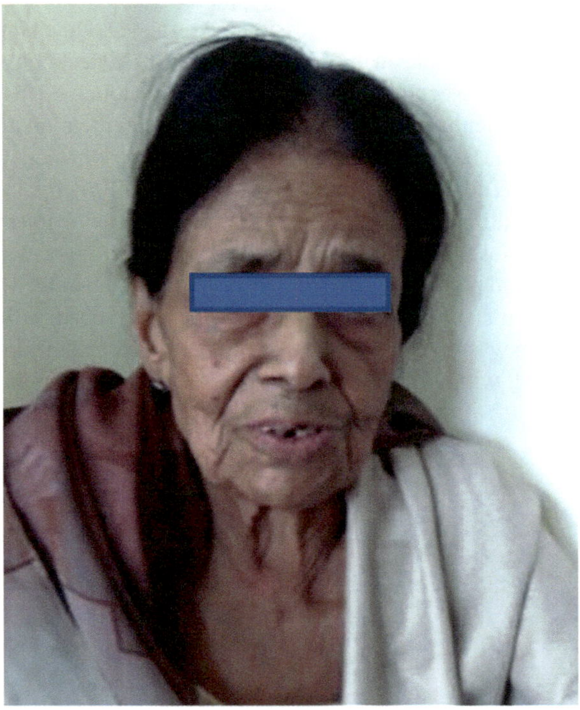

Fig. 2 Frail lady with retrosternal goiter with unacceptable surgical risk

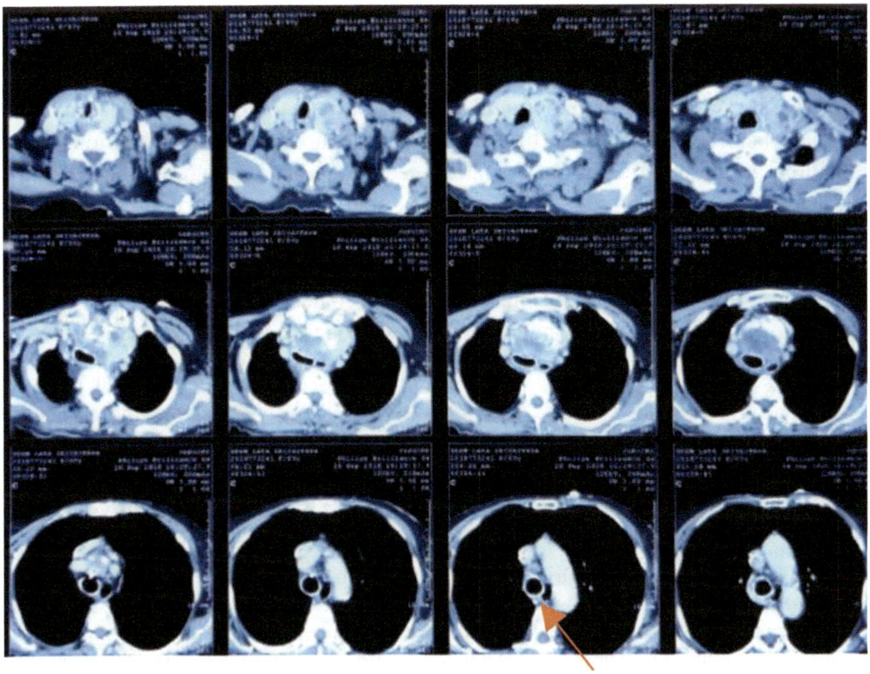

Fig. 3 Silicone endo-luminal stent in the trachea (arrow)

Discussion

Chronic obstructive airway disease, retrosternal extension, and long-standing goiter were found to be associated with the development of acute, life-threatening airway compromise in patients with benign thyroid disease. Tracheal compromise leading to significant airway compromise in patients with large goiters or retrosternal goiters is a serious situation which can lead to sudden asphyxia and death. Acute airway compromise is best treated by endotracheal intubation if patients fail conservative measures, followed by emergency thyroidectomy. Though surgical removal, either by cervical delivery or via a sternotomy relieves the patient of the airway compromise there may be certain situations where immediate surgery may not be possible. Stent placement with acceptable complications is a viable option for severe tracheal stenosis by massive retrosternal goiter especially for those who cannot be operated [1]. In such patients, this procedure may be the final or even optimal solution offering stable short-term or long-term airway stability. In other patients who are candidates for surgery, stent placement acts a bridge to tide over the crisis till thyroidectomy is successfully done [2]. Placement of endoluminal stent offers a rapid and effective means of airway patency, thereby leading to dramatic improvement of symptoms and pulmonary function [3]. It has been shown that after placement of the tracheobronchial stent, dramatic improvements of life-threatening dyspnea in 70–100% of patients with airway stenosis can be achieved immediately [4]. However, one should be aware of the complications of airway stent that have been reported in 20% of patients [5]. The most common and serious complications are granulation tissue formation, secretion obstruction, migration, malposition, infection, slippage, and bleeding [6]. As sputum retention or copious secretion can be life-threatening the selection of stents that are less prone to sputum retention definitely seems advantageous. It has been reported that there is low incidence (4%) of sputum retention on metallic stents internally coated with silicone [7]. Thus, an endoscopically inserted silicone endoprosthesis may be a valid alternative to surgery for tracheal obstruction due to retrosternal goiter in patients in whom surgery represents an unacceptable risk.

References

1. Kadhim AL, Sheahan P, Timon C. Management of life-threatening airway obstruction caused by benign thyroid disease. J Laryngol Otol. 2006;120:1038–41.
2. Piao M, Yuan Y, Wang Y, Feng C. Successful management of trachea stenosis with massive substernal goiter via thacheobronchial stent. J Cardiothorac Surg. 2013;8:212.
3. Badr EM, Osama YD. The role of endoluminal self-expanding stents in the management of pediatric tracheal stenosis. Int J Pediatr Otorhinolaryngol. 2008;72:1371–6.
4. Saad CP, Murthy S, Krizmanich G, Mehta AC. Self-expandable metallic airway stents and flexible bronchoscopy: long-term outcomes analysis. Chest. 2003;124:1993–9.
5. Tanigawa N, Sawada S, Okuda Y, Kobayashi M, et al. Symptomatic improvement in dyspnea following tracheobronchial metallic stenting for malignant airway obstruction. Acta Radiol. 2000;41:425–8.
6. Francisco VM, Stephanie MA, Ricardo LC. Endoscopically placed expandable metal tracheal stents for the management of complicated tracheal stenosis. Am J Otolaryngol. 2003;24:34.
7. Kim WK, Shin JH, Kim JH, Song JW, et al. Management of tracheal obstruction caused by benign or malignant thyroid disease using covered retrievable self-expandable nitinol stents. Acta Radiol. 2010;51(7):768–74.

Post-thyroidectomy Tracheomalacia in Large Goiters

Case A 50-year-old post-menopausal lady presented with complaints of rapid growth for 1 year in her neck swelling (Fig. 1) which was there for 25 years. She also gave a history of exertional breathlessness for 4 years and noisy breathing for 1 year which is increasing in severity. She also gave a history of change in voice for 1 year. On examination, there was a large multilobulated thyroid swelling in the anterior aspect of the neck extending from submandibular region, and ear lobule to supra sternal notch, laterally extending beyond bilateral SCM with restricted mobility. Trachea was not palpable. Imaging revealed severe tracheal deviation and compression (Fig. 2). She underwent total thyroidectomy after a fiber optic intubation. At operation following thyroid removal tracheal collapse was observed and with confirmation of tracheomalacia, tracheostomy was done. Post-operatively she developed symptomatic hypocalcemia and was managed with intravenous calcium followed by oral calcium and active vitamin D supplements. The operative specimen weighed 500 gm and HPE (Fig. 3) was reported as benign multinodular goiter. Tracheostomy tube was removed on the seventh post-operative day. At the time of discharge, she had no symptoms of respiratory distress and her tracheostomy opening has been covered with an occlusive dressing.

Amit Agarwal is the lead author of this chapter.

A. Agarwal et al., *Case Studies in Thyroid and Parathyroid Tumors*,
https://doi.org/10.1007/978-981-99-0938-4_62

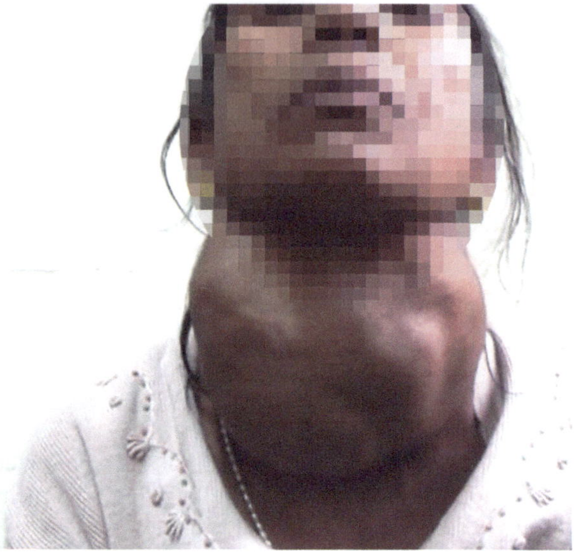

Fig. 1 Pre-operative picture of large goiter

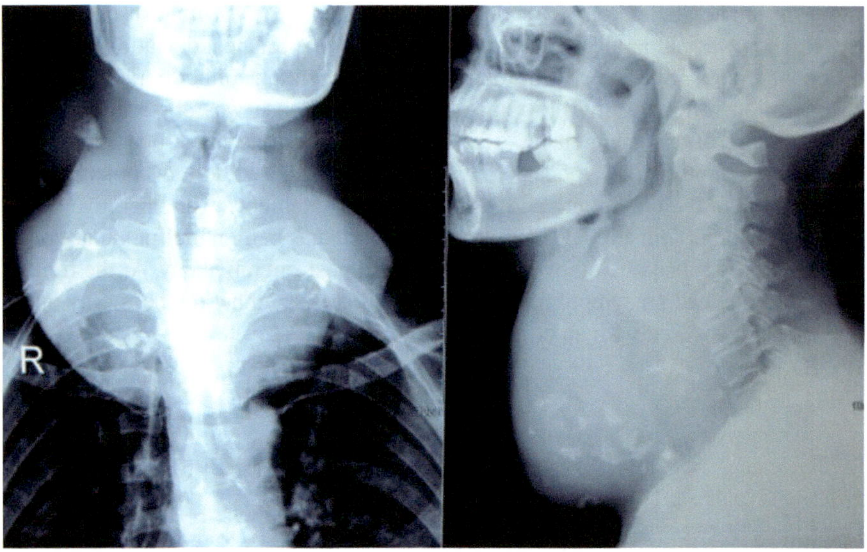

Fig. 2 Plain x-ray neck showing airway compression and deviation

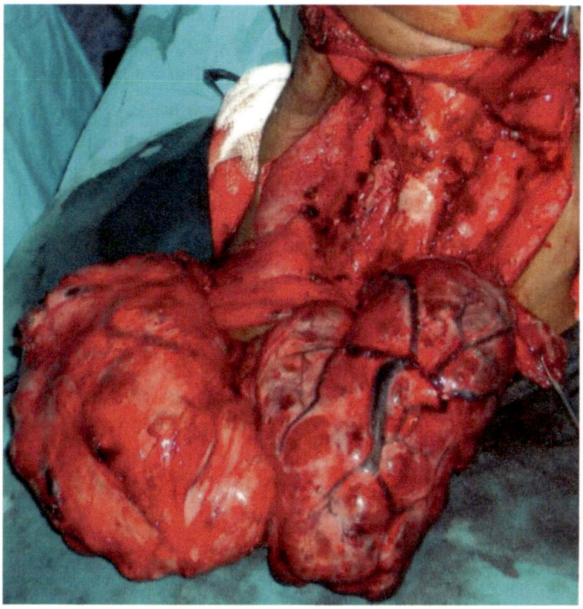

Fig. 3 Operative view of collapsed trachea following thyroidectomy

Discussion

Post-thyroidectomy tracheomalacia is a rare but life-threatening complication. It results from longstanding compression by a large goiter or thyroid cancer wherein the cartilaginous rings of the trachea are considerably weakened or destroyed, leading to softening and floppiness of the trachea. Such a trachea is prone to collapse after the external compression is relieved by thyroidectomy, resulting in postoperative airway compromise. Usually happens where the cross-sectional area of the trachea is reduced to less than half. The incidence of tracheomalacia has been reported to vary widely from 0% to 10.3% in the literature likely because of differences in the subjective perception of a soft trachea by each surgeon [1, 2]. A question often asked is can we predict tracheomalacia? There has been considerable debate about possible risk factors for the development of tracheomalacia and whether they can be sought preoperatively. Clinical findings thought to be associated with tracheomalacia are a preoperative history of stridor, radiological evidence of tracheal deviation or compression, retrosternal goiter, and difficulty in intubation by the anesthetist. It is worth noting that the absence of airway symptoms preoperatively does not necessarily spare the patient any postoperative respiratory problems. However, ease of Intubation is unrelated to the extent of abnormalities seen on imaging studies of the neck. The typical manifestation of post-thyroidectomy tracheomalacia is acute postoperative stridor and airway compromise that cannot be explained by any other cause. It is usually accompanied by a barking cough and expiratory stridor or wheezing. Patients with severe tracheal collapse are unable to maintain arterial oxygen saturation, even with the increasing fractionated inspired oxygen concentration

(FiO_2). When this is the case, immediate postoperative re-intubation or tracheostomy is necessary, measures that quickly relieve the respiratory distress. At operation, one should document the following: Identification of RLN, complete hemostasis, and evidence of tracheomalacia. There is no consistent criterion for confirming a diagnosis of post-thyroidectomy tracheomalacia in the literature, although many reports describe it as a softening and floppiness of the trachea. Worth noting is the subjective nature of a "soft trachea." Patients with some extent of soft trachea might be diagnosed intra-operatively as having tracheomalacia and thus kept intubated postoperatively. Another surgeon may see a similar case as insignificant, and this difference in diagnosis represents the potential statistical error introduced by varying sensitivity for each surgeon. There is no single foolproof criterion for confirming a diagnosis of tracheomalacia. However, for the intra-operative diagnosis of tracheomalacia, we have taken one or more of the following criteria: (1) Soft and floppy trachea on palpation by the surgeon at the end of thyroidectomy. However, because of the splinting effect of the endotracheal tube in situ, it may be difficult to appreciate a soft trachea. We therefore ask the anesthesiologist to gradually withdraw the tube for a short distance and then feel the trachea without the tube in site. This maneuver may also help the surgeon recognize an obvious collapse of the tracheal wall. (2) fiber-optic inspection of trachea to see collapse [3]. (3) Obstruction to spontaneous respiration during gradual withdrawal of the ETT after thyroidectomy. (4) Difficulty in negotiating the suction catheter beyond the ETT after gradual withdrawal. (5) After closure of the wound, tracheomalacia can be suspected: if there is absence of peritubal leak on deflation of ETT cuff, volume pressure loop on ventilator or development of respiratory stridor along with falling hemoglobin oxygen saturation (SpO_2) on pulse oximetry despite the administration of increasing FiO_2. The management of post-thyroidectomy tracheomalacia has not been standardized because of the rarity of the condition. Proposed approaches to management are diverse, including: tracheostomy, prolonged endotracheal intubation [4], tracheopexy, internal stent, and external splinting with Marlex mesh. Most published studies are case reports or small case series. Among the various options offered, tracheostomy is recommended by many authors. Another recent option suggested is the use of noninvasive positive pressure ventilation with bi-level positive airway pressure mode delivering positive airway pressure both during inspiratory and expiratory phases [5]. It is a widely accepted treatment of acute respiratory failure that does not require emergent intubation, and is used mostly for patients with chronic obstructive pulmonary disease or cardiogenic pulmonary edema. It is also used as a means of auxiliary respiratory support after extubation to prevent post-extubation respiratory failure in patients with chronic respiratory disorders. The rapid improvement in respiratory function in such cases is most likely due to the positive airway pressure that props up the softened trachea and decreases the work of breathing. Because stridor and airway compromise develop soon after removal of the endotracheal tube, we recommend that NPPV is offered without delay following extubation. Noninvasive positive pressure ventilation is generally safe. Most complications are local and related to the tightly fitting mask. Local skin damage may occur as a result of the pressure effect of the mask and straps. This can be easily avoided by cushioning the patient's forehead and the bridge of the nose prior to attaching the mask. Leakage around the mask is common and can be managed by changing the mask or ventilator settings. Eye irritation, sinus pain, or sinus congestion may occur and require either a lower inspiratory pressure or use of a face mask rather than a nasal mask. Mild gastric distention occurs frequently, but is rarely clinically significant at usual levels of inspiratory pressure; routine use of a nasogastric tube is not warranted.

References

1. Green WE, Shepperd HW, Stevenson HM, et al. Tracheal collapse after thyroidectomy. Br J Surg. 1979;66:554.
2. Agarwal A, Mishra AK, Gupta SK, Arshad F, Agarwal A, Tripathi M, Singh PK. Tracheomalacia in longstanding goiters. World J Surg. 2007;31:832–7.
3. Palazzo FF, Allen JG, Greatorex RA. Laryngeal mask airway and fibre-optic tracheal inspection in thyroid surgery: a method for timely identification of tracheomalacia requiring tracheostomy. Ann R Coll Surg Engl. 2000;82(2):141–2.
4. Singh B, Lucente FE, Shaha AR. Substernal goiter: a clinical review. Am J Otolaryngol. 1994;15:409.
5. Chi SY, Wu SC, Hsieh KC, Sheen-Chen SM, Chou FF. Noninvasive positive pressure ventilation in the management of post-thyroidectomy tracheomalacia. World J Surg. 2011;35(9):1977–83.

Surgery Under Local Anaesthesia

Case

A frail 75-year-old female was referred to the endocrine surgery clinic for discussion of surgical management of her biochemically proven primary hyperparathyroidism (PHPT). She was found to have osteoporosis on a bone mineral density assessment (BMD; T: −3.8), conducted after a fracture of her left humerus. Her adjusted calcium was 2.71 mmol/L, with a parathyroid hormone (PTH) of 13.2 pmol/L. Her calcium:creatinine clearance ratio was 0.0413, excluding familial hypocalciuric hypercalcemia (FHH). She subsequently underwent dual localization studies. Her Technetium 99 m Sestamibi (MIBI) revealed a MIBI-avid focus at the lower pole of the right thyroid lobe, in keeping with a parathyroid lesion (Fig. 1a). Her ultrasound scan (US) confirmed this as a parathyroid adenoma measuring 1.7 in largest diameter was noted, inferior to the right thyroid lobe (Fig. 1b).

The patient was counseled for surgical treatment, in the form of a focused parathyroidectomy. However, she was found to be unfit for general anesthesia, due to her various comorbidity. Therefore, a decision for surgery under local anesthesia was made. On the day of surgery, she underwent US-guided skin marking of the location of the lesion. In the operating theatre, she was given a combination of a very mild sedation, monitored by the anesthesia team, as well as a unilateral superficial cervical plexus block, by using 20 mL of 0.25% bupivacaine, and infiltration of the incision site, by using 2 mL of 1% lidocaine with 1:200,000 adrenaline. Via a small incision (2.5 cm), and using the lateral approach, the left inferior parathyroid gland was visualized and deemed to be enlarged, at about 1.6 cm in size (Fig. 2). This gland was removed, and the intra-operative PTH (ioPTH) dropped sufficiently (i.e., pre-excision ioPTH 13.3 pmol/L to post-excision ioPTH 3.1 pmol/L).

The patient recovered very well from the procedure, and although she was medically fit to be discharged on the same day, she spent one night in the hospital due to

---

Rajeev Parameswaran is the lead author of this chapter.

A. Agarwal et al., *Case Studies in Thyroid and Parathyroid Tumors*,
https://doi.org/10.1007/978-981-99-0938-4_63

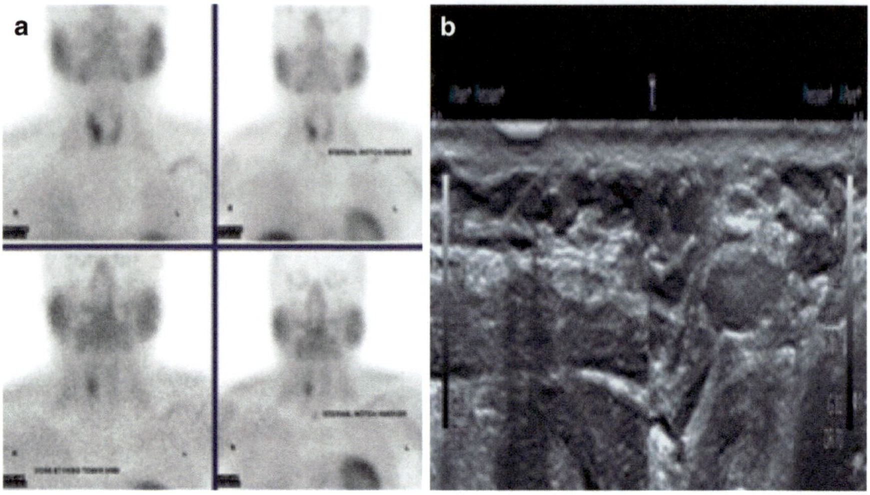

Fig. 1 (**a**) MIBI-avid focus at the lower pole of the right thyroid lobe. (**b**) Ultrasound scan (US) confirmed this as a parathyroid adenoma

Fig. 2 Operative specimen

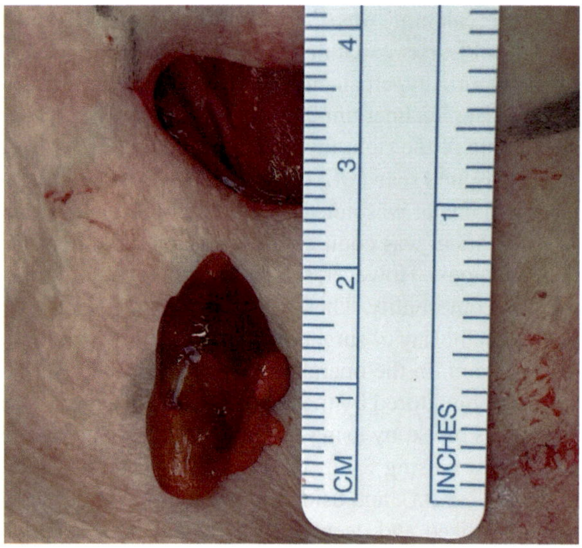

social circumstances. Her histology report described a parathyroid gland measuring 1.5 × 1.0 × 0.8 cm and weighing 0.8 g, with features compatible with a parathyroid adenoma. During her post-operative clinic visit, she was doing well and had no issues regarding her scar or voice. Her adjusted calcium measured 2.42 mmol/L, with a PTH 1.4 pmol/L, and she remains under follow-up by our endocrine medicine department who are managing her osteoporosis.

Discussion

When the procedure of a parathyroidectomy was first performed in 1925, this was done as an open, bilateral neck exploration using a sizeable incision. Currently, the first-choice treatment for parathyroid tumors localized on pre-operative imaging is a more focused approach, by means of a minimally invasive parathyroidectomy (MIP) [1, 2]. Apart from having a smaller scar, other advantages of this technique include lower cost, [3] shorter operating time, [4, 5] shorter stay in hospital, [2, 5] and improved patient satisfaction [6]. Most MIPs are performed under general anesthesia (GA), but the use of local anesthesia (LA) has been described and noted to have good outcomes [7–9].

Ambulatory parathyroidectomy has been in practice since the 1990s [10], but not many surgeons feel comfortable or appropriate for their cohort of patients. It has been reported that performance of MIP under LA is not only safe, with a similar rate of complications to performance under GA, but that it is also similarly effective in terms of achieving cure, even without the use of intra-operative PTH (ioPTH) [11]. This technique could particularly enable the performance of parathyroid surgery on elderly patients or those at too high a risk for GA [12]. Patient selection is therefore very important and treated in centers where ambulatory surgical practice is well established to ensure pathways for treating such patients. Patient selection criteria for MIPLA are highlighted in Table 1.

Different protocols are available, [9, 13] all require specific tailoring to both patient and local, institutional, requirements. It generally involves a combination of mild sedation (e.g., by intravenous remifentanil/propofol) and monitored anesthesia care, as well as regional anesthesia. The LA includes both a unilateral superficial cervical plexus block (e.g., by using 20 mL of 0.25% bupivacaine), as well as intra-operative infiltration of the surgical site after US-guided marking of the skin (e.g., by using 2 mL of 1% lidocaine with 1:200,000 adrenaline) [11]. This enables for employment of the lateral approach [14]. Some surgeons prefer to use a midline approach for lower parathyroids and lateral approach for superior parathyroids. However, a lateral approach may give the added advantage of exploring the parathyroids along the length of the thyroid and in a more posterior position.

Table 1 Patient selection criteria for MIPLA

Criteria for selection of patients for MIPLA
Confirmed hyperparathyroidism
Solitary adenoma on imaging
Concordant imaging or MIBI strongly suggestive of single gland disease
Previous neck surgery or thyroid disease requiring surgery
Favorable anatomy of the neck (avoid in short neck or where extension not possible)
Patients not on any anticoagulants
No known allergies to local anesthesia
No history of confusion or dementia in patient
Safe to be discharged (with someone to look after at home or place of residence)
Availability of IoPTH to ensure cure

Table 2 Published series showing failure rates and complications

Study (Reference)	No of patients	Cure	Complications
Benhami et al. (2018) [17]	129	98%	Persistent (5.4%) Recurrence (4.6%) Conversion (5%)
Sen et al. (2019) [22]	30	100% (6 months)	Conversion (6.7%) Temporary RLNP (3%)
Rajeev et al. (2013) [11]	85	100% (6 months)	None
Bergenfelz et al. (2005) [23]	25	–	Conversion (12%) Temporary RLNP (4%)
Shindo et al. (2008) [8]	186	99% (6 months)	Conversion (9.5%) Pneumothorax (1%) Temporary RLNP (0.5%) Hematoma (0.5%)
Cohen et al. (2005) [24]	239	98.6%	Conversion 3%

MIPLA is not a procedure without complications. Failure rates and complications vary between the cohorts but generally range between 0% and 10% (Table 2). A crucial factor is the experience of surgeon and there is clear evidence to suggest the fact that surgeons who performed more than 100 parathyroid surgeries per year had the highest rate of ambulatory surgery and lowest complication rates [15]. Conversion to an open procedure ranges between 0% and 10% and the rates may be smaller if localization is accurate [16]. Long-term cure reported in the literature with MIP is around 98% to 99% [11, 17]. Recurrences or persistent disease seen with MIP is around 2.5% to 8% in comparison to 1.9% seen in open parathyroidectomy [18, 19]. There is no statistical difference between MIPLA and open parathyroidectomy in terms of risk of recurrent laryngeal nerve palsy (0.1% vs 1.9%) [16] or hematoma [20, 21].

References

1. Sackett WR, et al. Worldwide trends in the surgical treatment of primary hyperparathyroidism in the era of minimally invasive parathyroidectomy. Arch Surg. 2002;137(9):1055–9.
2. Mihai R, et al. Minimally invasive parathyroidectomy without intraoperative parathyroid hormone monitoring in patients with primary hyperparathyroidism. Br J Surg. 2007;94(1):42–7.
3. Goldstein RE, et al. Effect of minimally invasive radioguided parathyroidectomy on efficacy, length of stay, and costs in the management of primary hyperparathyroidism. Ann Surg. 2000;231(5):732–42.
4. Palazzo FF, Sadler GP. Minimally invasive parathyroidectomy. BMJ. 2004;328(7444):849–50.
5. Udelsman R. Surgery in primary hyperparathyroidism: the patient without previous neck surgery. J Bone Miner Res. 2002;17(Suppl 2):N126–32.
6. Burkey SH, et al. Will directed parathyroidectomy utilizing the gamma probe or intraoperative parathyroid hormone assay replace bilateral cervical exploration as the preferred operation for primary hyperparathyroidism? World J Surg. 2002;26(8):914–20.
7. Miccoli P. Parathyroid surgery: we only need a minimal surgical approach. J Endocrinol Investig. 2005;28(6):570–3.

8. Shindo ML, Rosenthal JM, Lee T. Minimally invasive parathyroidectomy using local anesthesia with intravenous sedation and targeted approaches. Otolaryngol Head Neck Surg. 2008;138(3):381–7.
9. Rajeev P, et al. Safety and efficacy of minimally-invasive parathyroidectomy (MIP) under local anaesthesia without intra-operative PTH measurement. Int J Surg. 2013;11(3):275–7.
10. Chen H, Sokoll LJ, Udelsman R. Outpatient minimally invasive parathyroidectomy: a combination of sestamibi-SPECT localization, cervical block anesthesia, and intraoperative parathyroid hormone assay. Surgery. 1999;126(6):1016–22.
11. Rajeev P, et al. Safety and efficacy of minimally-invasive parathyroidectomy (MIP) under local anaesthesia without intra-operative PTH measurement. Int J Surg (Lond, Engl). 2013;11(3):275–7.
12. Fang WL, et al. The management of high-risk patients with primary hyperparathyroidism - minimally invasive parathyroidectomy vs. medical treatment. Clin Endocrinol. 2008;68(4):520–8.
13. Sen S, et al. Focused parathyroidectomy under local anesthesia - a feasibility study. Ind J Endocrinol Metab. 2019;23(1):67–71.
14. Agarwal G, et al. Minimally invasive parathyroidectomy using the 'focused' lateral approach II. Surgical technique. ANZ J Surg. 2002;72(2):147–51.
15. Stavrakis AI, et al. Surgeon volume as a predictor of outcomes in inpatient and outpatient endocrine surgery. Surgery. 2007;142(6):887–99.
16. Schneider DF, et al. Is minimally invasive parathyroidectomy associated with greater recurrence compared to bilateral exploration? Analysis of more than 1,000 cases. Surgery. 2012;152(6):1008–15.
17. Benhami A, et al. Ambulatory surgery under local anesthesia for parathyroid adenoma: feasibility and outcome. J Visc Surg. 2018;155(4):253–8.
18. Chapuis Y, et al. Values of ultrasonography, sestamibi scintigraphy, and intraoperative measurement of 1-84 PTH for unilateral neck exploration of primary hyperparathyroidism. World J Surg. 1996;20(7):835–40.
19. Norman J, Lopez J, Politz D. Abandoning unilateral parathyroidectomy: why we reversed our position after 15,000 parathyroid operations. J Am Coll Surg. 2012;214(3):260–9.
20. Bergenfelz A, et al. Unilateral versus bilateral neck exploration for primary hyperparathyroidism: a prospective randomized controlled trial. Ann Surg. 2002;236(5):543.
21. Westerdahl J, Bergenfelz A. Unilateral versus bilateral neck exploration for primary hyperparathyroidism: five-year follow-up of a randomized controlled trial. Ann Surg. 2007;246(6):976–81.
22. Sen S, et al. Focused parathyroidectomy under local anesthesia - a feasibility study. Indian J Endocrinol Metabol. 2019;23(1):67–71.
23. Bergenfelz A, et al. Conventional bilateral cervical exploration versus open minimally invasive parathyroidectomy under local anaesthesia for primary hyperparathyroidism. Br J Surg. 2005;92(2):190–7.
24. Cohen MS, et al. Outpatient minimally invasive parathyroidectomy using local/regional anesthesia: a safe and effective operative approach for selected patients. Discussion. New York, NY: Elsevier; 2005.

Stridor Following Thyroidectomy

Case

A 67-year-old woman presented with recurrent nodular goiter with hyperthyroidism with a history of having had a subtotal thyroidectomy in 1997 and redo-completion surgery in 2002. Preoperative nasoendoscopy revealed normally functioning cords and her thyroid function tests showed subclinical hyperthyroidism at the time of surgery. Computed tomography (CT) of the neck showed a large compressive goiter with an aberrant right subclavian artery (Fig. 1a, b). This raised the possibility of a nonrecurrent laryngeal nerve (NRLN).

She underwent surgery under general anesthesia and intraoperative neuromonitoring. The larger left lobe was tackled first and showed an intact recurrent laryngeal nerve (RLN) at the end of the procedure.

A nonrecurrent laryngeal nerve was tracked on the left side but previous 2 thyroidectomies made it difficult to isolate the nerve at the superior pole of the recurrence, which resulted in inadvertent injury. Ansa to RLN anastomosis was performed using 7–0 prolene. The patient was successfully extubated and returned to the ward. However, on day 4 she developed acute stridor, with cord evaluation showing bilateral palsy necessitating an urgent tracheostomy. Speech therapy and tracheostomy care was initiated. Her left cord was paretic but functioning and after 2 months she was weaned off her tracheostomy completely, with return of speech and swallowing functions.

Rajeev Parameswaran is the lead author of this chapter.

A. Agarwal et al., *Case Studies in Thyroid and Parathyroid Tumors*,
https://doi.org/10.1007/978-981-99-0938-4_64

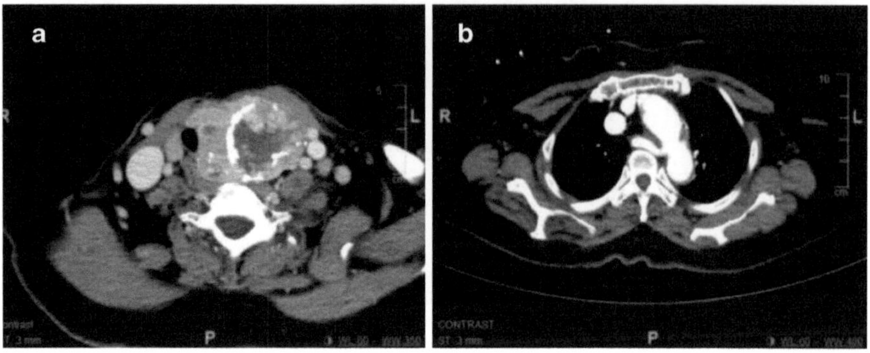

Fig. 1 (**a**, **b**) CT scan showing a large recurrent left thyroid nodule with tracheal compression and arteriogram showing an aberrant right subclavian artery, indicating the likely presence of non-recurrent laryngeal nerve

Discussion

Stridor is a very rare but very serious complication after thyroid surgery, necessitating immediate action. The most common causes of post-thyroidectomy stridor are bleeding and subsequent hematoma formation, recurrent laryngeal nerve (RLN) dysfunction, and laryngeal edema.

Bleeding following thyroidectomy is a serious complication that usually occurs within the first 24 to 48 h after surgery. It has a reported incidence of 0–5% [1]. Bleeding can occur in either the superficial or deep layers, and it can cause a degree of airway obstruction which is not only related to the total amount of blood loss, but also to its speed [2]. Difficulty breathing can occur when there is an ongoing bleeding and blood or hematoma accumulates to the point that the skin flaps swell. In this scenario, stridor could be a relative late sign. In case of bleeding in the thyroid bed, there could be more instantaneous signs of airway compromise and development of a stridor. The first step in managing airway obstruction from a suspected bleeding, is to open the surgical wound, whereby ensuring both superficial and deep layers are opened [3]. If this does not result in resolution of the airway compromise, emergency intubation must be considered, or, if this is found to be impossible, an emergency tracheostomy should be performed.

The incidence of unilateral RLN injury is not uncommon, with reported rates of transient RLN palsy ranging from 5% to 8%, and those of permanent RLN palsy from 0.3% to 3% [1]. However, while this injury could result in a hoarse and a breathy voice, the other cord usually compensates to a large extent, and it should not contribute to the development of a stridor. A stridor can develop when there is a bilateral vocal cord paralysis, from injuries to both RLNs. This is much rarer (0.4% of cases), and occurs most commonly with reoperations [4]. While a bilateral RLN palsy can be suspected during the operation when a nerve monitoring device is used, it does usually become apparent by the development of instant dyspnea and a stridor due to the closure of the glottis upon extubating [5]. As a short-term management option, immediate reintubation is usually possible; however, the formation of a tracheostomy may be required if reintubating is impossible, for instance, if both vocal cords are adducted [6]. For patients who have permanent bilateral vocal cord paralysis, sufficient laryngeal airflow with minimal vocal sequelae can sometimes be restored by performance of a partial posterior cordectomy, to avoid having a long-term tracheostomy [7].

Another potential cause of stridor is post-thyroidectomy laryngeal edema, which has a reported incidence of approximately 3% [1, 8]. This edema is most likely to direct intubation trauma, which could have caused a local contusion or a small hematoma contributing to the laryngeal edema and thereby induce an airway obstruction and thus an audible stridor. While the need for a careful intubation is principal, other preventative measures could be the administration of intraoperative steroids to reduce a stress response. If stridor from laryngeal edema does occur, the first treatment option consists of administration of a combination of steroid hormones and bronchodilators. However, if the results are insufficient, tracheostomy could be necessary [1].

An exceedingly rare cause of stridor following thyroidectomy, specifically for those patients who have had longstanding extrinsic tracheal compression by a goiter, with a 50% reduction in tracheal lumen with subsequent loss of tracheal cartilage rigidity, is post-thyroidectomy tracheomalacia and tracheal collapse [9]. In this setting, after the compressive goiter is removed by thyroidectomy, the trachea could be prone to collapsing, and could thus cause a postoperative respiratory obstruction and stridor. This post-thyroidectomy stridor will become evident only when the tracheal diameter is reduced to less than 3.5 mm [10]. Reported incidences vary extremely, from 0% to as high as 10%, [9–11] which could be due to the lack of a universally accepted definition. It has been suggested that a reduction in the ratio of tracheal cartilage to soft tissue, could be predictive [12]. Other proposed contributing factors are the loss of longitudinal elastic fibers in the pars membranacea, and cartilage fragmentation [11]. The exact pathophysiology of tracheomalacia remains unclear however, and it is generally considered a heterogenous phenomenon, which is difficult to predict prior to performance of the thyroid surgery. Early recognition of tracheomalacia prior to extubating is therefore paramount, in order to accommodate early intervention. Proposed criteria indicating the potential presence of this complication include a soft and floppy appearing trachea after removal of the thyroid gland, or an observed collapse of the trachea following gradual withdrawal of the endotracheal tube [10]. In these cases, formation of an intraoperative tracheostomy can be necessary, and this is generally considered the first choice in management [11]. Other suggested management options for tracheomalacia include prolonged intubation, tracheopexy, and external splinting or fixation of tracheal cartilage [10].

Another, incredibly rare cause of stridor is paradoxical vocal cord dysfunction. Here, there is an abnormal adduction of the vocal cords during the inspiratory phase, which causes obstruction at the level of the larynx. The diagnosis of paradoxical vocal cord dysfunction can be made by direct observation of vocal cord function by doing fiberoptic laryngoscopy. Although this dysfunction is a temporary phenomenon, a patient could need reintubation [13].

References

1. Jin S, Sugitani I. Narrative review of management of thyroid surgery complications. Gland Surg. 2021;10(3):1135–46.
2. Lee HS, Lee BJ, Kim SW, Cha YW, Choi YS, Park YH, et al. Patterns of post-thyroidectomy hemorrhage. Clin Exp Otorhinolaryngol. 2009;2(2):72–7.
3. Iliff H, El-Boghdadly K, Ahmad I, Davis J, Harris A, Khan S, et al. Management of haematoma after thyroid surgery: systematic review and multidisciplinary consensus guidelines from the Difficult Airway Society, the British Association of Endocrine and Thyroid Surgeons and the British Association of Otorhinolaryngology, Head and Neck Surgery. Anaesthesia. 2022;77(1):82–95.
4. Rosato L, Avenia N, Bernante P, De Palma M, Gulino G, Nasi PG, et al. Complications of thyroid surgery: analysis of a multicentric study on 14,934 patients operated on in Italy over 5 years. World J Surg. 2004;28(3):271–6.
5. Lukinović J, Bilić M. Overview of thyroid surgery complications. Acta Clin Croat. 2020;59(Suppl 1):81–6.
6. Sanapala A, Nagaraju M, Rao LN, Nalluri K. Management of bilateral recurrent laryngeal nerve paresis after thyroidectomy. Anesth Essays Res. 2015;9(2):251–3.
7. Finck C. Laryngeal dysfunction after thyroid surgery: diagnosis, evaluation and treatment. Acta Chir Belg. 2006;106(4):378–87.
8. Sanjeeva KK, Chandra B, Balakrishna MA, Ramesh DB. Clinico-epidemiological study and treatment outcome of multinodular goitre at a tertiary care hospital. J Clin Diagn Res. 2015;9(6):PC22-5.
9. White ML, Doherty GM, Gauger PG. Evidence-based surgical management of substernal goiter. World J Surg. 2008;32(7):1285–300.
10. Agarwal A, Mishra AK, Gupta SK, Arshad F, Tripathi M, Singh PK. High incidence of tracheomalacia in longstanding goiters: experience from an endemic goiter region. World J Surg. 2007;31(4):832–7.
11. Findlay JM, Sadler GP, Bridge H, Mihai R. Post-thyroidectomy tracheomalacia: minimal risk despite significant tracheal compression. Br J Anaesth. 2011;106(6):903–6.
12. Kandaswamy C, Balasubramanian V. Review of adult tracheomalacia and its relationship with chronic obstructive pulmonary disease. Curr Opin Pulm Med. 2009;15(2):113–9.
13. Harbison J, Dodd J, McNicholas WT. Paradoxical vocal cord motion causing stridor after thyroidectomy. Thorax. 2000;55(6):533–4.

Implications of Bethesda Cytology Category 4

Case
A 60-year-old male patient was referred to the endocrine surgery clinic with a finding of incidental thyroid nodule on a surveillance computed tomography (CT)-scan of his chest for follow-up of bilateral pulmonary nodules (Fig. 1). In the clinic, he denied any problems with swallowing or breathing, denied feeling any pressure in his throat, and did not notice any change in his voice. His thyroid screen was within normal range (free T4: 11.5 pmol/L [8.0–16.0] and TSH: 2.32 mIU/L [0.45–4.50]).

An ultrasound scan (US) confirmed a right-sided well-defined hypoechoic solid nodule with prominent internal vascularity, measuring 2.1 cm in largest diameter (Fig. 2). A fine needle aspiration (FNA) of this nodule was undertaken, and cytology showed follicular cells in atypical microfollicular forms, which did not show significant nuclear atypia. This FNA was therefore graded as suspicious for a follicular neoplasm (Bethesda IV). The risk of malignancy associated with this finding was discussed with the patient, and he was counseled for a diagnostic right hemithyroidectomy.

He underwent an uneventful right hemithyroidectomy and was discharged on post-operative day 1. His final histology report showed a benign follicular adenoma with a maximum diameter of 2.5 cm. Postoperatively, he did not develop any issues regarding his wound or voice nor any signs of hypothyroidism.

Rajeev Parameswaran is the lead author of this chapter.

A. Agarwal et al., *Case Studies in Thyroid and Parathyroid Tumors*,
https://doi.org/10.1007/978-981-99-0938-4_65

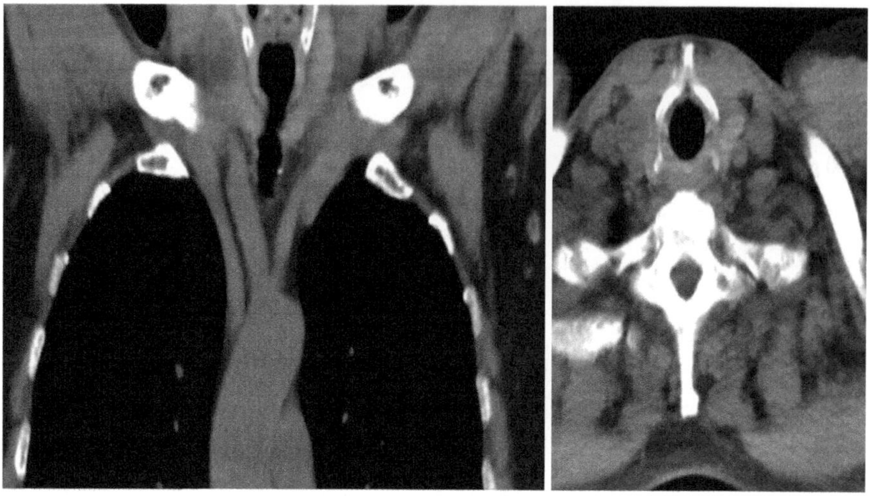

Fig. 1 CT scan showing the presence of an incidental right thyroid nodule

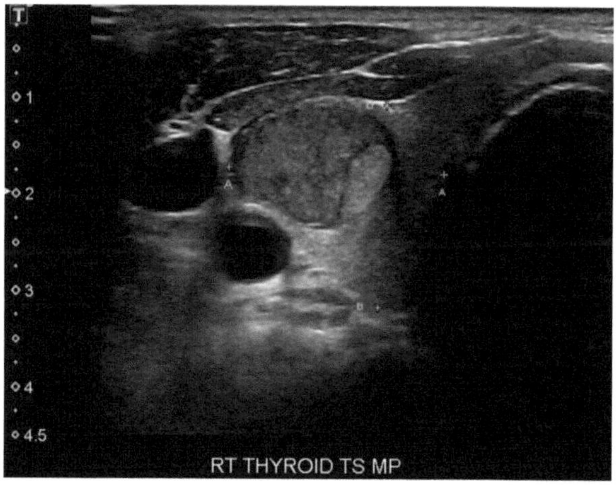

Fig. 2 US thyroid showing a hypoechoic lesion in the right thyroid lobe, with features of increased vascularity, and FNAC showing the presence of a follicular neoplasm

Discussion

Thyroid nodule risk-stratification based on ultrasound scan (US) appearance has become part of routine practice, with most clinicians using the TIRADS system [1] in order to select nodules that warrant further investigation with fine needle aspiration cytology biopsy (FNA). This modality provides information about the location and size of the nodule, stratifies nodules based on risk of malignancy, and guides towards the need of an FNA [2–4]. Where the strength of the US stratification using TIRADS lies in the selection of those nodules needing FNA, the TIRADS classification does not seem reliable to influence/change therapeutic decisions based on cytology appearance, as it has been shown that the risk of malignancy within same cytologic category cannot be stratified further based on the TIRADS-category [5].

The cytologic results of the FNA are classified according to The National Cancer Institute Thyroid Fine-Needle Aspiration State of the Science Conference ("Bethesda Conference") [6]. When the FNA results show a follicular neoplasm (Bethesda IV), these are generally called indeterminate; a category which also includes cytology suggesting a follicular lesion of undetermined significance or atypia of undetermined significance (FLUS/AUS, Bethesda III). Indeterminate thyroid nodules are diagnosed in up to 30% of fine-needle aspirations. Specifically, for Bethesda IV, signs of cell crowding and/or microfollicle formation without nuclear features of papillary thyroid cancer (architectural atypia) are seen on cytology.

While these lesions could be benign follicular adenomas (including autonomous nodules), follicular thyroid cancers (FTC), follicular variant papillary cancers (fvPTC), or NIFTP are also options. The risk of malignancy in these cases is highly variable, as the overall risk of malignancy for this group reportedly ranges from 24% to 50% [6]. Consequently, managing these indeterminate nodules has been a challenge, as traditional options for patients with indeterminate cytology include a repeat FNA for cytology or diagnostic thyroid surgery. The key issue here is that the differentiating characteristic between a benign and malignant follicular nodule is the absence or presence of capsular or vascular invasion, which can only be assessed on a surgical histology specimen.

Generally, the therapeutic steps after identifying a Bethesda IV lesion vary with national or local practices, as well as with the availability of molecular testing.

The formation of a thyroid nodules has its basis in an escape of the normal feedback mechanisms which should regulate cell proliferation. This unregulated cell division can be the result of mutations in both oncogenes and tumor suppressor genes [7]. Point mutations of RAS and rearrangements of PPARγ/PAX8 genes are most commonly found mutations in FTC, while mutations in components of the PI3K pathway, such as in PTEN or PIK3CA, have also been reported, though these are thought to be less common [8]. More recently, several molecular markers and tests have become available with potential to aid decision-making for patients with indeterminate thyroid nodules, including mutational analysis (e.g., ThyroSeq v3 – aimed at identification of particular molecular markers of malignancy, such as BRAF and RAS mutational status), mRNA genomic expression (e.g., Afirma genomic sequencing classifier [GSC] – usage of high-density genomic data for molecular classification), and a combination of microRNA (miRNA) gene expression and mutational analysis (e.g., ThyraMIR/ThyGen X) [4, 9–11]. According to the ATA guidelines, molecular testing should be considered for cytology samples showing a follicular neoplasm, as for those patients whose molecular testing shows a benign pattern, observation rather than performance of a diagnostic lobectomy could be considered. Conversely, for most patients with a suspicious pattern, thyroid surgery is required [12].

However, in most practices, these tests are yet to be fully adopted as a routine, especially since they have a restricted availability and carry high costs. Ongoing efforts to resolve these issues are likely to lead to fundamental changes in the approach to nodules with suspicious cytology, but the timescale for such changes remains unpredictable. In those settings in which molecular testing is not available, repeat FNA could be considered prior to contemplating surgical steps. However, it is important to assess the levels of thyroid-stimulating hormone (TSH) first, as there is an increased possibility of an hyperfunctioning nodule in the presence of (subclinical) hyperthyroidism [12]. Thus, thyroid scintigraphy should be obtained prior to repeating the FNA. Repeat FNA might not be necessary for a nodule that is hyperfunctioning on radioiodine imaging, as hyperfunctioning nodules rarely are malignant [13, 14]. Nonetheless, repeat FNA should be performed for those patients with nonfunctioning nodules. Importantly, the performance of a repeat FNA should not replace clinical judgment, as sound clinical decision-making remains imperative to form surgical decisions. Generally, if the repeat FNA suggests benign disease, conservative management could be considered. Conversely, if the repeat FNA continues to show follicular neoplasm, a diagnostic thyroid lobectomy should be discussed to obtain a histological diagnosis [4].

References

1. Russ G, Bonnema SJ, Erdogan MF, Durante C, Ngu R, Leenhardt L. European thyroid association guidelines for ultrasound malignancy risk stratification of thyroid nodules in adults: the EU-TIRADS. Eur Thyroid J. 2017;6(5):225–37.
2. Haugen BR. 2015 American Thyroid Association Management guidelines for adult patients with thyroid nodules and differentiated thyroid cancer: what is new and what has changed? Cancer. 2017;123(3):372–81.
3. Russ G, Royer B, Bigorgne C, Rouxel A, Bienvenu-Perrard M, Leenhardt L. Prospective evaluation of thyroid imaging reporting and data system on 4550 nodules with and without elastography. Eur J Endocrinol. 2013;168(5):649–55.
4. Alexander EK, Kennedy GC, Baloch ZW, Cibas ES, Chudova D, Diggans J, et al. Preoperative diagnosis of benign thyroid nodules with indeterminate cytology. N Engl J Med. 2012;367(8):705–15.
5. de Jong MC, McNamara J, Winter L, Roskell D, Khan S, Mihai R. Risk of malignancy in thyroid nodules with indeterminate (THY3f) cytology. Ann R Coll Surg Engl. 2022;104(9):703–9.
6. Cibas ES, Ali SZ. The 2017 Bethesda system for reporting thyroid cytopathology. Thyroid. 2017;27(11):1341–6.
7. Rao SN, Bernet V. Indeterminate thyroid nodules in the era of molecular genomics. Mol Genet Genomic Med. 2020;8(9):e1288.
8. Xing M. Molecular pathogenesis and mechanisms of thyroid cancer. Nat Rev Cancer. 2013;13(3):184–99.
9. Patel KN, Angell TE, Babiarz J, Barth NM, Blevins T, Duh QY, et al. Performance of a genomic sequencing classifier for the preoperative diagnosis of cytologically indeterminate thyroid nodules. JAMA Surg. 2018;153(9):817–24.
10. Steward DL, Carty SE, Sippel RS, Yang SP, Sosa JA, Sipos JA, et al. Performance of a multigene genomic classifier in thyroid nodules with indeterminate cytology: a prospective blinded multicenter study. JAMA Oncol. 2019;5(2):204–12.
11. Chudova D, Wilde JI, Wang ET, Wang H, Rabbee N, Egidio CM, et al. Molecular classification of thyroid nodules using high-dimensionality genomic data. J Clin Endocrinol Metab. 2010;95(12):5296–304.

12. Haugen BR, Alexander EK, Bible KC, Doherty GM, Mandel SJ, Nikiforov YE, et al. 2015 American Thyroid Association Management guidelines for adult patients with thyroid nodules and differentiated thyroid cancer: the American Thyroid Association guidelines task force on thyroid nodules and differentiated thyroid cancer. Thyroid. 2016;26(1):1–133.
13. Boelaert K, Horacek J, Holder R, Watkinson J, Sheppard M, Franklyn J. Serum thyrotropin concentration as a novel predictor of malignancy in thyroid nodules investigated by fine-needle aspiration. J Clin Endocrinol Metabol. 2006;91(11):4295–301.
14. Fiore E, Rago T, Provenzale M, Scutari M, Ugolini C, Basolo F, et al. Lower levels of TSH are associated with a lower risk of papillary thyroid cancer in patients with thyroid nodular disease: thyroid autonomy may play a protective role. Endocr Relat Cancer. 2009;16(4):1251–60.

Part VII

Malignant Thyroid Diseases

Rapidly Enlarging Thyroid Mass

Case

A 68-year-old male presented with a rapidly enlarging neck mass with pressure symptoms that included dysphonia, dysphagia, and Horner's syndrome (as shown in Fig. 1a). Clinical examination revealed a large thyroid mass with no associated lymphadenopathy. Serum biochemistry revealed subclinical hypothyroidism (TSH -15mIU/L) and normal thyroid autoantibodies. Fine needle cytology showed the presence of mononuclear and atypical cells. Ultrasound and CT neck showed a large thyroid mass as shown in Fig. 1b. Core biopsy performed showed the presence of DLBCL and Ann Arbor Stage was IIE. He was commenced on (R–CHOP; rituximab, cyclophosphamide, doxorubicin, vincristine, and prednisolone) regime followed by adjuvant EBRT. His thyroid mass subsided following combined chemoradiotherapy. The patient continues to be disease free with no palpable neck mass and no signs of HS at 1 year.

Rajeev Parameswaran is the lead author of this chapter.

A. Agarwal et al., *Case Studies in Thyroid and Parathyroid Tumors*,
https://doi.org/10.1007/978-981-99-0938-4_66

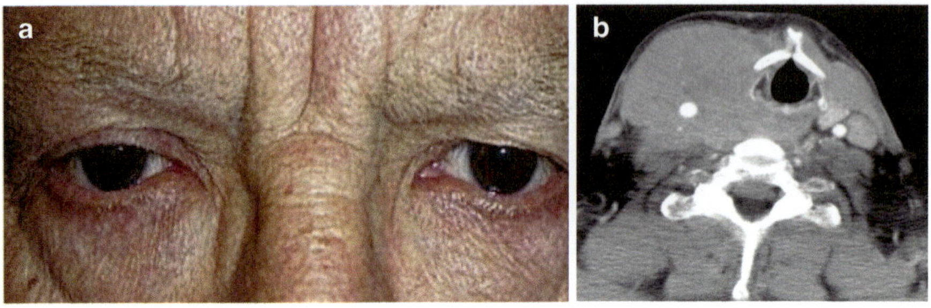

Fig. 1 (**a**, **b**) Patient with Horner's syndrome and CT showing the presence of the large thyroid mass

Discussion

Primary thyroid lymphomas (PTL) are rare malignancies seen in the thyroid gland, accounting for about 2% of all extranodal lymphomas and about 5% of all thyroid neoplasms. These neoplasms usually arise on a background of longstanding Hashimoto's thyroiditis (HT) [1], with a risk being about 40 to 80 times higher than the general population [2, 3]. The transformation from thyroiditis to lymphoma only occurs in a very small proportion of patients [2], probably due to chronic antigenic stimulation of lymphocytes [4]. It is believed that primary thyroid lymphomas arise from mucosa-associated lymphoma tissue (MALT) [5] and hence the initial description of these lesions as MALT lymphomas [6]. However, these lesions are now included under the entity "marginal zone B-cell lymphoma of MALT-type" (MZBL) as proposed by the WHO Classification for Neoplastic Diseases of the Lymphoid Tissues [7] and Revised European-American Classification of Lymphoid Neoplasms (REAL) [8]. Currently, primary thyroid lymphomas are classified into 2 broad categories: extranodal marginal zone B-cell lymphoma (EMZBCL) and diffuse large B-cell lymphoma (DLBCL).

Diffuse B-cell lymphoma accounts for over 50% of cases of PTL, followed by EMZBCL lymphomas in nearly quarter of case, followed by rarer types such as follicular lymphoma, Hodgkin's lymphoma, T-cell type, etc. [9, 10]. DLBCL behaves in a more aggressive manner in comparison to the indolent behavior of EMZBCL or follicular types. Most commonly patients present with an enlarging neck mass of a short duration and patients experience a range of compressive symptoms such as dysphagia, dyspnea, or hoarseness [11, 12]. Other presentations include Horner's syndrome [13], pain over the thyroid gland [10, 14], and B-symptoms such as fever, night sweats [14]. Clinical examination usually reveals a hard thyroid mass and about a third of patients may have a history of hypothyroidism secondary to Hashimoto's thyroiditis [10, 11].

Investigations include ultrasound scan of the thyroid, fine needle aspiration cytology, core biopsy or excision biopsy, and staging CT scan. Ultrasound scan may show features based on the nature of presentation such as nodular or diffuse enlargement [15]. Though fine needle cytology can help diagnose lymphoma in about

Table 1 Ann Arbor staging of lymphoma

Stage	Location of disease
I E	No disease seen
II E	Regional lymph nodes
III E	Disease on both sides of the diaphragm
IV E	Systemic disease

80–100% of cases, problem is that of high rate of false negatives [16], especially in a background of lymphocytic infiltration commonly associated with HT. When FNA is performed without immunotyping or immunohistochemistry, the diagnosis can be difficult, especially MZBL [11, 17]. The alternative therefore would be to perform a core biopsy or open biopsy, especially to distinguish thyroiditis from low-grade marginal zone lymphoma and diagnose aggressive variants. Open biopsies especially are useful in examining tissue for detailed histology, immunostaining, and evaluating any genetic rearrangements [16]. Stage of disease is evaluated with a CT scan of the head, neck, chest, abdomen, and pelvis and staging done using the Ann Arbor staging [18] (Table 1).

The treatment of PTL is primarily radiotherapy (RT) or combined multimodal therapy (CMT) with no or limited role for surgery [19]. RT is more effective for MZBL than DLBCL especially in localized disease using doses ranging from 30 to 50 Gy [20, 21]. Reported 5-year cause-specific survival rates are around 80 to 100% for MZBL compared to 55% to DLBCL [22, 23]. In patients with aggressive or disseminated disease usually associated with DLBCL disease, CMT is usually required [24, 25]. The common agents used for multimodal therapy are cyclophosphamide, vincristine & prednisolone (CVP), cyclophosphamide, doxorubicin, vincristine, and prednisolone (CHOP) and more recently include rituximab, an anti-CD20 monoclonal antibody (R-CHOP) [17, 25, 26]. CMT was associated with improved survival rates and decreased relapse rates [27, 28]. Factors associated with poor prognosis include increasing age and stage, DLBCL type, large size, rapid progression, mediastinal disease, and presence of B-symptoms [9, 16, 29].

References

1. Pedersen RK, Pedersen NT. Primary non-Hodgkin's lymphoma of the thyroid gland: a population based study. Histopathology. 1996;28(1):25–32.
2. Holm LE, Blomgren H, Löwhagen T. Cancer risks in patients with chronic lymphocytic thyroiditis. N Engl J Med. 1985;312(10):601–4.
3. Abbasgholizadeh P, Naseri A, Nasiri E, Sadra V. Is Hashimoto thyroiditis associated with increasing risk of thyroid malignancies? A systematic review and meta-analysis. Thyroid Res. 2021;14(1):26.
4. Kossev P, Livolsi V. Lymphoid lesions of the thyroid: review in light of the revised European-American lymphoma classification and upcoming World Health Organization classification. Thyroid. 1999;9(12):1273–80.

5. Isaacson P, Wright DH. Malignant lymphoma of mucosa-associated lymphoid tissue. A distinctive type of B-cell lymphoma. Cancer. 1983;52(8):1410–6.
6. Isaacson PG. Lymphoma of the thyroid gland. Curr Top Pathol. 1997;91:1–14.
7. Swerdlow SH, Campo E, Harris NL, Jaffe ES, Pileri SA, Stein H, et al. WHO classification of tumours of haematopoietic and lymphoid tissues: international agency for research on cancer. Lyon: IARC; 2008.
8. Sander CA, Flaig MJ, Kaudewitz P, Jaffe ES. The revised European-American Classification of Lymphoid Neoplasms (REAL): a preferred approach for the classification of cutaneous lymphomas. Am J Dermatopathol. 1999;21(3):274–8.
9. Graff-Baker A, Roman SA, Thomas DC, Udelsman R, Sosa JA. Prognosis of primary thyroid lymphoma: demographic, clinical, and pathologic predictors of survival in 1,408 cases. Surgery. 2009;146(6):1105–15.
10. Watanabe N, Noh JY, Narimatsu H, Takeuchi K, Yamaguchi T, Kameyama K, et al. Clinicopathological features of 171 cases of primary thyroid lymphoma: a long-term study involving 24553 patients with Hashimoto's disease. Br J Haematol. 2011;153(2):236–43.
11. Sarinah B, Hisham A-N. Primary lymphoma of the thyroid: diagnostic and therapeutic considerations. Asian J Surg. 2010;33(1):20–4.
12. Sitges-Serra A. The rapidly growing thyroid mass. Br J Surg. 2006;93(6):647–9.
13. Donaldson JF, Rodriguez-Gomez IA, Parameswaran R. Rapidly enlarging neck masses of the thyroid with Horner's syndrome: a concise clinical review. surgeon (Edinburgh). 2014;13(2):110–5.
14. Alzouebi M, Goepel JR, Horsman JM, Hancock BW. Primary thyroid lymphoma: the 40 year experience of a UK lymphoma treatment centre. Int J Oncol. 2012;40(6):2075–80.
15. Ota H, Ito Y, Matsuzuka F, Kuma S, Fukata S, Morita S, et al. Usefulness of ultrasonography for diagnosis of malignant lymphoma of the thyroid. Thyroid. 2006;16(10):983–7.
16. Stein SA, Wartofsky L. Primary thyroid lymphoma: a clinical review. J Clin Endocrinol Metab. 2013;98(8):3131–8.
17. Matsuzuka F, Miyauchi A, Katayama S, Narabayashi I, Ikeda H, Kuma K, et al. Clinical aspects of primary thyroid lymphoma: diagnosis and treatment based on our experience of 119 cases. Thyroid. 1993;3(2):93–9.
18. Carbone PP, Kaplan HS, Musshoff K, Smithers DW, Tubiana M. Report of the committee on Hodgkin's disease staging classification. Cancer Res. 1971;31(11):1860–1.
19. Klyachkin ML, Schwartz RW, Cibull M, Munn RK, Regine WF, Kenady DE, et al. Thyroid lymphoma: is there a role for surgery? Am Surg. 1998;64(3):234–8.
20. Harrington KJ, Michalaki VJ, Vini L, Nutting CM, Syrigos KN, A'Hern R, et al. Management of non-Hodgkin's lymphoma of the thyroid: the Royal Marsden Hospital experience. Br J Radiol. 2005;78(929):405–10.
21. Blair TJ, Evans RG, Buskirk SJ, Banks PM, Earle JD. Radiotherapeutic management of primary thyroid lymphoma. Int J Radiat Oncol Biol Phys. 1985;11(2):365–70.
22. Laing RW, Hoskin P, Hudson BV, Hudson GV, Harmer C, Bennett MH, et al. The significance of MALT histology in thyroid lymphoma: a review of patients from the BNLI and Royal Marsden Hospital. Clin Oncol (R Coll Radiol). 1994;6(5):300–4.
23. Tsang RW, Gospodarowicz MK, Pintilie M, Wells W, Hodgson DC, Sun A, et al. Localized mucosa-associated lymphoid tissue lymphoma treated with radiation therapy has excellent clinical outcome. J Clin Oncol. 2003;21(22):4157–64.
24. Vigliotti A, Kong JS, Fuller LM, Velasquez WS. Thyroid lymphomas stages IE and IIE: comparative results for radiotherapy only, combination chemotherapy only, and multimodality treatment. Int J Radiat Oncol Biol Phys. 1986;12(10):1807–12.
25. Miller TP, Dahlberg S, Cassady JR, Adelstein DJ, Spier CM, Grogan TM, et al. Chemotherapy alone compared with chemotherapy plus radiotherapy for localized intermediate- and high-grade non-Hodgkin's lymphoma. N Engl J Med. 1998;339(1):21–6.

26. Portlock CS, Rosenberg SA. Combination chemotherapy with cyclophosphamide, vincristine, and prednisone in advanced non-Hodgkin's lymphomas. Cancer. 1976;37(3):1275–82.
27. Doria R, Jekel JF, Cooper DL, Thyroid lymphoma. The case for combined modality therapy. Cancer. 1994;73(1):200–6.
28. Ha CS, Shadle KM, Medeiros LJ, Wilder RB, Hess MA, Cabanillas F, et al. Localized non-Hodgkin lymphoma involving the thyroid gland. Cancer. 2001;91(4):629–35.
29. Onal C, Li YX, Miller RC, Poortmans P, Constantinou N, Weber DC, et al. Treatment results and prognostic factors in primary thyroid lymphoma patients: a rare cancer network study. Ann Oncol. 2011;22(1):156–64.

Papillary Carcinoma in a Retrosternal Component of Goiter

Case

A 20-year-old male presented to the National Chest hospital Welisara with some dyspnea and discomfort in the chest and a mediastinal mass was detected on CT scan. Guided biopsy was inconclusive and a decision was made to excise the lump via R Thoracotomy (Fig. 1) done for a mediastinal mass (Fig. 2).

The histology proved that it was a papillary carcinoma in a mediastinal component of goiter. He was referred for revision total thyroidectomy. The picture shows the R thoracotomy seen on review (Fig. 1).

Total thyroidectomy was done via a cervical incision. The goiter was small involving mainly the right lobe. The connection between the thoracic component and the goiter was tenuous explaining why it was thought to be a mediastinal mass initially.

Ranil Fernando is the lead author of this chapter.

A. Agarwal et al., *Case Studies in Thyroid and Parathyroid Tumors*,
https://doi.org/10.1007/978-981-99-0938-4_67

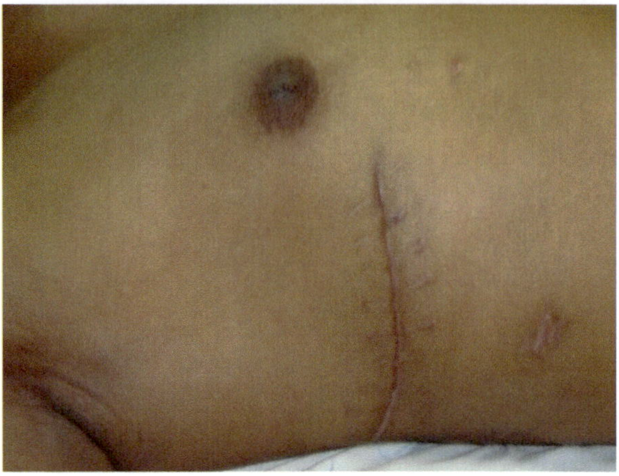

Fig. 1 Right Thoracotomy scar

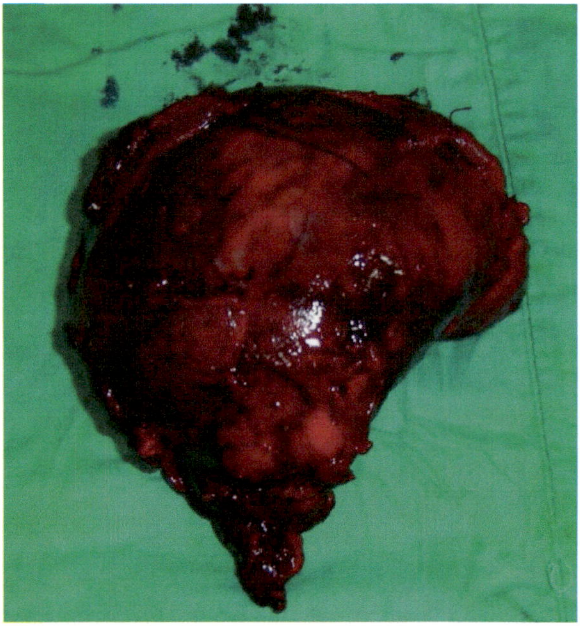

Fig. 2 Mediastinal mass specimen

Ulcerated Thyroid Cancer Causing Anaemia

Case

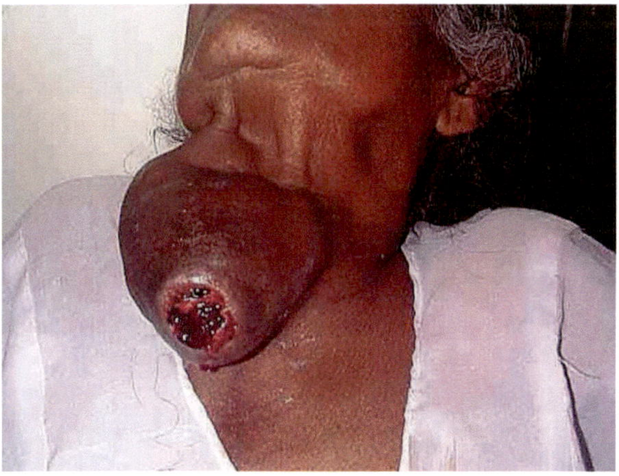

A 78-year-old lady presented with malaise, lethargy, and difficulty in doing simple tasks. She did not particularly complain of the goiter or the ulcer, as she has had the goiter for 15 years and the ulcer for about 2 years.

She was found to be anemic on assessment. FNAC confirmed it to be a papillary carcinoma.

Total thyroidectomy was done after correcting her anemia. Histologically as the lesion was a classical papillary carcinoma of the thyroid. She received radio iodine treatment postoperatively.

This is a very unusual presentation of thyroid cancer.

Ranil Fernando is the lead author of this chapter.

A. Agarwal et al., *Case Studies in Thyroid and Parathyroid Tumors*,
https://doi.org/10.1007/978-981-99-0938-4_68

Thyroglossal Cyst (TGC) and Papillary Thyroid Cancer

Case 1: Papillary Thyroid Cancer in Thyroglossal Cyst with PHPT
A 43-year-old lady presented to the OPD with anterior neck swelling with ulceration (Fig. 1). Patient had this anterior neck swelling for 20 years for which she was advised surgery but she did not opt for the same. She planned to seek medical help after the development of ulceration in the swelling. After clinical diagnosis of infected/malignant thyroglossal cyst, imaging and cytology was advised. CECT (Fig. 2a) showed lesion with infiltration into the left belly of digastric and mylohyoid muscle and left submandibular gland infiltration with infiltration of strap muscles with nodule in the right lobe of thyroid measuring 7.5 × 5.2 mm. Cytology from the lesion was Bethesda V: Suspicious for papillary thyroid carcinoma. On CECT discussion preoperatively contrast-enhancing lesion (Fig. 2b) was visible separate from thyroid? enlarged parathyroid (red arrow), hence total calcium and intact PTH were done which were found to be high (s. calcium 10.7 and intact PTH: 357), hence a diagnosis of primary hyperparathyroidism was made. Thereafter patient was planned for total thyroidectomy with sistrunks procedure and parathyroidectomy. Right superior parathyroid was found to be enlarged weighing 1000 mg. There was 50% fall in IOPTH (Miami's criteria). The cyst was adhered to hyoid

Roma Pradhan is the lead author of this chapter.

A. Agarwal et al., *Case Studies in Thyroid and Parathyroid Tumors*,
https://doi.org/10.1007/978-981-99-0938-4_69

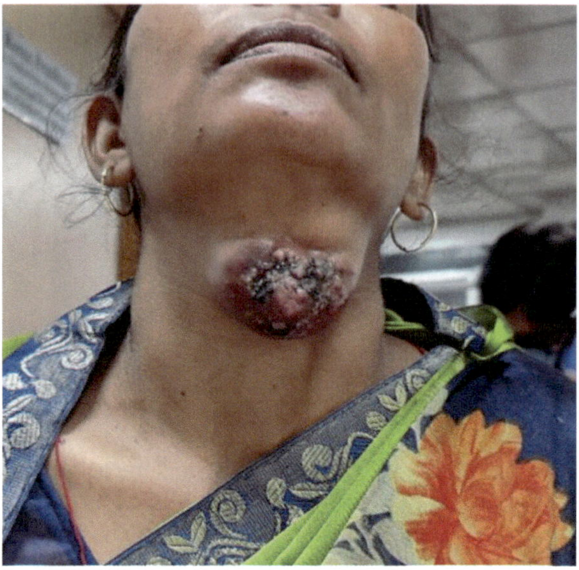

Fig. 1 Clinical picture

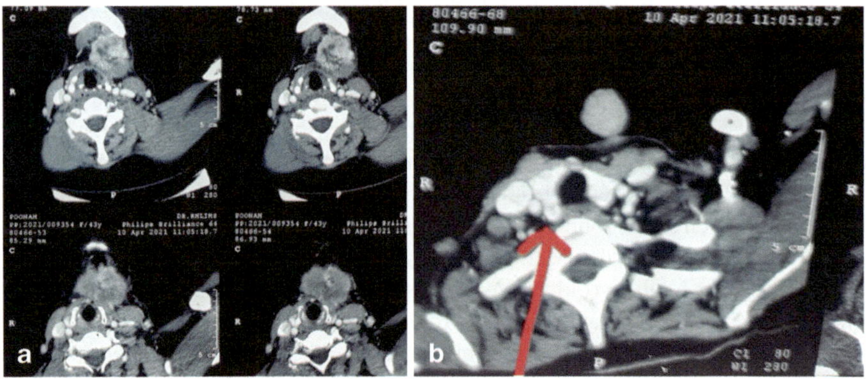

Fig. 2 (**a**) CECT showing the thyroglossal cyst lesion, (**b**) parathyroid lesion (red arrow)

cartilage and left submandibular gland, which was removed along with the specimen. Total Thyroidectomy was performed along with sistrunks procedure (Fig. 3). Postoperatively patient developed biochemical and clinical hypocalcemia which was managed by oral calcium and active vitamin D3. Histopathology showed papillary thyroid cancer in thyroglossal cyst with involvement of submandibular gland without any tumor in thyroid gland with BRAF positivity. The patient received 125 mCi radioactive iodine treatment after surgery.

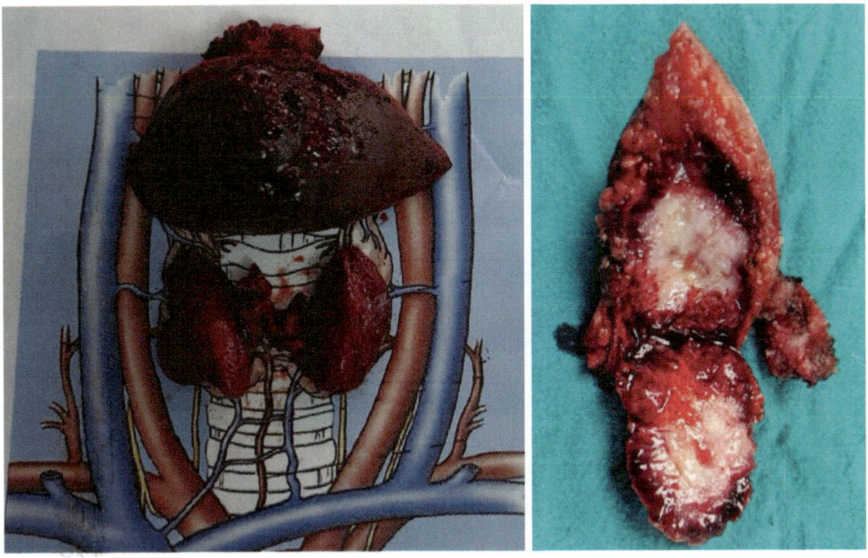

Fig. 3 Postoperative specimen

Case 2: Thyroglossal Cyst with Incidental Micro Papillary Thyroid Carcinoma

A 31-year-old lady presented with anterior neck swelling for 1 year with a history of discharge from the swelling on and off (Fig. 4). On examination patient had swelling in midline which moves with deglutition and also with protrusion of tongue. Ultrasound neck showed hypoechoic collection in midline in submental region along with a hypoechoic lesion measuring 7.3 × 8.9 × 7.2 mm in the left lobe of thyroid with areas of calcification (Fig. 5). Guided fnac done from the lesion was inconclusive. After discussion with the patient she was planned for sistrunk's procedure along with hemithyroidectomy. Intraoperatively few black nodes were found in central compartment hence a decision of total thyroidectomy with hemi cclnd was taken. Postoperatively patient recovered well with no clinical hypocalcemia. Histopathology showed a lesion of size 1.2 cm with one lymph node involved.

Case 3: Thyroglossal Cyst with Intracystic PTC

A 35-year-old lady presented with midline neck swelling (Fig. 6) since 3 years. Neck examination showed a swelling just below the chin measuring 4 × 3 cm, cystic consistency, irreducible, moving with deglutition and protrusion of tongue. USG showed a large, lobulated 6 × 4.8 × 4.2 cm, well-defined, mixed solid cystic, taller than wide, with echogenic foci and calcification within, separate from thyroid in the midline.- TIRADS V lesion hence CECT neck was advised. A well-defined peripherally enhancing cystic lesion measuring 4.3 × 3.2 × 4.5 cm in the midline, superiorly up to the base of the tongue, inferiorly up to the superior border of the thyroid gland, extending posteriorly up to left paraglottic space with the

Fig. 4 Clinical picture

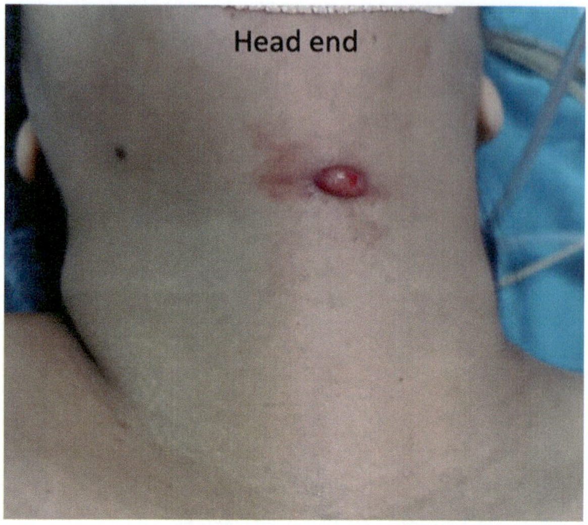

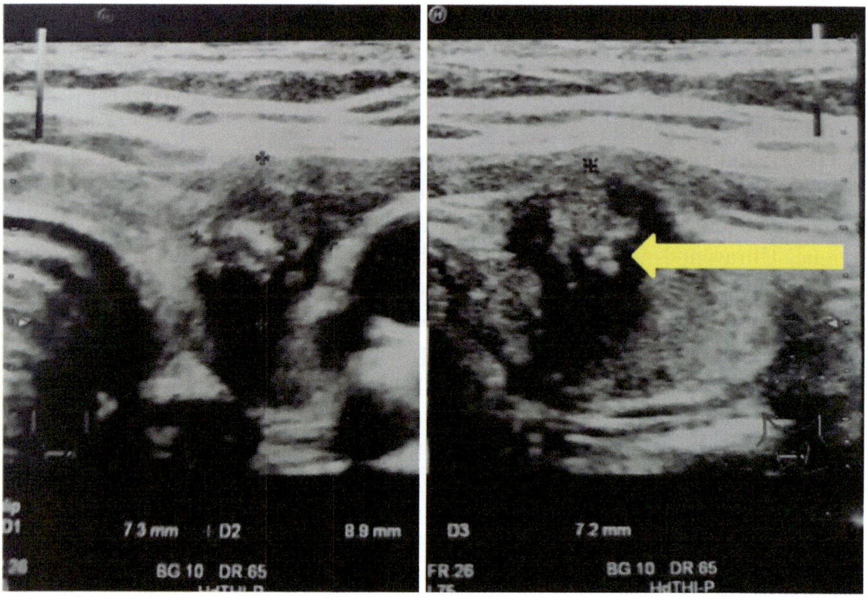

Fig. 5 Hypoechoic lesion with microcalcification

impression of malignant transformation. Guided fnac was suggestive of papillary thyroid cancer. Hence with diagnosis of TGC carcinoma patient was planned for sistrunks procedure along with total thyroidectomy. Cyst was dissected by sharp dissection from pharynx (Fig. 7) Postoperative recovery was smooth and the patient was discharged on fifth post-operative day. HPE was intracystic ptc with unremarkable thyroid.

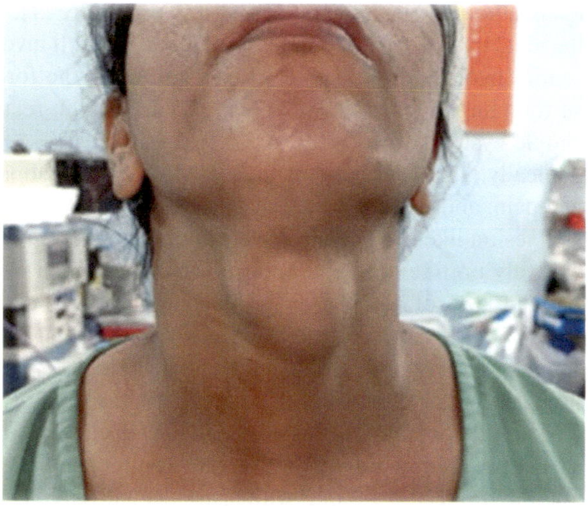

Fig. 6 Clinical picture with upper midline swelling

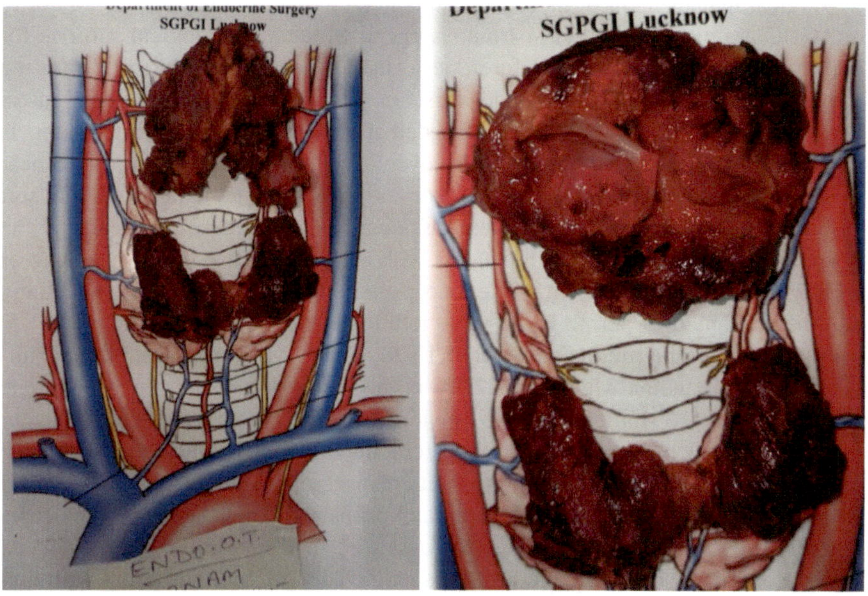

Fig. 7 Postoperative specimen picture

Discussion

The thyroid gland arises from foramen caecum and descents down to the neck. Any anomaly in the descent may leave a space in the tract and gives rise to thyroglossal duct cyst (TGDC). The thyroid tissue is normally located in the wall of the cyst and has a potential to harbor malignancy and most of the cases are detected in histopathology specimen after sistrunk procedure [1]. Sistrunk's procedure (SP) is the ideal treatment for benign thyroglossal cysts. It involves en bloc cystectomy and central hyoidectomy, with tract excision up to the foramen cecum along with the surrounding soft tissue. SP has reduced the high recurrence rate associated with simple cyst excision (up to 60%) to less than 10% [2]. In a review published [3] clinically, 95.1% of patients presented with an asymptomatic neck swelling, 1.8% had pain, and 3.1% reported dysphagia. None of the patients presented with ulcerated lesion like our patient. In 1/fifth of the patients the diagnosis was made preoperatively on fine needle cytology. The mean tumor size was 1.7 cm in the review. Around 80% of patients of TGDC carcinoma are diagnosed as histopathological surprise after sistrunks surgery. Hence proper imaging with high-resolution ultrasound or CT scan of neck should be done to look for any mural mass with calcification. Preoperative fnac is debatable and has a sensitivity of 56% to 62% [4] and fnac doesn't rule out malignancy especially if the clinical suspicion is high. On the other side a preoperative diagnosis if carcinoma clearly defines the management with Total thyroidectomy along with sistrunks and saves patient another surgery. Hence a preoperative discussion of possibility of harboring a malignancy should be done.

Surgical management of thyroglossal duct carcinoma is controversial. Majority of TGDC are diagnosed after sistrunks surgery, hence a pathological surprise for both patient and surgeon. Therefore due to lack of sufficient information on the subject, no well-defined guideline exist in the management of such cases. Controversy exists as to the treatment needed after sistrunks if TGDC carcinoma is a pathological surprise. Incidentally discovered well-differentiated thyroid cancer in a TGDC in a low-risk patient with tumor less than 4 cm in diameter without soft tissue extension, without distant metastases can be adequately taken care by the Sistrunk procedure. However, in patients with advance disease like our patient, or with lymph node involvement and extracapsular extension, a total thyroidectomy may be warranted to permit radioactive iodine ablation. However, one study [5] seems to support the routine addition of TT to SP due to the high rate of concomitant thyroid carcinoma which was 62.3% in this series; moreover, the average rate calculated from 16 studies with five or more cases was 46.3% [5]. This is higher than the 35% risk of incidental thyroid carcinoma discovered at autopsy [6]. Hence recommendations have been suggested with respect to indications for total thyroidectomy. These include finding a concomitant primary thyroid cancer, which occurs in 11% to 33% of cases, invasion into cyst wall, and tumors larger than 1 cm. Complete removal of all thyroid tissue also allows long-term monitoring with thyroglobulin levels and radioiodine ablation therapy if needed.

Furthermore, it is demonstrated here that co-existing thyroid cancers may escape sonographic detection, and that the size of TCC is not a reliable predictor of their presence or absence. The thyroglossal cyst patients must undergo an ultrasound of thyroid in order to detect any thyroid lesion and if found then thyroid nodule must be treated according to the established guidelines. We discussed about the concomitant lesion in thyroid of our case 2 and took a combined decision with the patient regarding management. In the third case, total thyroidectomy was planned in view of cyst lesion more than 1 cm.

Thyroglossal duct cyst carcinomas are rare findings in thyroglossal duct cyst. Overall prognosis is excellent, with a survival rate of 99.4% and a recurrence rate of 4.3% among cases reported in the literature.

References

1. Wei S, LiVolsi VA, Baloch ZW. Pathology of thyroglossal duct: an institutional experience. Endocr Pathol. 2015;26(01):75–9.
2. Chrisoulidou A, Iliadou P, Doumala E, et al. Thyroglossal duct cyst carcinomas: is there a need for thyroidectomy? Hormones (Athens). 2013;12:522–8.
3. Rayess HM, Monk I, Svider PF, Gupta A, Raza SN, Lin HS. Thyroglossal duct cyst carcinoma: a systematic review of clinical features and outcomes. Otolaryngol Head Neck Surg. 2017;156(5):794–802.
4. Bardales RH, Suhrland MJ, Korourian S, Schaefer RF, Hanna EY, Stanley MW. Cytologic findings in thyroglossal duct carcinoma. Am J Clin Pathol. 1996;106:615–9.
5. Bakkar S, Biricotti M, Stefanini G, Ambrosini CE, Materazzi G, Miccoli P. The extent of surgery in thyroglossal cyst carcinoma. Langenbeck's Arch Surg. 2017;402(5):799–804. https://doi.org/10.1007/s00423-016-1460-x.
6. Harach HR, Franssila KO, Wasenius VM. Occult papillary carcinoma of the thyroid. A "normal" finding in Finland. A systemic autopsy study. Cancer. 1985;56:531–8.

CT Imaging in Thyroid Cancer

Case
A 70-year-old lady presented with a history of painless anterior neck swelling for 1 year with the rapid increase in the preceding 1 month. She had no compressive features. On examination, she had a 4 × 3 cm firm to hard nodule arising from the right lobe of thyroid and was having restricted mobility. There was no retrosternal extension and no deep cervical lymphadenopathy. USG was reported as: Rt lobe of thyroid enlarged with multiple solid well-defined hypoechoic nodules with calcification and increased peripheral vascularity without any extrathyroidal extension and no cervical lymphadenopathy. FNAC was reported as papillary thyroid

Amit Agarwal is the lead author of this chapter.

A. Agarwal et al., *Case Studies in Thyroid and Parathyroid Tumors*,
https://doi.org/10.1007/978-981-99-0938-4_70

carcinoma and IDL examination showed normal B/L Vocal cords mobility. CECT Neck was reported as a 4 × 3.5 cm, in-homogenous lesion arising from the right lobe of thyroid (Fig. 1) with few hypodense areas and with loss of fat planes with strap muscles. She underwent Total Thyroidectomy + CLND. Operative findings were: enlarged right lobe with single nodule adhered to sternothyroid muscle and so was sacrificed. Right RLN was densely adhered to the central compartment LN (Fig. 2) and had to be separated with great difficulty by sharp dissection. HPE was reported as papillary thyroid carcinoma with extension into muscles (Fig. 3) and positive central compartment nodes (3/9).

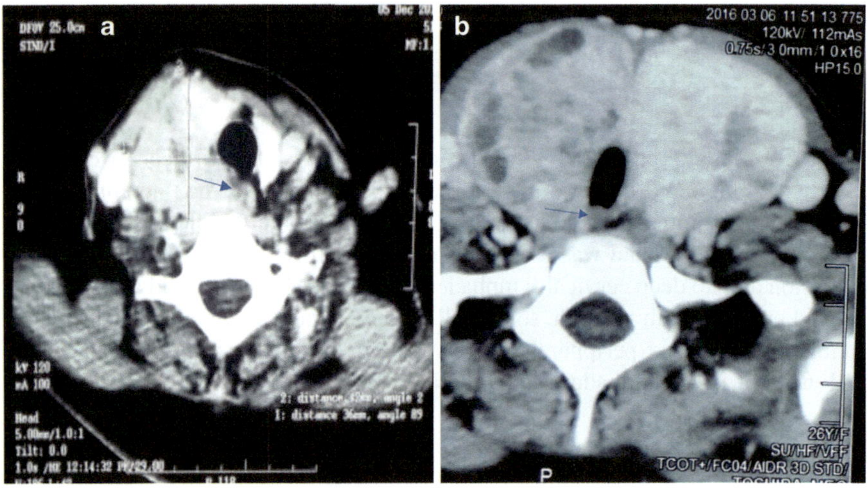

Fig. 1 (**a**) CECT of the patient showing effacement of T-O groove (arrow). (**b**) CECT of another case of PTC without RLN invasion showing normal T-O groove fat (arrow)

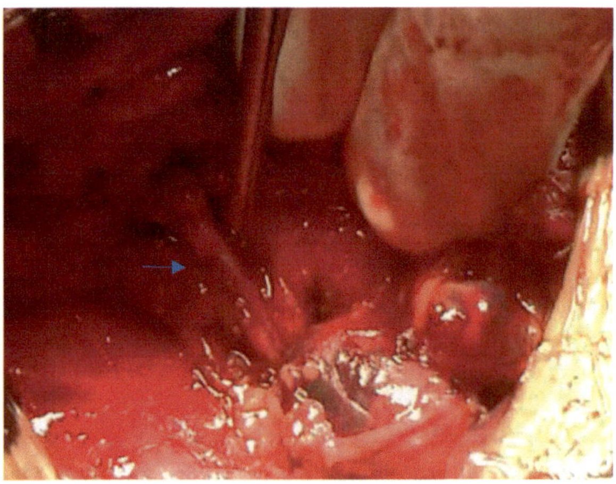

Fig. 2 Central LN invading the RLN (arrow)

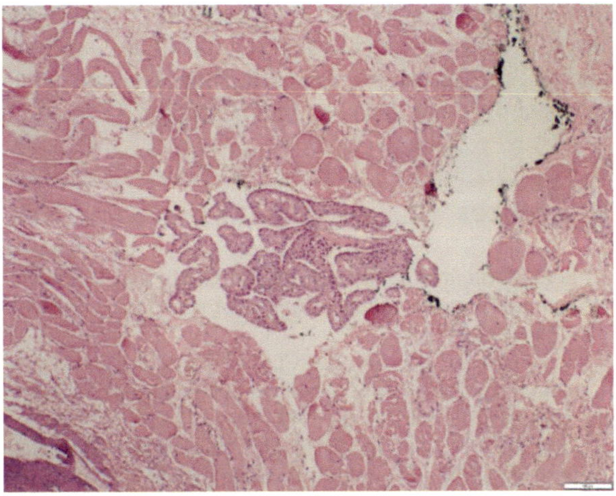

Fig. 3 Photomicrograph showing infiltration of skeletal muscles with tumor

Discussion

Extrathyroidal invasion of adjacent soft tissue structures has been reported to occur in less than 5% of cases of well-differentiated carcinoma of the thyroid [1]. The reason to image with cross-sectional modalities such as CT or MRI is concern for local invasion that may change the approach from curative to palliative, help plan the extent of surgery, and help in counseling the patient in case of need to sacrifice the RLN. The RLN is the structure most commonly involved in locally invasive thyroid cancer. Normal RLN lies posterior to the thyroid lobe, and most of the track of the RLN usually lies in the fatty tissue in the tracheoesophageal groove. Only 2 studies have reported the criteria and sensitivity of CT in assessing RLN invasion [2, 3]. While reading a CT a 3-step checklist can be followed: (1) *looking at central structures* around which the thyroid normally drapes such as trachea, esophagus, RLN, larynx, and pharynx, (2) *Structures immediately surrounding thyroid gland* such as vascular structures (IJV, carotid artery), strap muscles, prevertebral space., (3) *Assessment of deep cervical LN. Invasion of the trachea* can be deemed present when at least one of the following CT criteria is fulfilled: tumor in contact with 180° or more of the tracheal circumference (grades 3 and 4); deformity of the tracheal lumen at the level of the mass; and focal irregularity, thickening, or bulging in the mucosal portion adjacent to the mass. *Invasion of the esophagus* can be diagnosed when at least one of the following CT criteria is fulfilled: tumor in contact with 180° or more of the esophageal circumferences (grades 3 and 4) and loss of the normal esophageal structures (wall and lumen). *Invasion of the CCA or IJV* is diagnosed if the tumor was in contact with 180° or more of the circumferences of the vessel (grades 3 and 4). Invasion of IJV is suspected if it is occluded or effaced by tumor. Invasion of the RLN is diagnosed when at least two of the following three criteria were fulfilled: completely effaced fatty tissue was present in the tracheoesophageal groove for more than three axial images; more than 25% of the circumference of the tumor abutted the capsule at the posterior portions of the thyroid (posterior extra-capsular invasion); and ipsilateral vocal cord palsy was present on the basis of CT findings such as paramedian cord, anteromedial deviation of the arytenoid cartilage, enlarged pyriform sinus, or enlarged laryngeal ventricle.

References

1. Segal K, Shpitzer T, Hazan A, Bachar G, Marshak G, Popovtzer A. Invasive well-differentiated thyroid carcinoma: effect of treatment modalities on outcome. Otolaryngol Head Neck Surg. 2006;134:819–22.
2. Seo YL, Yoon DY, Lim KJ, Cha JH, Yun EJ, Choi CS, Bae SH. Locally advanced thyroid cancer: can CT help in prediction of extrathyroidal invasion to adjacent structures? AJR Am J Roentgenol. 2010;195(3):W240–4.
3. Takashima S, Takayama F, Wang J, Kobayashi S, Kadoya M. Using MR imaging to predict invasion of the recurrent laryngeal nerve by thyroid carcinoma. AJR. 2003;180:837–42.

Papillary Thyroid Cancer in a Pregnant Patient

Case
A 32-year-old pregnant female (*G.A. = 18w4d*) presented to us with a history of anterior neck swelling for 6 months which was insidious in onset but now progressively increasing in size, painless with no history of dysphagia/dyspnea/hoarseness of voice; no history suggestive of hyperthyroidism/hypothyroidism. She also gave a past history of ATT intake for pulmonary T.B. 12 years back. On examination both lobes of thyroid were found to be enlarged with one nodule palpable in the middle of either lobe (Fig. 1). Isthmus was normal and there was no cervical LAP.

SL. NO1	Investigation	Value	Interpretation
1.	CBC/RFT/LFT	WNL	WNL
2.	FT4	15.24 pmol/L	WNL
3.	TSH	1.95 mIU/L	WNL
4.	IDL	B/L VC mobile	

USG Thyroid showed a well-defined hypoechoic lesion, 2.2 cm × 2.2 cm × 0.9 cm in either lobes with internal septations and punctate microcalcifications and increased central vascularity+. Both nodules were reported as *TIRADS-IVc* (Fig. 2). No significant cervical LAP. FNAC from B/L thyroid nodules was reported as papillary thyroid cancer. After counseling the patient and in keeping with her wishes a

Amit Agarwal is the lead author of this chapter.

A. Agarwal et al., *Case Studies in Thyroid and Parathyroid Tumors*,
https://doi.org/10.1007/978-981-99-0938-4_71

Total Thyroidectomy was done in second trimester. Decision to avoid central compartment dissection was taken to avoid the possibility of post-operative hypocalcemia. At operation left lobe adherent was found to be adherent to straps muscles. There was no central or lateral compartment LN enlargement.

The cut surface on grossing of the specimen showed fleshy nodules of size 2.5 cm × 1.8 cm at the upper pole in the left lobe and a fleshy nodule of size 2.0 cm × 1.5 cm at the lower pole in the right lobe (Fig. 3). Histopathology was reported as bilateral papillary thyroid cancer without invasion or involvement of strap muscles. Early post-operative recovery was uneventful and she was started on prophylactic calcium and Vitamin D supplements. She was given thyroxine suppression, keeping TSH near the lower limit of the range and delaying the WBRAI until after the delivery. She was discharged on post-operative day 3. Subsequently, she delivered a healthy baby and 8 months later underwent WBRAI Scanning. Pre-therapy WBRI scan showed uptake only in the cervical level VII lymph node and she was given 50 mCi of I-131 given orally. The post-therapy scan was the same as pre-therapy scan.

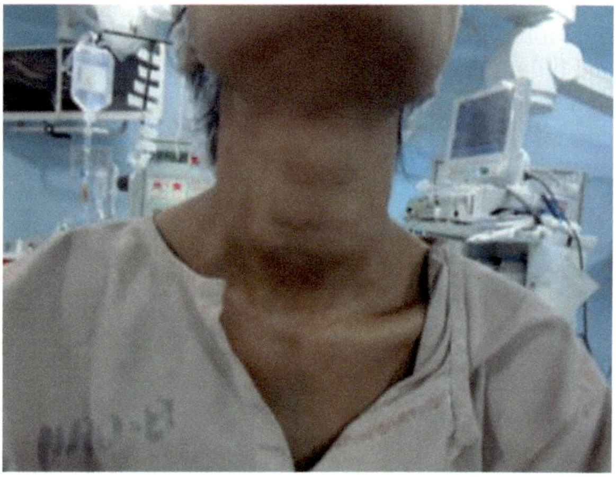

Fig. 1 Pregnant patient with bilateral thyroid nodules

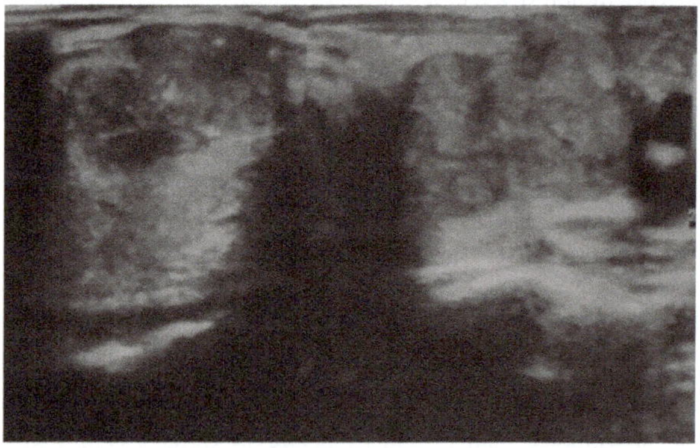

Fig. 2 USG thyroid showing bilateral nodules with punctate micro-calcifications (TIRADS 4C)

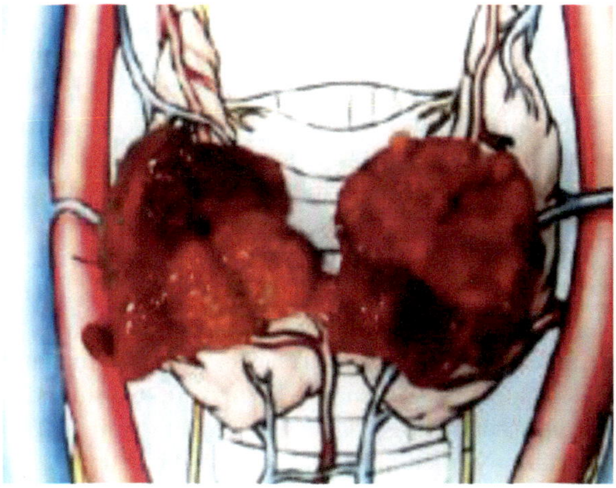

Fig. 3 Gross specimen showing nodules in both lobes

Discussion

Several studies have examined the prevalence of thyroid nodules during pregnancy using neck ultrasonography [1, 2]. Prevalence ranged between 3% and 30% and correlated with increasing age and parity. It has been postulated that pregnancy is associated with an increase in the size of preexisting thyroid nodules, as well as new thyroid nodule formation. In relation to nodule growth, one study showed a doubling in nodule size and volume during pregnancy [3]. Additionally, up to 20% of women with a thyroid nodule detected in the first trimester of pregnancy developed another nodule before delivery. However, the prevalence of thyroid cancer in thyroid nodules discovered during pregnancy in these studies is likely over-reported. Family history of thyroid cancer and exposure to head, neck and/or cranial radiation or ionizing radiation should be recorded. Neck ultrasound remains the most accurate and safe imaging modality for detecting thyroid nodules, assessing their pattern and features, and surveying cervical lymph nodes in pregnancy. Studies to date have shown that FNA is a safe procedure and may be performed in any trimester as pregnancy does not seem to modify cellular appearance at the microscopic level. For most patients with possible or confirmed well-differentiated thyroid carcinoma (WDTC) discovered by cytology in early pregnancy, the following should be done:

1. Cancer should be initially assessed
2. Surgical and Adjuvant Treatment: If sonographic evidence of substantial growth, tracheal or vessel invasion, or lymph node involvement is detected, surgery should be considered in the second trimester. Several studies have assessed the impact of thyroidectomy on the pregnant woman and fetus, with most surgeries taking place in the second trimester [4–6]. More recently, a retrospective study compared the clinicopathological features and outcomes of 24 women with DTC who underwent surgery during the second trimester of pregnancy, to those of 21 women who underwent surgery within 1 year of delivery. No surgical complications, no miscarriages or birth defects were reported in either group, leading the authors to

conclude that surgery can safely be carried out in the second trimester [7]. Similarly, in a study of 29 pregnant patients with PTC, 24 underwent total thyroidectomy with only one patient undergoing prophylactic LN dissection, with no maternal or fetal complications [8]. Thus, no maternal or fetal complications were reported in any of these studies. Women who have surgery for WDTC during pregnancy should be followed-up conservatively with regular monitoring and TSH suppressive therapy. In view of evidence that subclinical hyperthyroidism does not lead to any maternal or neonatal adverse outcomes [9], it is reasonable to maintain the same degree of TSH suppression in pregnancy as preconception, but taking into account a close to 30% increase in thyroid hormone replacement requirement during pregnancy [10]. Careful monitoring of thyroid function tests should be undertaken to avoid hypothyroidism and overt hyperthyroidism. Serum TSH should be checked every 4 weeks until 16–20 weeks of gestation, and subsequently at least once between weeks 26 and 32.

3. On rare findings of a more aggressive type of thyroid malignancy (e.g., medullary, poorly differentiated, or anaplastic) surgery in the second trimester should be considered.
4. If low-risk DTC surgery can be safely deferred to until after delivery. However, then it should be regularly monitored for evidence of highly aggressive behavior for which intervention during gestation may become necessary. If a low-risk cancerous nodule is being followed with a nonoperative approach during pregnancy, starting levothyroxine in doses of 50–75 mcg, targeting a serum TSH level less than 2.0 mU/L can be considered.

References

1. Kung AW, Chau MT, Lao TT, et al. The effect of pregnancy on thyroid nodule formation. J Clin Endocrinol Metab. 2002;87:1010–4.
2. Sahin SB, Ogullar S, Ural UM, et al. Alterations of thyroid volume and nodular size during and after pregnancy in a severe iodine-deficient area. Clin Endocrinol (Oxford). 2014;81:762–8.
3. Struve CW, Haupt S, Ohlen S. Influence of frequency of previous pregnancies on the prevalence of thyroid nodules in women without clinical evidence of thyroid disease. Thyroid. 1993;3:7–9.
4. Tan GH, Gharib H, Goellner JR, et al. Management of thyroid nodules in pregnancy. Arch Intern Med. 1996;156:2317–20.
5. Doherty CM, Shindo ML, Rice DH, et al. Management of thyroid nodules during pregnancy. Laryngoscope. 1995;105:251–5.
6. Vini L, Hyer S, Pratt B, et al. Management of differentiated thyroid cancer diagnosed during pregnancy. Eur J Endocrinol. 1999;140:404–6.
7. Uruno T, Shibuya H, Kitagawa W, et al. Optimal timing of surgery for differentiated thyroid cancer in pregnant women. World J Surg. 2014;38:704–8.
8. Boucek J, de Haan J, Halaska MJ, et al. Maternal and obstetrical outcome in 35 cases of welldifferentiated thyroid carcinoma during pregnancy. Laryngoscope. 2018;128:1493–500.
9. Casey BM, Dashe JS, Wells CE, et al. Subclinical hyperthyroidism and pregnancy outcomes. Obstet Gynecol. 2006;107:337–41.
10. Loh JA, Wartofsky L, Jonklaas J, et al. The magnitude of increased levothyroxine requirements in hypothyroid pregnant women depends upon the etiology of the hypothyroidism. Thyroid. 2009;19:269–75.

Child with DTC

Case 1

A 11-year-old boy presented with an anterior neck swelling for 4 years which was progressively increasing in size but without pressure symptoms and no symptoms of hypothyroidism or hyperthyroidism. He gave a history of occasional cough with breathlessness on exertion. Examination of neck showed right thyroid lobe solitary thyroid nodule 3 × 3.5 cm, hard in consistency, left thyroid lobe was enlarged, but no nodule was palpable. He also had bilateral multiple level 2, 3, 4 and 5 nodes, rounded and firm in consistency, largest 1 × 1.5 cm in right level 3, nontender. Investigations revealed TSH (Thyrotropin) 3.26 miu/l Thyroglobulin TG > 300 ng/ml (ATG <20.0 IU/ML), USG Neck: ill-defined infiltrative lesion replacing right lobe and isthmus with multiple punctate calcifications, extra-thyroidal extension with abutment to right ICA; ill-defined lesions in left lobe. Bilateral multiple enlarged level IIA, IIB, III, IV, V, and VI nodes. FNAC thyroid and lymph nodes showed papillary thyroid carcinoma. Chest X-ray showed bilateral miliary mottling

---

Amit Agarwal is the lead author of this chapter.

A. Agarwal et al., *Case Studies in Thyroid and Parathyroid Tumors*,
https://doi.org/10.1007/978-981-99-0938-4_72

in both lung fields (Fig. 1). CECT neck showed 42 × 26 × 18mm heterogenous mass lesion involving right thyroid lobe with multiple enhancing lymph nodes at bilateral level I, II, III, IV, V and VI and numerous tiny nodular lesions in both lung fields suggestive of lung metastases (Fig. 2). The child was taken up for total thyroidectomy + CCLND + B/L SLND. At operation right lobe was found to be enlarged and adherent to trachea but could be separated. Multiple enlarged LNs in central compartment (largest 2 × 2 cm). CCLND done till brachiocephalic artery. Right and left RLN preserved, Rt RLN densely adherent to central compartment lymph nodes but could be shaved off. Both left-sided parathyroids identified but de-vascularized, hence auto transplanted in the right SCM. Multiple enlarged LNs on both sides from level II to V. B/L SLND done (level II–V). Right lateral LN mass was densely adherent to IJV, dissected with difficulty. Grossing: weight- 20 g (TT specimen), Right lobe—3.5 × 3 × 1.5, Left lobe—3 × 2 × 1; c/s: fleshy, greyish white right lobe, isthmus and left lobe normal (Fig. 3). Post op period developed symptomatic hypocalcemia managed by intravenous calcium followed by oral calcium and vitamin D supplements. Histopathology revealed: Papillary thyroid carcinoma (solid variant); right CCLND: metastatic carcinoma (2/3) left CCLND: metastatic carcinoma (6/7); right SLND: metastatic carcinoma (11/26); left SLND: metastatic carcinoma (10/51). He was referred for WBRAI scan. Serum thyroglobulin levels were >300 ng/ml with ATG of 252 IU/ML. Pretherapy WBRAI scan showed uptake in thyroid bed, right level II lymph node and bilateral lung metastases (Fig. 4). He was given 100 mCI of I-131 orally under medical supervision. Post therapy scan was the same as pre-therapy (Fig. 5). Second WBRAI was done after 1 year and showed increased uptake in right level II, bilateral lungs. Scanning was again repeated after 9 months and pre-therapy scan showed increased uptake in right level II, bilateral lung nodules (macronodular) and the child was treated with 100 mCi again. His serum TG remained >300 ng/ml even after 200 mCi.

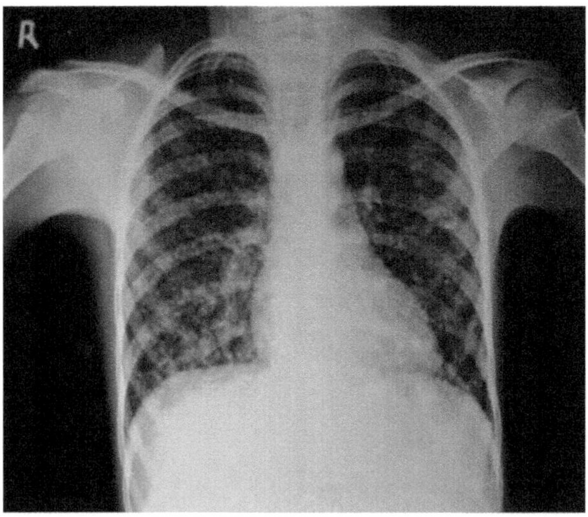

Fig. 1 Chest-x-ray showing diffuse mottling suggestive of metastases

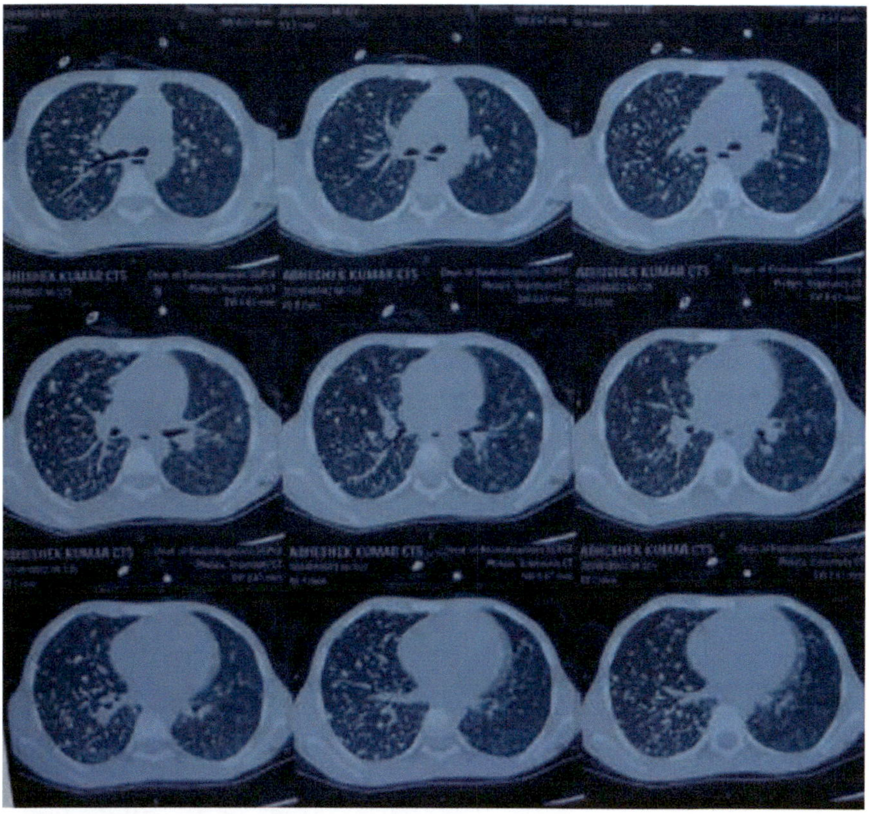

Fig. 2 CECT thorax showing diffuse lung metastases

Fig. 3 Surgical specimen of total thyroidectomy with central compartmental dissection with bilateral selective LN dissection. Cut-surface of right lobe shows solid architecture

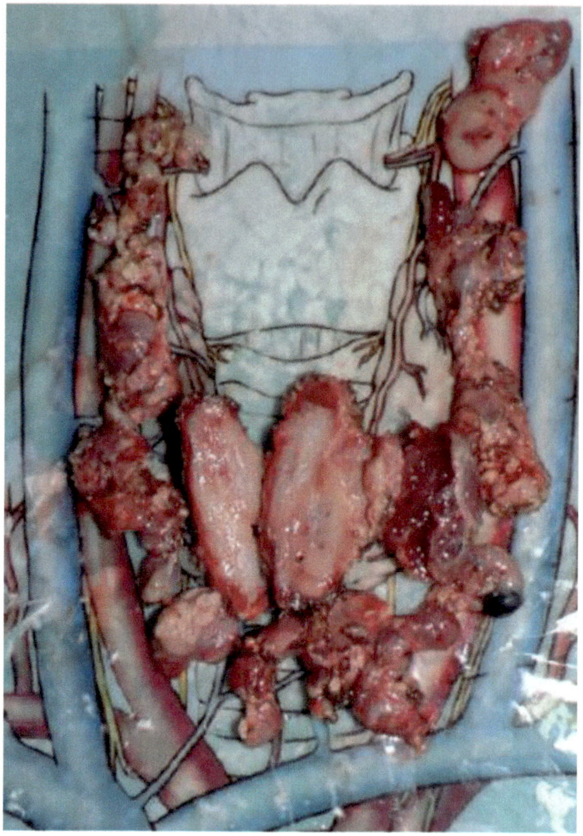

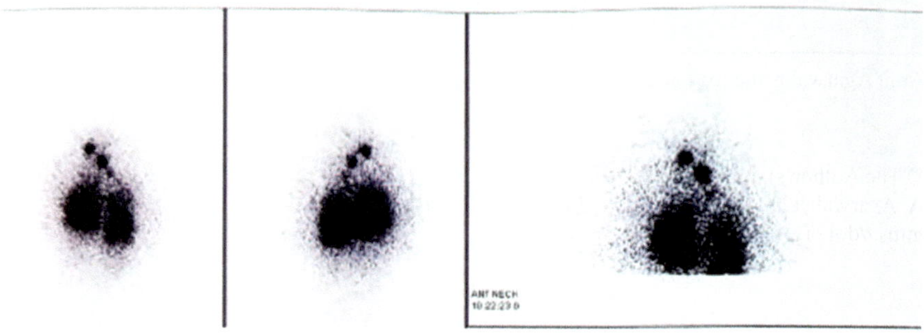

Fig. 4 Pre-therapy WBRAI scan shows uptake in level II LN and bilateral lung metastases

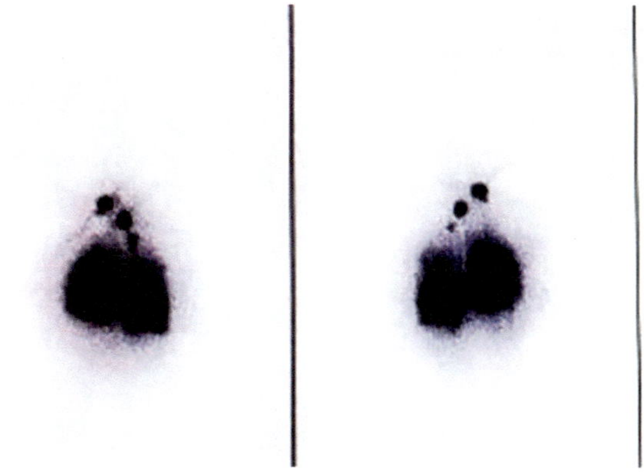

Fig. 5 Post-therapy scan showing similar status

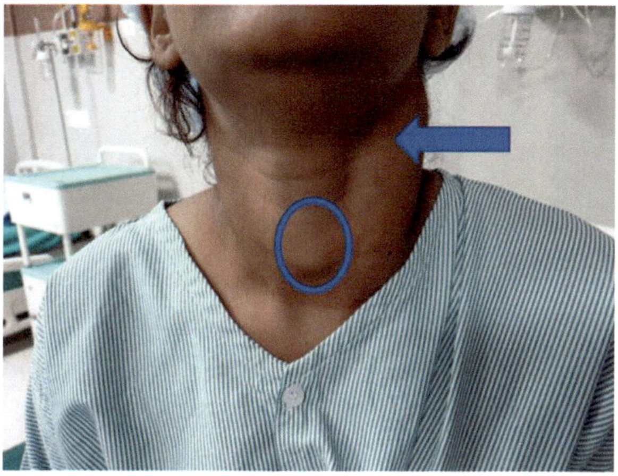

Fig. 6 Clinical image showing left nodule and left lateral nodes (blue arrow)

Case 2

An 18-year-old girl presented with a history of anterior neck swelling (Fig. 6) since the age of 5 years. There was recent appearance of left lateral neck swelling which made her visit our outpatient clinic. There was no history of voice change or hemoptysis. Fine needle aspiration cytology was papillary thyroid carcinoma. Contrast-enhanced CT scan was done showing indentation of the trachea at the second and third tracheal ring (Fig. 7) with no breach of the cartilage. The patient was planned for surgery. Total thyroidectomy with central compartment lymph nodes dissection with left selective lymph node dissection was done. The tumor was easily separable from the trachea without the involvement of the cartilage. The indent on the trachea can be appreciated in Fig. 8. The histopathology was suggestive of classical PTC with BRAF negative. The patient received 125mci of I 131 therapy and post-therapy scan revealed lung metastasis. After the second dose RAI patient showed complete disappearance of lung metastasis and the patient is doing fine after 24 months with no biochemical or structural disease.

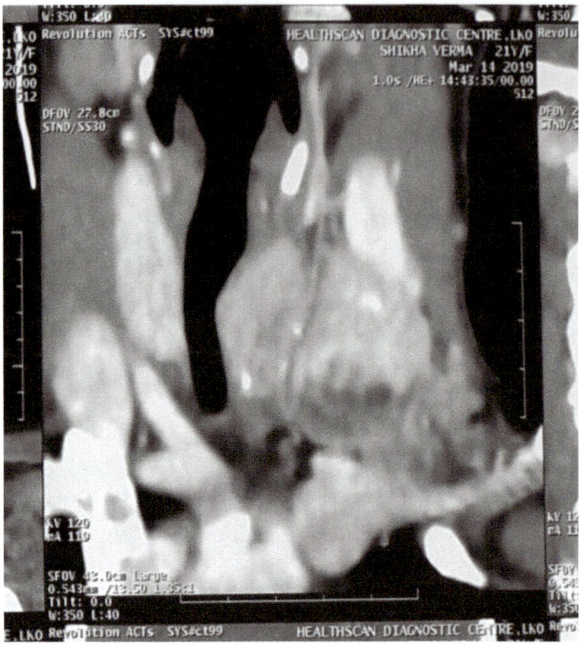

Fig. 7 CECT showing indentation of trachea

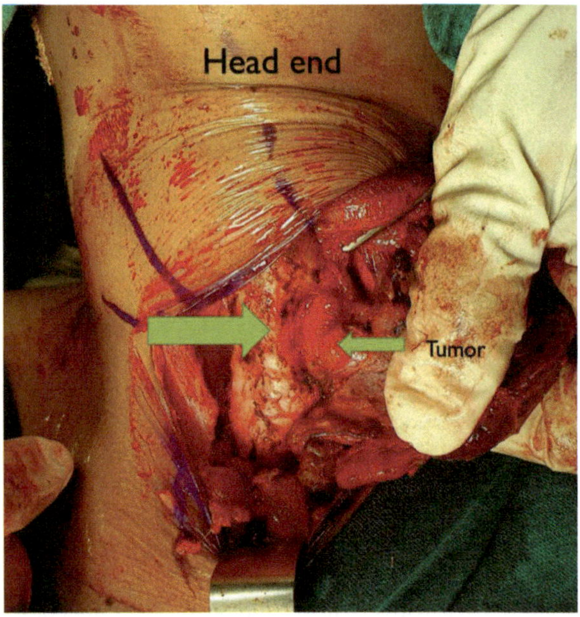

Fig. 8 Intraoperative image showing tracheal indentation without tracheal wall involvement

Discussion

In children less than 10 years of age, the incidence of DTC is one per 1,000,000, whereas in children from 10 to 14 years of age, the incidence of DTC is one per 200,000 [1]. One of the largest growing groups of children at risk for thyroid cancer is childhood cancer survivors who have had head and neck irradiation. Rare genetic syndromes are associated with thyroid cancer. Cowden's syndrome, Gardener's syndrome, Werner syndrome, and congenital hypothyroidism may also be associated with pediatric DTC. The genetic landscape of pediatric DTC is different. Unlike adults, BRAF mutations are infrequent, whereas RET/PTC rearrangements are more frequent in children [1]. The RET/PTC1 type rearrangement is more common in children with tumors with classic papillary architecture whereas RET/PTC 3 type mutation is associated with the solid variant of papillary carcinoma. In children, 40% of PTC are typical PTC, 30% are the follicular variant, 10% to 35% are the solid variant, and 20% to 30% are the mixed variant [2] [124 OF EMCNA]. The solid variant is thought to occur more commonly in radiation-induced tumors. Unlike adults, because about 30% of pediatric thyroid nodules are malignant, and US-guided FNA can be performed in nodules less than 1 cm, it is recommended to biopsy smaller lesions in children. The UICC/AJCC classification of the DTC which has been developed for adults is also not valid for children as very few pediatric patients belong to low-risk category. The thyroid cancer types in children are PTC in 60%, follicular variant of PTC in 23%, FTC in 10%, and medullary thyroid cancer (MTC) in 5% (1). Compared to adults, children with DTC present with more extensive disease (5–14). In general, the following observations about pediatric DTC can be made [3]: (1) About 40–90% of children present with disease that is metastatic to lymph nodes, compared with 20–50% of adults. (2) About 15% of children present with distant metastatic disease, most commonly to the lungs. In more than 50% of these cases, lung tumors are micrometastases. (3) The prevalence of distant metastases, most commonly lung, is 20–30% in children vs. 2% in adults (5–14, 17). (4) Multifocal disease is more common in children than adults and is seen in about 40% of childhood PTC cases. It is believed that the proliferation of individual clones, not metastases, accounts for the multifocal nature of disease. (5) DTC with onset at less than 10 yr. of age appears to have higher recurrence (30%) and mortality rates than presentation at older ages. (6) Most tumors respond well to RAI therapy; fortunately, even in the presence of metastatic disease, long-term follow-up data show 30-yr survival rates of 90–99% for children with DTC. Pulmonary metastases can remain stable for extended periods. Whereas empiric activity selection is convenient and practical, blood-dose limiting-based or lesion-based dosimetry should be considered for children with metastatic disease to the lungs and other sites. As far as treatment is concerned, large cohort studies [4–6] on pediatric thyroid cancers collectively show that DTC recurrence risk can be reduced by (1) performing total thyroidectomy vs. lobectomy; (2) performing compartment lymph node dissection vs. selective or no lymph node dissection; and (3) administering WBRAI Therapy. Surgery should be performed by high-volume thyroid surgeons and surgeons should preferably be using surgical loupes for better identification of small parathyroids to avoid the dreaded complication of permanent hypocalcemia.

References

1. Rivkees SA, Mazzaferri EL, Verburg FA, Reiners C, Luster M, Breuer CK, Dinauer CA, Udelsman R. The treatment of differentiated thyroid cancer in children: emphasis on surgical approach and radioactive iodine therapy. Endocr Rev. 2011;32(6):798–826.
2. Dinauer C, Gary L. Francis thyroid cancer in children. Endocrinol Metab Clin N Am. 2007;36:779–806.
3. Francis GL, Waguespack SG, Bauer AJ, Angelos P, Benvenga S, Cerutti JM, Dinauer CA, Hamilton J, Hay ID, Luster M, Parisi MT, Rachmiel M, Thompson GB, Yamashita S. Management guidelines for children with thyroid nodules and differentiated thyroid cancer. Thyroid. 2015;25:716–59.
4. Demidchik YE, Demidchik EP, Reiners C, Biko J, Mine M, Saenko VA, Yamashita S. Comprehensive clinical assessment of 740 cases of surgically treated thyroid cancer in children of Belarus. Ann Surg. 2006;243:525–32.
5. Handkiewicz-Junak D, Wloch J, Roskosz J, Krajewska J, Kropinska A, Pomorski L, Kukulska A, Prokurat A, Wygoda Z, Jarzab B. Total thyroidectomy and adjuvant radioiodine treatment independently decrease locoregional recurrence risk in childhood and adolescent differentiated thyroid cancer. J Nucl Med. 2007;48:879–88.
6. Hay ID, Gonzalez-Losada T, Reinalda MS, Honetschlager JA, Richards ML, Thompson GB. Long-term outcome in 215 children and adolescents with papillary thyroid cancer treated during 1940 through 2008. World J Surg. 2010;34:1192–202.

Tall Cell Variant PTC

Case

A 35-year-old gentleman came with a history of swelling in the front of his neck for one and a half years which was gradually increasing in size. He also gave a history of breathlessness and stridor for one and a half months and hemoptysis, 2–3 episodes per month. He was a chronic tobacco smoker, chronic alcoholic but has been abstaining for the last 8 years. On examination, he had a 4 × 4 cm hard solitary thyroid nodule without any deep cervical lymphadenopathy. The FNAC from the thyroid nodule was reported as papillary thyroid cancer. Indirect laryngoscopy showed B/L VC were mobile. CECT showed a 44 × 42 mm necrotic soft tissue mass lesion in the left side of the neck involving the left thyroid gland extending to infra-glottic larynx, infiltration noted over the left thyroid gland and cricoid cartilage and trachea with airway narrowing (Fig. 1). He underwent total Thyroidectomy + Tracheostomy + tracheal resection and crico-tracheal anastomosis. Operative findings included adherent strap muscles to the surface of the left lobe of thyroid and growth arising from the left lobe of thyroid and isthmus extending to the intraluminal part of the trachea by invading the cricoid and upper 2 tracheal rings. Total thyroidectomy was performed with en-bloc resection of cricoid and tracheal rings (Fig. 2) (preserving normal posterior wall of trachea); crico-tracheal anastomosis performed with intermittent 3–0 vicryl sutures (Fig. 3). On histology: "the sections from left lobe and isthmus show a tumour disposed in papillary pattern with central fibrovascular core. These cells show nuclear

Amit Agarwal is the lead author of this chapter.

A. Agarwal et al., *Case Studies in Thyroid and Parathyroid Tumors*,
https://doi.org/10.1007/978-981-99-0938-4_73

stratification, clearing, grooving, psuedoinclusions in few and granular eosinophilic cytoplasm. Most of these cells are tall (Figs. 4 and 5), have abundant eosinophilic cytoplasm. The tumour is seen infiltrating the skeletal muscles and trachea. The inferior margin of trachea is also involved. Foci of lymphovascular invasion are seen. The right lobe appears free of tumour." The patient subsequently received 125 mci RAI since his TG was elevated (166 ng/ml) and RAI scan showed uptake in thyroid remnant and left cervical LN (level II). On follow-up his TG started rising and he became RAI refractory. PET scan revealed hypermetabolic cervical, mediastinal lymphadenopathy with multiple pulmonary nodules suggestive of metastatic disease. He is currently on TKI and his TG values are 53.3 ng/ml.

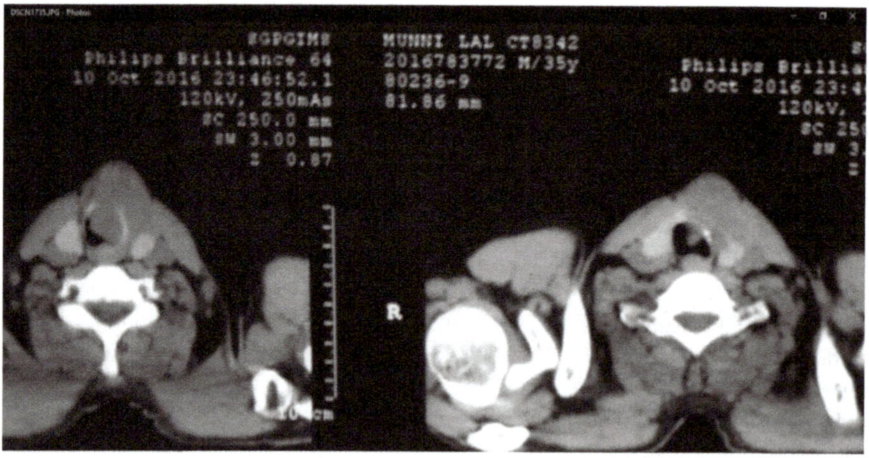

Fig. 1 CECT showing intra-luminal invasion of the trachea

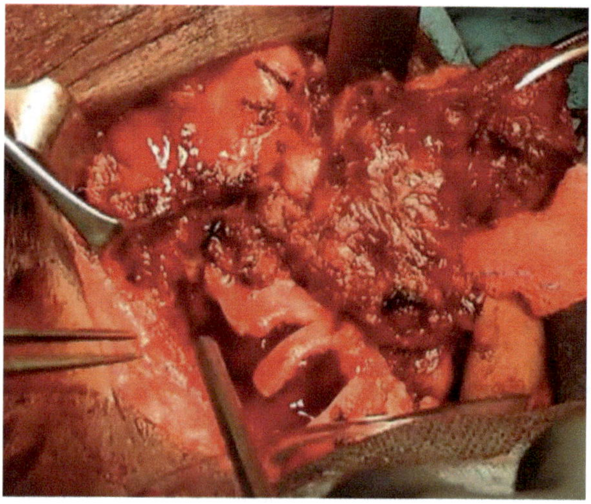

Fig. 2 Thyroid cancer invading the cricoid and first 2 tracheal rings

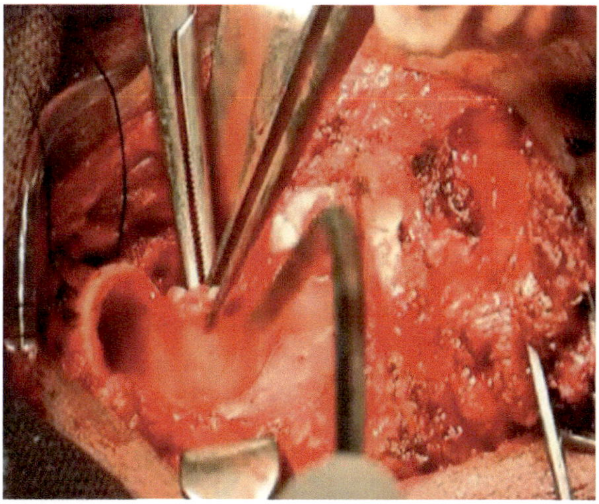

Fig. 3 Crico-tracheal anastomosis in progress

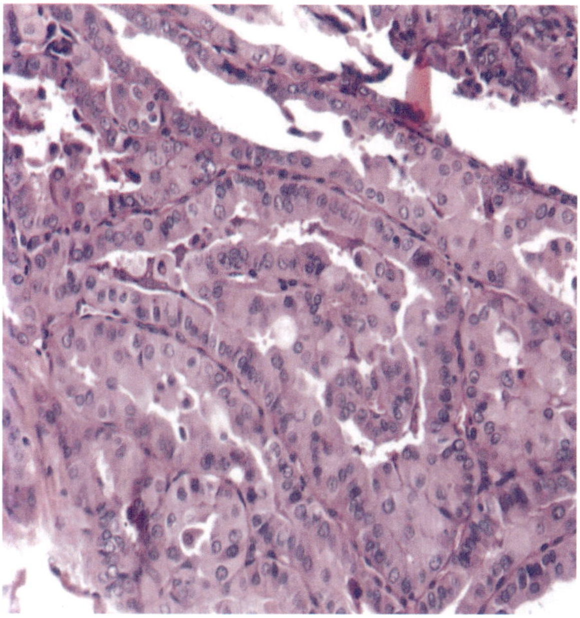

Fig. 4 Papillary carcinoma, tall cell variant having elongated columnar cells arranged parallelly. H&E, 20× Magnification

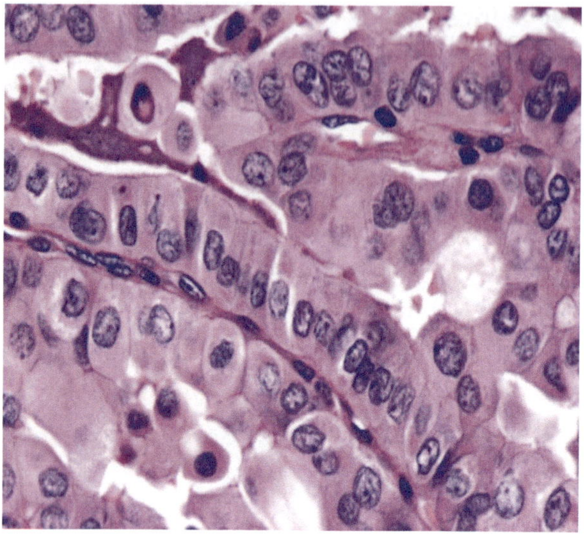

Fig. 5 Microphotograph of papillary carcinoma, tall cell variant—The height of the cell is >3 times the width. H&E, 40× Magnification

Discussion

Though the majority of PTCs are well differentiated with an excellent long-term outcome, there are a small group of tumors with distinct histology which behave more aggressively and have frequent recurrences and locoregional and distant metastases. The most common aggressive variant is the tall cell variant (TCV). Though there has been disagreement about the percentage of tall cells needed to make the diagnosis of TCV, a recent World Health Organization (WHO) [1] definition of TCV is a tumor that is composed "of cells that are two to three times as tall as they are wide, and that show abundant eosinophilic (oncocytic-like) cytoplasm. Because tall-cell areas are frequently present in otherwise conventional papillary carcinomas, tall cells must account for ≥30% of all tumour cells for the diagnosis of the tall-cell variant." TCV is more commonly seen in women, occurs in older patients, presents with larger tumor size, more frequent extrathyroidal involvement, 20% of them are RAI refractory and they have a shorter survival [2]. Vuong et al. [3] in a recent meta-analysis found that even PTCs with only 10% tall cells were associated with a poor clinical outcome. They suggest that the presence of tall cells in a small percentage, even only 10%, must be reported. On cytology, TCV can be recognized by the soap-bubble appearance. On histology, besides the striking tall cell feature, these tumors also exhibit stretched elongated follicles in histologic sections, a finding termed as "tram-track appearance." TCV also shows higher prevalence of BRAF, TERT mutations, and RET/PTC rearrangements. Regarding treatment, TCV tumors have to be treated aggressively with total thyroidectomy with or without neck dissection and RAI therapy.

References

1. Lloyd R, Osamura R, Klöppel G, Rosai J. WHO classification of tumours of endocrine organs. 4th ed. Lyon: International Agency for Research on Cancer; 2017.
2. Coca-Pelaz A, Shah JP, Hernandez-Prera JC, et al. Papillary thyroid cancer-aggressive variants and impact on management: a narrative review. Adv Ther. 2020;37(7):3112–28.
3. Vuong HG, Kondo T, Pham TQ, et al. Prognostic significance of diffuse sclerosing variant papillary thyroid carcinoma: a systematic review and metaanalysis. Eur J Endocrinol. 2017;176:433–41.

Recurrent Papillary Thyroid Cancer

Case

A 53-years-old woman presented to us with a recurrent thyroid swelling. She had undergone 2 previous surgeries - left hemithyroidectomy 8 years back (reported as PTC) and excision of a recurrent mass 4 years back (reported as follicular variant PTV). At presentation she had left vocal cord palsy and asymmetrical exophytic swelling in front of the neck, 8.5 × 7.5 cm in size arising from the right lobe of thyroid, all borders well defined, with the bosselated surface with erythema of skin over the mid 1/3 of swelling and engorged superficial veins over the anterior chest with two surgical scars seen over lower neck & in the mid portion of swelling. CECT Neck and upper mediastinum revealed non-visualization of left lobe of thyroid and a large exophytic lobulated heterogeneously enhancing mass 7.5 × 5.2 × 4.8 cm in right lower anterolateral neck in s/c plane, arising from isthmus and right thyroid lobe, focally infiltration into adjoining right SCM and B/L straps. TG: >300 ng/ml (0–52). ATG: <20 IU/ml, FNAC was PTC. Total thyroidectomy with intra-operative neuromonitoring was done and a solid mass of size 10 cm × 5 cm × 5 cm deep to skin and superficial to straps muscles was excised along with right hemithyroidectomy. Histopathology was reported as a follicular variant of PTC. WBRAI Scan showed uptake in thyroid bed with right level VI LN. 150 mCi of I-131 was given orally under supervision. Post-therapy scan was same as pre-therapy scan.

Amit Agarwal is the lead author of this chapter.

A. Agarwal et al., *Case Studies in Thyroid and Parathyroid Tumors*,
https://doi.org/10.1007/978-981-99-0938-4_74

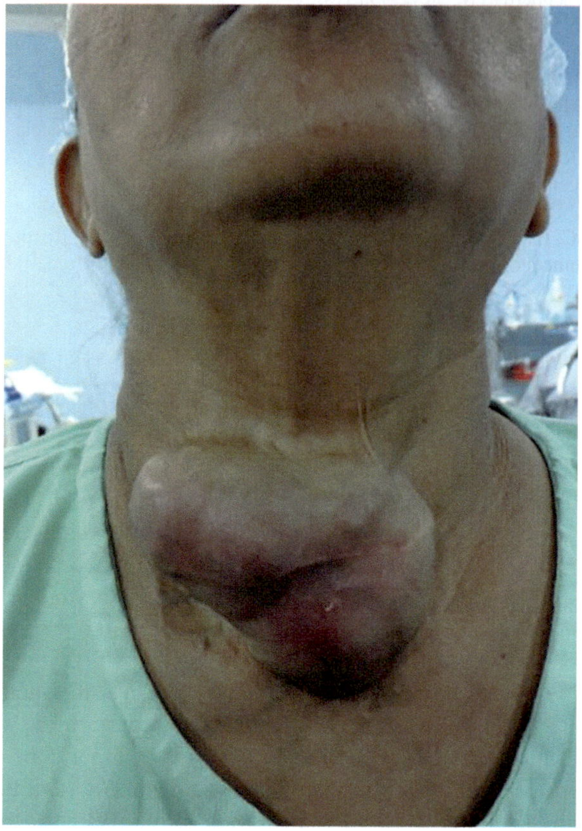

Discussion

The frequency of locoregional recurrence is anywhere from 5% to 20% in PTC [1], and more than one-third of reoperations for persistent or recurrent disease are related to insufficient initial thyroid surgery. The impact of the development of recurrent disease on long-term survival has been controversial. It is felt that the development of locoregionally recurrent disease increases the risk of death from differentiated thyroid cancer fivefold. Risk factors for loco-regional recurrences include: stage III tumors (>4 cm), incomplete surgical removal (hemithyroidectomy in a case of multifocal disease, leaving behind disease in a case of extra-thyroidal extension), and presence of positive central compartment lymph nodes [2]. As reported by Leboulleux and colleagues [3], when a tumor is less than 4 cm but there are more than 10 metastatic lymph nodes or more than 3 lymph nodes with extra-capsular extension, the risk of persistent disease is 20% to 45%. The overall 5-, 10-, and 15-year survival rates for the patients with T1 through T3 disease are 96%, 93%, and 87%, respectively, while those with T4 disease are 70%, 54%, and 45% respectively.

Diagnosis of recurrence involves the following:

1. Clinical examination and imaging: to establish whether it is a:
   (a) Thyroid bed recurrence thyroid remnant recurrence, soft tissue recurrence, or recurrence in intact thyroid lobe, or
   (b) LN recurrence (central compartment LN or Lateral LN)
2. Serum thyroglobulin: To identify a small recurrence, thyrotropin-stimulation serum thyroglobulin measurements along with antithyroglobulin antibodies are needed. While the normal level of thyroglobulin differs for each patient, it is generally accepted that a level above 2 ng/mL is associated with recurrent disease. In patients with abnormal Tg, either as a persistent abnormal or a new finding, it is both the trend in values over time and the magnitude of the elevation that is of clinical relevance. In general, serum Tg levels correlate with volume of disease as well as with the site of the metastatic disease [4].
3. Ultrasound imaging: In regard to the evaluation of the primary site after surgery, the paralaryngeal and paratracheal region will typically have homogenous, slightly hyperechoic scar tissue present with the common carotid artery closely approximated to the upper aerodigestive tract. Recurrent disease will appear as a hypoechoic mass in the operative bed showing irregular border and microcalcification.
4. FNAC: Recurrent structural disease that measures 8 to 10 mm or larger on anatomic imaging in the central and lateral neck, respectively, should be considered for cytology biopsy, and Tg aspirate rinsing analysis.
5. Cross-sectional imaging: Several areas of potential recurrence are not visualized on ultrasound, including the tracheal esophageal groove, retropharyngeal region and superior mediastinum. Hence CECT is indicated in all recurrent thyroid cancer cases to provide a road map as well for surgery.
6. Whole-body RAI scan: In high-risk patients ^{131}I uptake scan, when combined with a stimulated thyroglobulin, offers a sensitivity for identifying recurrent disease approaching 100% [5].
7. PET-CT (FDG PET): Should be considered when there is elevated thyroglobulin and no iodine uptake on whole-body imaging. It should be remembered that PET–CT scan is not useful as a screening tool because the false-negative rates are relatively high (15–30%).

Treatment of Recurrent Disease Surgery is the preferred treatment modality of resectable recurrent thyroid carcinoma with preservation of the recurrent laryngeal nerve and parathyroids when possible. However, thyroid remnant recurrences are more amenable to resection as compared to soft tissue recurrence (90% in a thyroid remnant versus 45% in the soft tissue recurrence) [6]. In general, the goal of revision surgery should be to remove any remaining native thyroid tissue, to resect locally recurrent cancer in the thyroid bed, to clear the involved nodal basins in a compartmental fashion, and to dissect nodal basins likely to harbor microscopic regional metastases. The intent of such an approach is to reduce the need for future surgery and to avoid having to explore a compartment again. For nodal regions that have been previously dissected, there may be very low nodal yield; dissection in these areas may necessarily be more targeted/selective.

True local recurrence or thyroid bed recurrence (newly formed disease found within soft tissue, often densely attached or invading these structures) makes surgical resection more difficult and potentially involving sacrifice of important structures such as RLN, tracheal cartilage [7]. The surgical approach to the **thyroid bed soft tissue recurrence** should include identification and protection of the recurrent laryngeal nerves. In the previously operated thyroid bed, the nerve is often contained within fibrotic scar and can be somewhat difficult to identify. The surgical approach to the thyroid bed should be done through the prior incision site. Strategies to decrease the risk of injury to the recurrent laryngeal nerve include identifying the nerve low in the tracheoesophageal groove well below the thyroid bed, use of neuromonitoring, and use of surgical loupes [8].

Surgical approach to central compartment should be directed at full compartment dissection rather than berry picking. Thus, the central compartment dissection should contain all of the remaining lymphatic tissue from the carotid artery laterally to the trachea medially. Superiorly, the dissection should extend from just above the cricoid to the level of the clavicle inferiorly. If the tumor adheres to the nerve but can be dissected away, the nerve should be preserved. Resection of the nerve may be required if the tumor encompasses the nerve. The risk of recurrent laryngeal nerve injury resulting in permanent vocal cord paralysis ranges from 1% to 12%, which is higher than the risk in primary surgery of the central compartment. Similarly, the parathyroid glands in revision central compartment surgery are at high risk for devascularization and inadvertent removal. The incidence of permanent hypoparathyroidism after reoperation ranges from 1% to 4%.

Surgical Management of Laryngotracheal Invasion In regards to the thyroid bed, it is not uncommon for the recurrent disease to adhere to the tracheal or esophageal wall or to minimally invade the tracheal or esophageal wall. Laryngeal or tracheal invasion can be found in around 4% to 16% of patients and has been found to be an independent predictor of poor prognosis. Patients who underwent radical resection with complete tumor removal were able to achieve a 5-year survival rate of about 77% and a 10-year survival rate of about 60%,20 while those with residual disease after resection had 5-year survivals of just over 20%. Therefore, all attempts should be made to remove the invaded structure. The surgeon should seek out surgical resection options that offer the lowest perioperative morbidity and the highest long-term quality of life.

Role of External Beam Radiation External beam radiation to this area carries side effects and morbidity, and the overall effect on locoregional recurrence and survival has not been clearly shown to be positive. Thus, this treatment modality is often saved for the recurrent disease in which further surgical management (with or without radioactive iodine) will compromise function, diminish quality of life, or be likely ineffective.

Non-operative Management Patients who have small structural recurrences, particularly small metastatic LN in a badly scarred neck or the patients are unfit for surgery can benefit from various non-operative modalities such as percutaneous ethanol injection, percutaneous laser ablation, high-frequency US ablation (HIFU), radio-frequency ablation,, cryotherapy, and microwave thermal ablation.

References

1. Kouvaraki MA, Lee JE, Shapiro SE, et al. Preventable reoperations for persistent and recurrent papillary thyroid carcinoma. Surgery. 2004;136(6):1183–91.
2. Stojadinovic A, Shoup M, Nissan A, et al. Recurrent differentiated thyroid carcinoma: biological implications of age, method of detection and site and extent of recurrence. Ann Surg Oncol. 2002;9(8):789–98.
3. Leboulleux S, Rubino C, Baudin E, et al. Prognostic factors for persistent or recurrent disease of papillary thyroid carcinoma with neck lymph node metastases and/or extension beyond the thyroid capsule at initial diagnosis. J Clin Endocrinol Metab. 2005;90(10):5723–9.
4. Robbins RJ, Srivastava S, Shaha A, et al. Factors influencing the basal and recombinant human thyrotropin-stimulated serum thyroglobulin in patients with metastatic thyroid carcinoma. J Clin Endocrinol Metab. 2004;89:6010–6.
5. Pacini F, Molinaro E, Castagna G, et al. Recombinant human thyrotropin–stimulated serum thyroglobulin combined with neck ultrasonography has the highest sensitivity in monitoring differentiated thyroid carcinoma. J Clin Endocrinol Metab. 2003;88:3668–78.
6. Hessel A, Chalian AA, Clayman GL. Surgical management of recurrent thyroid cancer. Neuroimaging Clin N Am. 2008;18(3):517–25, viii.
7. Grant CS. Recurrence of papillary thyroid cancer after optimized surgery. Gland Surg. 2015;4(1):52–62.
8. Scharpf J, Tuttle M, Wong R, Ridge D, Smith R, Hartl D, Levine R, Randolph G. Comprehensive management of recurrent thyroid cancer: an American Head and Neck Society consensus statement: AHNS consensus statement. Head Neck. 2016;38(12):1862–9.

Warthin-Like Variant of Papillary Thyroid Carcinoma

Case

A 42-year-old female was being evaluated for generalized weakness and found to have anterior neck mass. On examination, she had a diffusely enlarged thyroid with nodules in both lobes: size 3 × 2 cm in the left lobe and 2 × 2 cm in the right lobe. USG neck: Rt lobe 2.2 × 2.1 cm, left lobe 3.3 × 1.9 cm with ill-defined hypoechoic area noted in bilateral lobe with increased vascularity with TIRADS-5. She was taken up for total thyroidectomy with CCLND. At operation both lobes were grossly enlarged with increased surface vascularity; strap muscles were densely adhered to left lobe, central part excised with specimen. 2 left level II lymph nodes sent for FSB, reported as negative for malignancy. HPE was reported as Warthin-like variant in view of presence of lympho-plasmacytic infiltrate (Fig. 1 4x magnification, Fig. 2 10x magnification, Fig. 3 20x magnification) in the fibrovascular core which was lined by cuboidal to tall eosinophilic cells displaying nuclear grooving, clearing and crowding. Right lobe showed features of lymphocytic thyroiditis.

Amit Agarwal is the lead author of this chapter.

A. Agarwal et al., *Case Studies in Thyroid and Parathyroid Tumors*,
https://doi.org/10.1007/978-981-99-0938-4_75

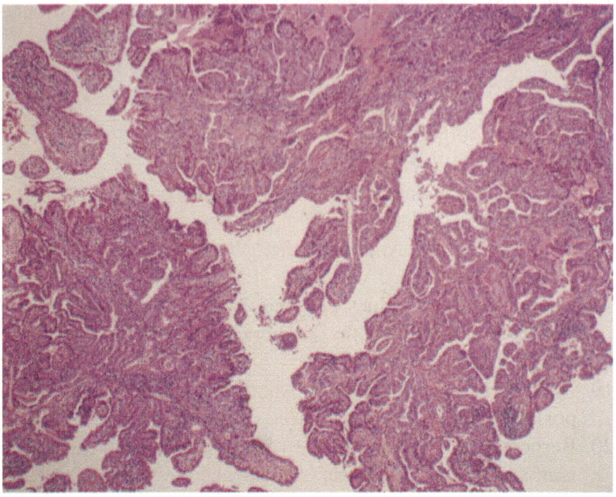

Fig. 1 Low power view of Warthin-like variant of papillary carcinoma showing heavy lymphomononuclear cell infiltrate in the cores of papillae lined by tumor epithelial cells (H&E stain; **4× Magnification**)

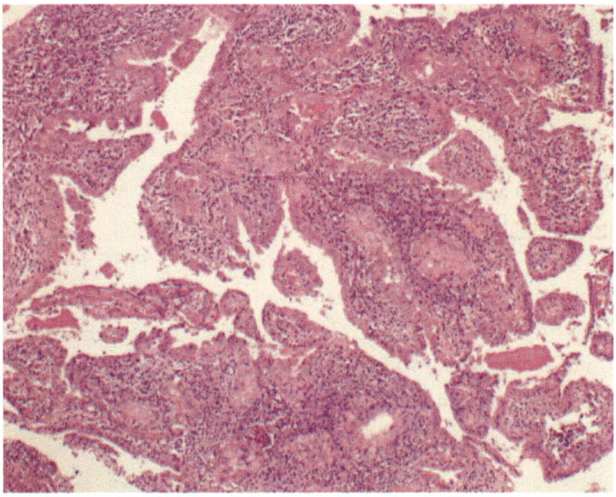

Fig. 2 Low power view of Warthin-like variant of papillary carcinoma showing heavy lymphomononuclear cell infiltrate in the cores of papillae lined by tumor epithelial cells (H&E stain; **10× Magnification**)

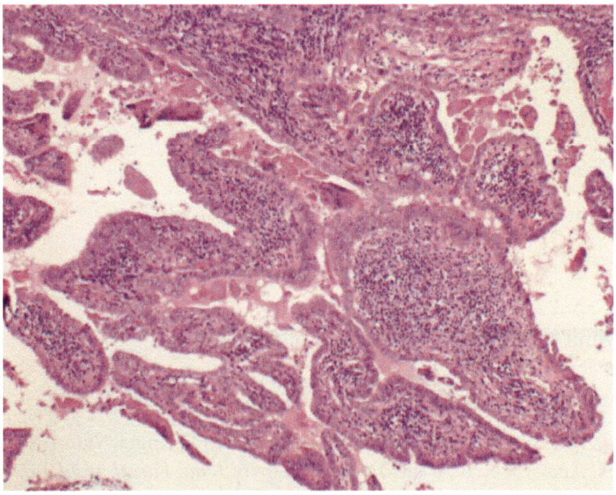

Fig. 3 Low power view of Warthin-like variant of papillary carcinoma showing heavy lymphomononuclear cell infiltrate in the cores of papillae lined by tumor epithelial cells (H&E stain; **20× Magnification**)

Discussion

Warthin-like variant of papillary carcinoma is an uncommon variant that was first described by Apel et al. [1] in 1995. This morphologic variant has distinct features of papillary architecture with prominent lymphocytic stroma in fibrovascular cores, resembling Warthin tumor of the salivary gland. The neoplastic cells lining the papillary folds have nuclear features of usual papillary carcinoma. The World Health Organization (WHO) has classified "Warthin-like tumor" under the oncocytic variant of PTC [2]. Thus, 4 essential histological features to diagnose these cases include: presence of papillary architecture, oncocytic change, nuclear features of PTC, and dense lymphoid infiltrates of the papillary core. Warthin-like PTC is more common in females and usually affects middle age group. Yeo et al. [3] in their study have concluded that WLPTC is similar to classic PTC coexisting with Hashimoto thyroiditis with regard to demographic, clinical, pathologic, and molecular features [4]. There are no typical US features and hence it can be misdiagnosed by US as a probably benign nodule or focal thyroiditis. Studies show that the overall and progression-free survival rates of these patients are similar to patients who have conventional papillary carcinoma [5–7]. Recognition of variants is important because different types of tumor have distinct cytological and nuclear features and prognosis.

References

1. Apel RL, Asa SL, LiVolsi VA. Papillary Hürthle cell carcinoma with lymphocytic stroma. "Warthin-like tumor" of the thyroid. Am J Surg Pathol. 1995;19:810–4.
2. Wajahat M, Jeelani T, Gupta K, Bashir N. Warthin like papillary carcinoma - a rare variant of papillary carcinoma thyroid. Hum Pathol Case Rep. 2018;13:21–3.
3. Yeo MK, Bae JS, Lee S, Kim MH, Lim DJ, Lee YS, et al. The warthin-like variant of papillary thyroid carcinoma: a comparison with classic type in the patients with coexisting Hashimoto's thyroiditis. Int J Endocrinol. 2015;2015:456027. https://doi.org/10.1155/2015/456027, Epub 2015 Apr 23. PMID: 25983754; PMCID: PMC4423001.
4. Maffini F, Lorenzini D, Lepanto D, De Fiori E, Fumagalli C, Rappa A, et al. A case of Warthin-like papillary thyroid carcinoma with diffuse sclerosing stroma and a novel RET mutation: a new entity or a combined tumour? Ecancermedicalscience. 2019;13:965.
5. Kim J, Lim BJ, Hong SW, Pyo JY. Preoperative cytologic diagnosis of warthin-like variant of papillary thyroid carcinoma. J Pathol Transl Med. 2018;52:105–9.
6. Kim EY, Lee KH, Park YL, Park CH, Kim DH, Chae SW, et al. Warthin-like papillary thyroid carcinoma accompanying classical papillary carcinoma: report of three cases and systematic review of the literature. Int J Clin Exp Pathol. 2017;10:7223–31.
7. Baloch ZW, LiVolsi VA. Warthin-like papillary carcinoma of the thyroid. Arch Pathol Lab Med. 2000;124:1192–19.

Papillary Thyroid Cancer Presenting with Lung Metastases

Case

A 40-year-old lady presented with a history of swelling in the front of her neck for 12 years which had gradually increased in size. She had undergone right hemithyroidectomy in 2007 in another center. She had developed back ache and on evaluation was found to have lytic lesion in sacrum. Biopsy from sacral lesion had revealed metastatic PTC. Subsequent FDG PET showed an avid tumor in the left lobe of thyroid, lung, and sacrum. She had received Zoledronic infusion and palliative RT to sacrum in 2009. On examination, she had a collar scar which was well healed and a left lobe thyroid swelling measuring 4 × 3 cm. Pulmonary function tests showed restrictive disease. Chest X ray showed macronodular lung metastases in lower zones (Fig. 1). CECT showed large lesion in left upper lobe near hila and multiple nodules in both lobes (Fig. 2). She underwent completion total thyroidectomy (+CCLND) (Fig. 3). She had respiratory distress after 6 h of surgery and had to be shifted to Post-Op ICU, was intubated and put on SIMV ventilator support. She was successfully weaned off the ventilatory support after 3 days and discharged. Subsequently, she received high dose of RAI therapy with close monitoring of her pulmonary function tests.

Amit Agarwal is the lead author of this chapter.

A. Agarwal et al., *Case Studies in Thyroid and Parathyroid Tumors*,
https://doi.org/10.1007/978-981-99-0938-4_76

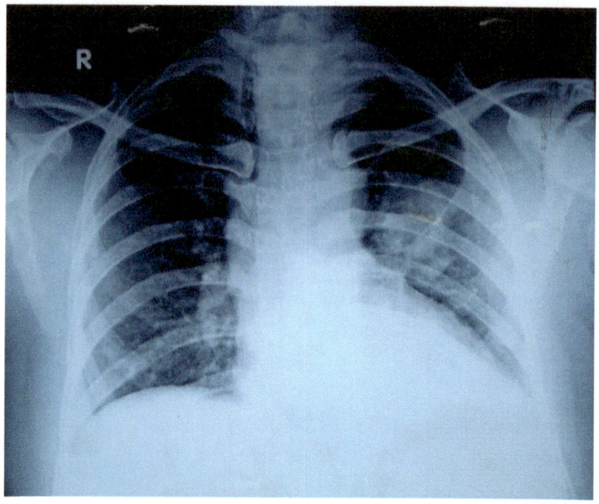

Fig. 1 Chest x-ray showing macronodular lung metastases in lower zones

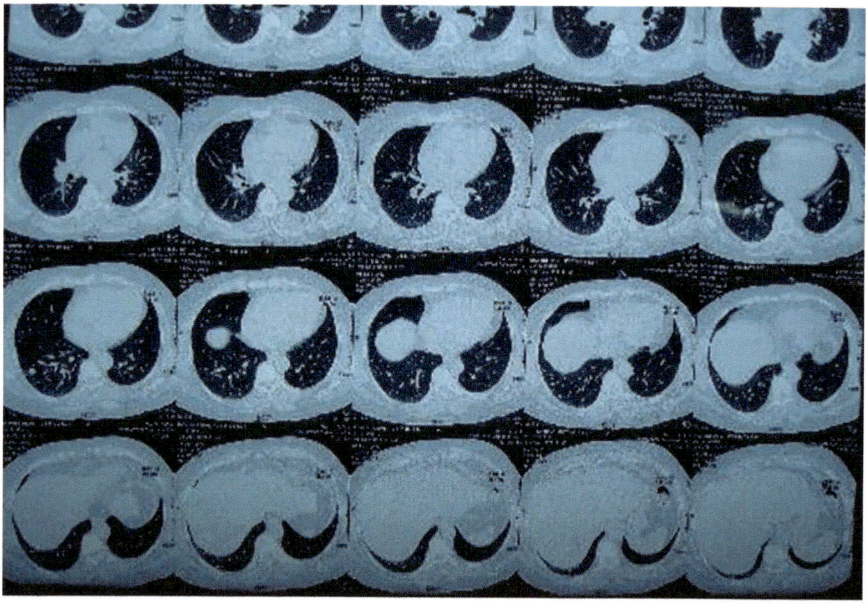

Fig. 2 CECT thorax showing bilateral lung metastases, especially in lower lobes

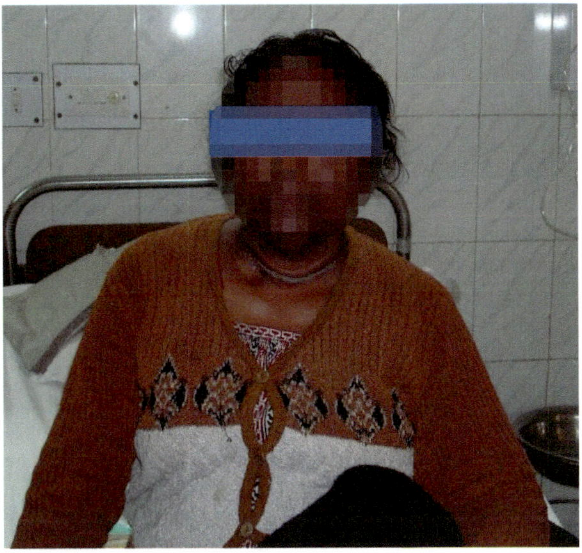

Fig. 3 Patient having undergone total thyroidectomy

Discussion

1% to 8% of papillary and 8% to 33% of patients with follicular thyroid carcinoma present with distant metastases at the time of diagnosis [1, 2]. In the study by Schlumberger et al. [3] among the 64 patients detected by chest x-ray, 35 were detected at the time of thyroid cancer diagnosis. According to their radiographic and scanning features, pulmonary metastases fall into two main classes [4]: micronodular and macronodular. Micronodular metastases, radiographically appear either as tiny miliary densities predominating on the lower lung fields or as diffuse reticular patterns. Corresponding RAI scan finding will be of homogeneously diffuse uptake. The radiological pattern of macronodular metastases is that of disseminated nodular masses of unequal size varying between 0.5 and 3 cm in diameter, again more pronounced in the lower lung fields and their RAI uptake is characterized by a heterogeneous pattern of uptake. Associated symptoms or signs are usually absent and rarely there may be a pleural effusion or involvement of mediastinal lymph nodes. Patients with cervical LN metastases are more likely to have pulmonary metastases. Aggressive variant of PTC like tall cell, solid variants are more likely to have synchronous lung metastases. General principle of treatment involves total thyroidectomy if the primary is resectable, followed by high-dose RAI therapy. Appropriate and optimal management of these patients with distant metastasis generally remains unsatisfactory due to lack of radio avidity [5] and such patients may require the use of TKI. Two problems arise in the overall surgical management of such patients: Firstly, if they have extensive lung metastases, they may require ventilatory care in the post-operative period; secondly, following RAI administration, they may develop lung fibrosis which may preclude giving further RAI doses. In a recent study [6] it has been shown that the patients with papillary thyroid carcinoma who are older, male with larger tumor size, or higher Tg level during follow-up had greater risk of developing lung metastases; prognosis of patients with papillary thyroid carcinoma with lung metastases at the time of diagnosis is the same as for those whose lung metastases are discovered later and survival analysis demonstrated no difference between lung metastases and multiorgan metastases.

References

1. Mazzaferri EL, Robbins RJ, Spencer CA, Braverman LE, Pacini F, Wartofsky L, Haugen BR, Sherman SI, Cooper DS, Braunstein GD, Lee S, Davies TF, Arafah BM, Ladenson PW, Pinchera A. A consensus report of the role of serum thyroglobulin as a monitoring method for low-risk patients with papillary thyroid carcinoma. J Clin Endocrinol Metab. 2003;88:1433–41.
2. Schelfhout LJ, Creutzberg CL, Hamming JF, Fleuren GJ, Smeenk D, Hermans J, van de Velde CJ, Goslings BM. Multivariate analysis of survival in differentiated thyroid cancer: the prognostic significance of the age factor. Eur J Cancer. 1988;24:331–7.
3. Schlumberger M, Tubiana M, De Vathaire F, Hill C, Gardet P, Travagli JP, Fragu P, Lumbroso J, Caillou B, Parmentier C. Long-term results of treatment of 283 patients with lung and bone metastases from differentiated thyroid carcinoma. J Clin Endocrinol Metab. 1986;63:960–7.
4. Mishra A, Mishra SK, Agarwal A, Das BK, Agarwal G, Gambhir S. Metastatic differentiated thyroid carcinoma: clinicopathological profile and outcome in an iodine deficient area. World J Surg. 2002;26:153–7.
5. Shaha AR, Shah JP, Loree TR. Differentiated thyroid cancer presenting initially with distant metastasis. Am J Surg. 1997;174:474–6.
6. Lin J-D, Chao T-C, Chou S-C, Hsueh C. Papillary thyroid carcinomas with lung metastases. Thyroid. 2004;14(12):1091–6.

Follicular Adenoma Developing Bone Metastases

Case
A 57-year-old lady presented with a history of swelling in front of her neck first noticed 1 year back painless, gradually increasing in size. Associated with malaise and weakness. No features of hypothyroidism or hyperthyroidism. No features of any local compression. No history suggestive of DM, HTN. No contributory family history of thyroid swelling. O/E swelling in the front of the neck 8 × 6 cm in the right lobe of thyroid which moves with deglutition. Lower border is reachable. Trachea is central B/L carotids palpable. Cervical LN are not palpable. FNAC was suggestive of follicular lesion. She consented for hemithyroidectomy which was performed uneventfully. Right lobe was found to be enlarged with single nodule replacing whole of the right lobe Rt RLN + EBSLN+ both parathyroid glands identified and saved. Grossing—Weight—90 g, Right lobe—6.5 × 6 × 4.5 cm, Isthmus—1 × 1.5 cm, Cut section—single pale fleshy nodule replacing whole of the right lobe. Histopathology was reported as follicular adenoma. She was then lost to

Amit Agarwal is the lead author of this chapter.

A. Agarwal et al., *Case Studies in Thyroid and Parathyroid Tumors*,
https://doi.org/10.1007/978-981-99-0938-4_77

follow-up until 3 years later when she presented again with fracture of humerus from trivial trauma (Fig. 1) and a mandibular swelling. FNAC from mandibular swelling was reported as follicular carcinoma of thyroid. Bone scan showed increased uptake in mandibular swelling and lower end of humerus. A review of the previous hemithyroidectomy histopathology report was sought. More sections were taken by the pathologists and were now revised to minimally invasive follicular carcinoma on finding a focus of vascular and capsular invasion (Fig. 2). Subsequently, she underwent completion total thyroidectomy and which was reported as normal thyroid without any evidence of malignancy. She had elevated serum thyroglobulin levels:Tg > 300 ng/ml. She was then referred to the Department of Nuclear Medicine. Diagnostic WBRI scan was done which showed right thyroid bed remnant and lytic lesion involving lower 1/3rd of left humerus and right mandible with soft tissue component. 200 mCi of I^{131} therapy was given orally under supervision and post-therapy scan was reported the same as pre-therapy WBRAI. Subsequently, orthopedic consultation was sought and she underwent CRIF (closed reduction with internal fixation) with humerus interlocking nailing under regional block. She then received further RAI therapy at 6 months interval amounting to cumulative dose of 1100 mCi of $I^{131.}$ The recent WBRAI diagnostic scan shows uptake in mandible and shaft of left humerus.

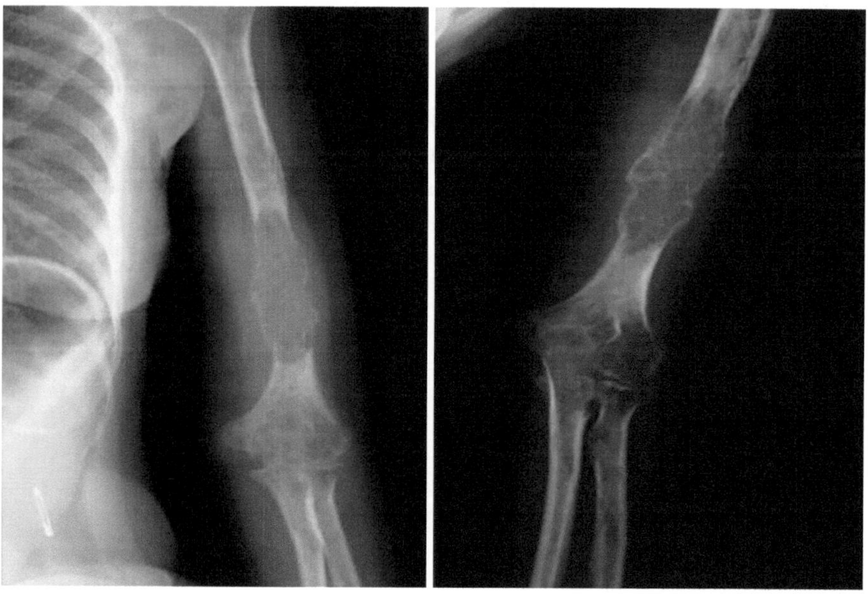

Fig. 1 Xray left arm showing pathological fracture of shaft of humerus

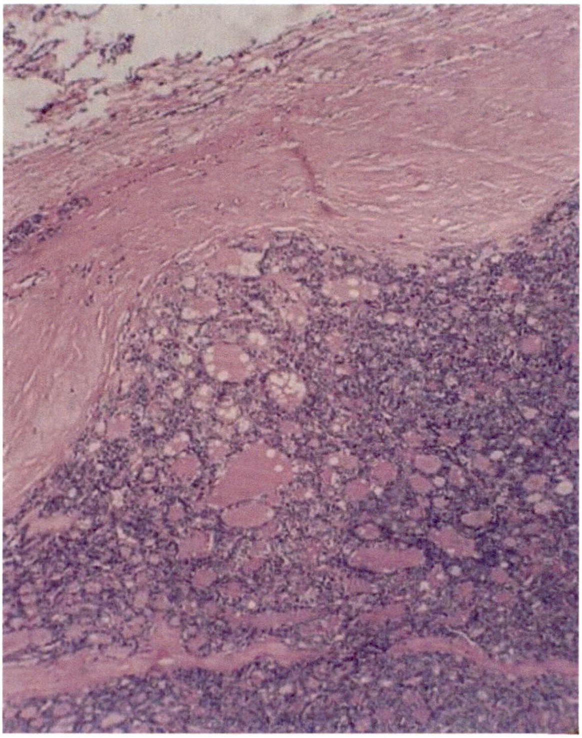

Fig. 2 Photomicrograph showing incomplete invasion of capsule, hence reported as follicular adenoma when limited sections were taken in the first surgery

Discussion

Unlike PTC, FTC cannot be diagnosed by FNAC because the distinction between FTC (which shows capsular and/or vascular invasion) and FA (which does not show invasion) requires pathological examination of tumor capsule after thyroidectomy. Follicular patterned lesions include FA, FTC, FVPTC, and NIFTP. On cytology, all these lesions will either be categorized as Bethesda class III (rate of malignancy being 5–15%) or class IV (rate of malignancy being 15–30%). Unlike PTC where BRAF is the most common oncogenic mutation, in FTC the primary mutations are the RAS point mutations (40–50%; NRAS, HRAS, and less commonly KRAS) as well as the PAX8PPARy rearrangements (30–40%). However, these mutations are not diagnostic of malignancy and they are also detected in FA.

Molecular Testing Novel genetic approaches are now available as commercial assays. However, these assays have been validated mostly with PTC. These assays are marketed mainly as rule-out tests with the objective of identifying benign nodules for avoiding lobectomy. These assays are: ThyroSeq V2 (sensitivity/specificity 70% and 77%), GEC (Affirma)—NPV of 94–95%, PPV of 37–38%, ThyraMIR and Thy GenX (sensitivity and specificity-n 89% and 85%).

Histology Unlike the classical PTC, where the histopathological diagnosis is straightforward, the pathological diagnosis of FTC is rather difficulty because of the need of examination of multiple sections/whole of the capsule; lack of standardized definition of types of FTC; and because of significant inter- or intra-observer variations. The diagnosis of CI or VI requires examination of multiple sections of tumor; some recommend at least ten sections [1] while others recommend examination of the entire tumor capsule; while still others recommend minimum of at least 4 blocks/cm [2]. Lang et al. demonstrated that the assessment accuracy for follicular neoplasm increased significantly when the number of blocks taken increased from two to ten per specimen [1]. They also characterized the features of atypical adenomas that help to differentiate them from encapsulated follicular carcinomas (MIFTC).

Growth pattern: high cellularity plus increased mitotic rate, increased nuclear size, disturbed architecture

1. Tumor capsule: Questionable infiltration (focal attenuation of capsule, cellular lump within capsule, splitting of capsule)
2. Blood vessels: Questionable invasion (tumor cells intruding into space without clearly identifiable vascular wall, isolated cellular aggregates within vascular space)

References

1. Lang W, Georgii A, Stauch G, Kienzle E. The differentiation of atypical adenomas and encapsulated follicular carcinomas in the thyroid gland. Virchows Arch As Pathol Anat Histol. 1980;385:125–41.
2. Lang BH, Shek TW, Wu AL, Wan KY. The total number of tissue blocks per centimetre of tumor significantly correlated with the risk of distant metastasis in patients with minimally invasive follicular thyroid carcinoma. Endocrine. 2017;55:496–502.

Minimally Invasive FTC

Case

A 54-year-old lady was admitted with complaints of swelling in the anterior aspect of the neck for 10 years which was painless and gradually progressing, without any compressive symptoms. On examination there was left lobe solitary thyroid nodule 6 × 6 cm, mobile, moving with deglutition and without any deep cervical lymphadenopathy. FNAC was reported as cellular colloid nodule. USG showed solitary left lobe nodule (TIRADS 3) and normal right lobe. She underwent left hemithyroidectomy (Fig. 1). Operative findings included a very vascular thyroid gland. HPE was reported as minimally invasive follicular carcinoma (Fig. 2). However, since there were more than 4 foci of vascular invasion, she was offered completion thyroidectomy. HPE of contralateral lobe was however benign. She was referred for WBRAI scanning which revealed increased tracer uptake in the thyroid bed. She was treated with high-dose RAI therapy. Subsequent follow-up WBRAI scan did not reveal any tracer uptake and her serum thyroglobulin level is <2 ng/ml at 7 years of follow-up.

Amit Agarwal is the lead author of this chapter.

A. Agarwal et al., *Case Studies in Thyroid and Parathyroid Tumors*,
https://doi.org/10.1007/978-981-99-0938-4_78

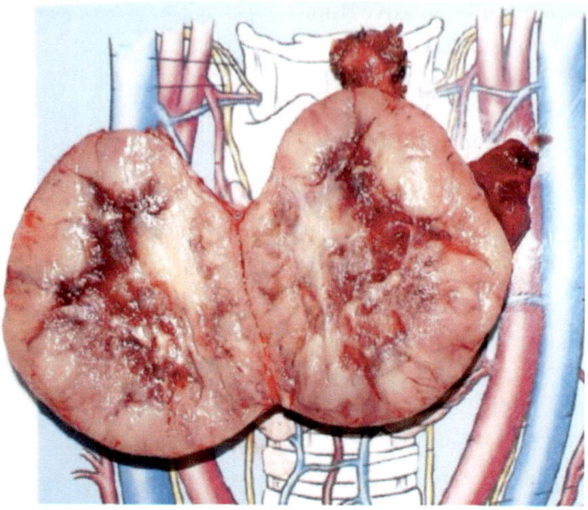

Fig. 1 Cut-section of left hemithyroidectomy: Left lobe was entirely replaced by a nodule with area of hemorrhage, cystic degeneration, and central scared area

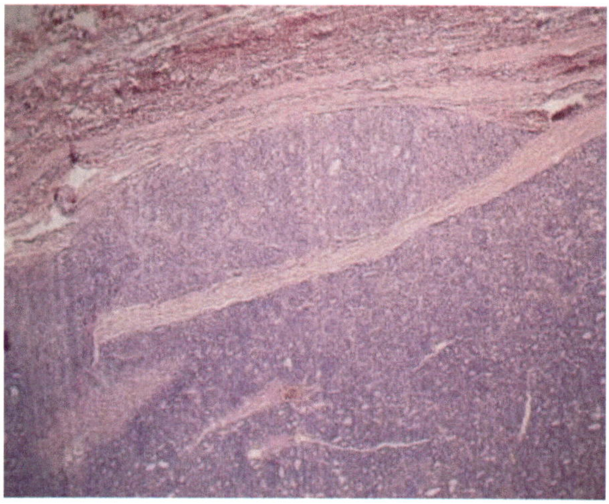

Fig. 2 Photomicrograph showing capsular breach in a case of follicular carcinoma, H&E, 4× Magnification

Discussion

Unlike PTC, FTC cannot be diagnosed by FNAC because the distinction between FTC (which shows capsular and/or vascular invasion) and FA (which does not show invasion) requires pathological examination of tumor capsule after thyroidectomy. Similarly, the pathological diagnosis of FTC is rather difficulty because of: the need of examination of multiple sections/whole of the capsule; lack of standardized definition of types of FTC. WHO defines the presence of capsular invasion when a tumor completely transgresses the tumor capsule, often mushrooming beyond the capsule [1]. True vascular invasion (VI) is defined as invasion into veins with tumor cells adherent to vessel wall, either covered by endothelium or within a thrombus or fibrin. WHO divided FTC into 3 main pathological categories[162]:

1. Minimally invasive: tumor with only CI
2. Encapsulated angioinvasive: without reference to no. of blood vessel
3. Widely invasive: gross invasion

ATA 2015 guidelines categorize [2]:

1. FTC with CI only
2. FTC with minimal VI (<4 blood vessel invasion)
3. FTC with extensive VI (>4 blood vessel invasion)

Other authors like Daniels [3] have recommended using the criteria:

1. CI alone,
2. minimal VI(<4) + −CI,
3. Extensive VI(>4) or extensive ETE.

It should be remembered that MIFTC is much more common (85%) than WIFTC (15%).

FTC are usually larger than PTC with a median diameter of 3.0 cm as against the median diameter of 1.8 cm for PTC. Similarly, multifocality and lymphatic invasion is rare in FTC. In fact if the histopathologist finds lymphatic invasion then the diagnosis is likely to be FVPTC rather than FTC. According to some authors [4, 5], hemithyroidectomy is considered sufficient if HPE is MIFTC with:

1. Only CI with no VI
2. <45 years old
3. Tumor <4 cm,
4. No LNM, no DM

All others should undergo completion thyroidectomy. In the study done at Mayo Clinic [6] determination of CSM was the presence of DM at diagnosis and VI.

RAI is strongly recommended only for FTC patients who fall into ATA high-risk category (MI, VI with >4 foci, extensive ETE).

References

1. 2017 WHO classification of tumours of endocrine organs, 4th ed. Lyon: IRAC.
2. Haugen BR, Alexander EK, Bible KC, et al. American thyroid association management guidelines for adult patients with thyroid nodules and differentiated thyroid cancer: the American Thyroid Association Guidelines Task Force on Thyroid Nodules and Differentiated Thyroid Cancer. Thyroid. 2016;26(1):1–133.
3. Daniels GH. Follicular thyroid carcinoma: a perspective. Thyroid. 2018;28(10):1229–42.
4. Huang CC, Hsueh C, Liu FH, Chao TC, Lin JD. Diagnostic and therapeutic strategies for minimally and widely invasive follicular thyroid carcinomas. Surg Oncol. 2011;20(1):1–6.

5. Collini P, Sampietro G, Pilotti S. Extensive vascular invasion is a marker of risk of relapse in encapsulated non-Hürthle cell follicular carcinoma of the thyroid gland: a clinicopathological study of 18 consecutive cases from a single institution with a 11- year median follow-up. Histopathology. 2004;44(1):35–9.
6. Van Heerden JA, Hay ID, Goellner JR, Salomao D, Ebersold JR, Bergstralh EJ, Grant CS. Follicular thyroid carcinoma with capsular invasion alone: a non-threatening malignancy. Surgery. 1992;112:1130–6.

Follicular Thyroid Cancer with Skull Metastasis

Case

A 62-year-old lady presented to the neurology OPD with swelling over the right parietal region and with protrusion of the right eye and decrease vision for 7 months. On examination, she had a 7 × 5 cm swelling over the right parietal region and protrusion of the right eye (Fig. 1) with decreased vision in bilateral eyes (CF at 2 m for right and left eye). Rest all cranial nerves were normal. A biopsy was done from parietal swelling which showed metastasis from thyroid with TTF and thyroglobulin positivity. Hence the patient was referred to endocrine surgery. The neck examination showed a nodule in the left lobe measuring 2 × 2 cm. ultrasound confirmed multiple nodules in bilateral lobes largest measuring 2.3 × 2 cm in the left lobe.

Hence with diagnosis of metastatic FTC, the patient underwent total thyroidectomy. Postoperative course was uneventful. After thyroxine withdrawal patient received 150 mCi of RAI. Her thyroglobulin reduced from 23,000 to 9900 after 150 mCi RAI treatment. Post therapy scan showed multiple bone metastasis in addition to the skull metastasis. Pain and visual improvement were seen after RAI treatment.

Roma Pradhan is the lead author of this chapter.

A. Agarwal et al., *Case Studies in Thyroid and Parathyroid Tumors*,
https://doi.org/10.1007/978-981-99-0938-4_79

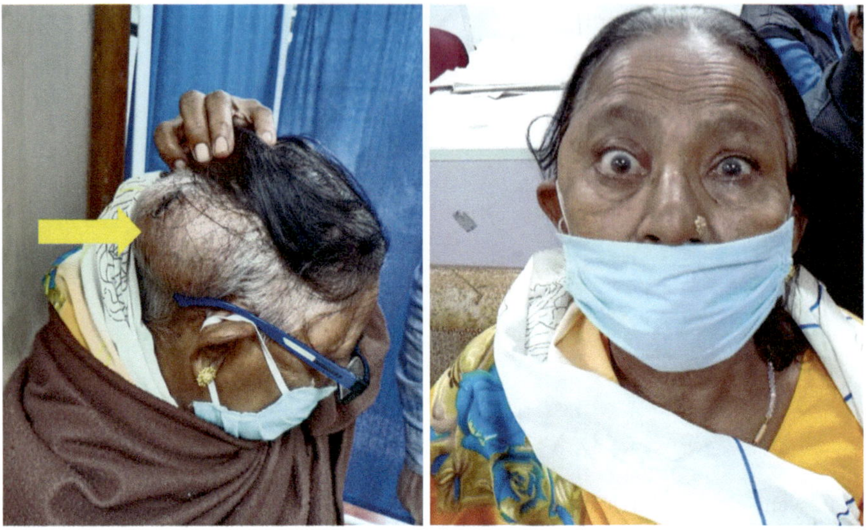

Fig. 1 Yellow pointer: parietal swelling with protrusion of the right eye

Discussion

10–15% of FTCs will disseminate hematogenously to bone and lungs and less commonly brain, liver, bladder, and skin. Bone metastases can occur in the vertebral bodies followed by the pelvis, femur, skull, and ribs. FTC facial bone metastasis can present in the gnathic bones, the paranasal sinuses, or the orbit. Metastasis to the facial skeleton may be the first clinical sign of an underlying malignancy and clinical presentation varies depending on the site of presentation as well as the primary site. Oral cavity and maxillofacial region metastasis is uncommon and represent 1–2% of all oral and maxillofacial malignancies. Primary sites of tumors metastatic to the facial skeleton are most commonly from the breast and lungs and thyroid malignancy represents only 2% of facial skeleton metastasis and 4.2–6.1% of all jaw metastases; 41% of facial skeleton metastasis from thyroid cancer occurs in the mandible and only 60% of these metastases are from well-differentiated thyroid cancer. There have been 41 reported cases in the literature of thyroid malignancy with metastasis to the mandible of which 21 reported cases were FTC [1, 2]. The majority of metastatic tumors to the mandible present with facial swelling and an osteolytic lesion but may also result in significant bleeding, infection, fractures, and disturbances in swallowing and mastication. Metastatic thyroid carcinomas are also reported in the orbit and paranasal sinuses. Surgical debulking of the metastatic foci may restore vision in cases of sudden onset vision loss. The thyroid gland is almost never implicated as the primary tumor in orbital metastases. Of 134 orbital métastases described in four separate series [3, 4]· only 3% were found to be of thyroid origin. In an extensive review of follicular thyroid carcinoma with metastases, no orbital spread was reported [5]. In addition to these four large series, only isolated cases of orbital metastases from thyroid carcinoma were reported. Hornblass et al. [6] described a case of orbital metastasis 6 years after the diagnosis of the initial thyroid lesion.

There are isolated case reports of thyroid malignancy presenting as a paranasal sinus mass (14.1%). Clinical manifestations include epistaxis, nasal obstruction, visual disturbances, and facial or intraoral swelling. The maxillary sinus is the most commonly involved sinus followed by the sphenoid sinus, ethmoid, and frontal sinus. The vertebral venous plexus, which allows retrograde spread of tumor emboli, could explain the etiology of paranasal sinus and orbital metastasis. Craniofacial resection or debulking with or without preoperative vascular embolization can be considered; however, the proximity of the metastatic tumor to the skull base may preclude surgical extirpation. Isolated facial skeleton metastasis may be treated with surgical resection, radioactive iodine, external beam radiation, or combinations of the three. However, treatment plans should be formulated with a multidisciplinary team involving surgical oncology, radiology, pathology, endocrinology, medical oncology, radiation oncology, reconstructive surgeons, and possibly palliative care.

References

1. Tamiolakis D, Tsamis I, Thomaidis V, Lambropoulou M, Alexiadis G, Venizelos I, et al. Jaw bone metastases: four cases. Acta Dermatovenerol Alp Panonica Adriat. 2007;16:21–5.
2. Kumar RVK, Chakravarthy C, Sekhar GR, Devireddy SK, Kumaravelu C, Kare A. Metastatic thyroid carcinoma presenting as Hypervascular lesion of the mandible: a case report and review of literature. J Oral Maxillofac Surg. 2010;68:2613–6.
3. Boughattas S, Chatti K, Degdegui M, Bouslama Z, Elaouni C. Uncommon case of orbital metastasis secondary to papillary thyroid carcinoma. Thyroid. 2005;15:1311–2.
4. Rocha Filho FD, Lima GG, Ferreira FV, Lima MG, Hissa MN. Orbital metastasis as primary clinical manifestation of thyroid carcinoma–case report and literature review. Arq Bras Endocrinol Metabol. 2008;52:1497–500.
5. Shaha AR, Shah JR, Loree TR. Differentiated thyroid cancer presenting initially with distant metastasis. Am J Surg. 1997;174:474–6.
6. Hornblass A, Kass LG, Reich R. Thyroid carcinoma to the orbit. Ophthalmology. 1987;94:1004–7.

Thyroxine Producing Metastases in Follicular Carcinoma of Thyroid

Case

A 48-year-old lady presented with swelling in front of her neck from 20 years and scalp swelling and right shoulder swelling for 4–5 months. She also gave a history of left lower limb pain for 1 year and having sustained a fracture of right humerus 6 months back from a trivial trauma. On examination there were multiple bony swellings over scalp, right shoulder, arm and back and a palpable 4 × 3 cm nodule from the right lobe of thyroid. There was no focal neurological deficit. On evaluation: Bone scan showed multiple bone metastases in skull, right humerus, sternum, D11 vertebra, sacrum & bilateral sacro-iliac joints, left iliac blade and left ischium. CECT Thorax and head showed 3.3 × 2.5 cm lytic lesion in frontal bone, 5.9 × 6 cm lesion in thyroid compressing and deviating trachea, multiple hypodense lesions in left thyroid lobe and multiple nodules in both lungs. FNAC from scalp swelling showed metastatic follicular carcinoma FNAC from thyroid, suggestive of follicular carcinoma. Her fT4 was normal (16.09) but her TSH was suppressed (0.2 miu/L). She was taken up for total thyroidectomy. Subsequently, she was kept on endogenous withdrawal of thyroxine for WBRAI. However, even after 4 weeks of withdrawal of thyroxine her TSH still was not elevated (2.60 miu/L). Her serum Tg levels were >300 ng/ml with ATG <20 IU/L. However, despite this she was given 150 mCi of $I\text{-}^{131}$ orally under supervision. Post therapy course was uneventful and she was discharged under permissible limits of radiation. Post therapy scan showed multiple skeletal metastasis with no uptake in thyroid bed (Fig. 1).

Amit Agarwal is the lead author of this chapter.

A. Agarwal et al., *Case Studies in Thyroid and Parathyroid Tumors*,
https://doi.org/10.1007/978-981-99-0938-4_80

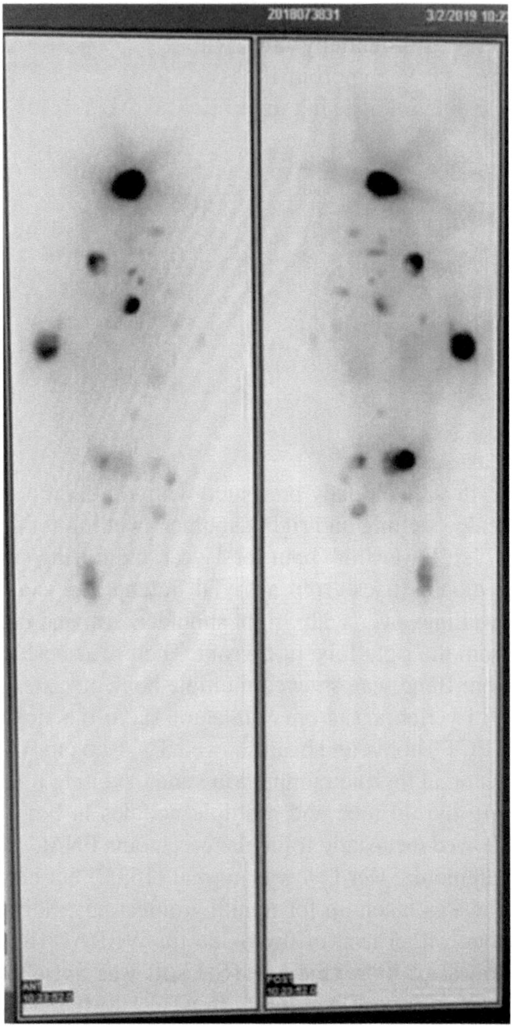

Fig. 1 WBRAI scan showing multiple skeletal metastases

Discussion

^{131}I for the treatment of metastatic differentiated thyroid cancer has been widely used for advanced differentiated thyroid cancer including follicular cancer [1]. Radioiodine uptake by thyroid remnants or thyroid cancer will be sufficient if serum TSH levels are more than 30 mU = L [2]. Endogenous TSH elevation is usually achieved by allowing patients to become hypothyroid. However, some patients with thyroid cancer cannot elevate their endogenous TSH to these levels or it is not desirable to make these patients hypothyroid. These include 3 class of patients: (1) those having hypothalamic or pituitary disorders [3], (2) those that have sufficient residual thyroid tissue or thyroxine-producing thyroid cancer tissue that prevents TSH from rising substantially after withdrawal of thyroxine therapy, and (3) those patients who have comorbid illnesses which may worsen during the period of profound hypothyroidism like-psychiatric illness, respiratory compromise, central nervous system complications (impending paraplegia, brain metastases), congestive heart failure and coronary artery disease. Three things in particular demonstrate that the metastases were responsible for production of thyroxine: no uptake of radioactive iodine in the neck, high Tg values and the confirmation of follicular metastases by FNAC of the scalp swelling. In the three situations mentioned above, it is advised to use rTSH which would ensure adequate RAI uptake by the metastases. Three studies [4–6] have established the safety of rhTSH-assisted radioiodine therapy administered under euthyroid conditions to patients who cannot raise their TSH levels under thyroid hormone withdrawal or who cannot be safely rendered hypothyroid.

References

1. Robeson WR, Ellwood JE, Margulies P, Margouleff D. Outcome and toxicity associated with maximum safe dose radioiodine treatment of metastatic thyroid cancer. Clin Nucl Med. 2002;27:556–66.
2. Schlumberger MJ. Papillary and follicular thyroid carcinoma. N Engl J Med. 1998;338:297–306.
3. Masiukiewicz US, Nakchbandi IA, Stewart AF, Inzucchi SE. Papillary thyroid carcinoma metastatic to the pituitary gland. Thyroid. 1999;9:1023–7.
4. Luster M, Lassmann M, Haenscheid H, Michalowski U, Incerti C, Reiners C. Use of recombinant human thyrotropin before radioiodine therapy in patients with advanced differentiated thyroid carcinoma. J Clin Endocrinol Metab. 2000;85:3640–5.
5. Jarzab B, Handkiewicz-Junak D, Roskosz J, Puch Z, Wygoda Z, Kukulska A, Jurecka-Lubieniecka B, Hasse-Lazar K, Turska M, Zajusz A. Recombinant human TSH-aided radioiodine treatment of advanced differentiated thyroid carcinoma: a single-Centre study of 54 patients. Eur J Nucl Med Mol Imaging. 2003;30:1077–86.
6. Robbins RJ, Driedger A, Magner J, U.S. and Canadian Thyrogen Compassionate Use Program Investigator Group. Recombinant human thyrotropin-assisted radioiodine therapy for patients with metastatic thyroid cancer who could not elevate endogenous thyrotropin or be withdrawn from thyroxine. Thyroid. 2006;16:1121–30.

Thyroglobulin Elevation with No Uptake on Radioiodine Scan (TENIS)

Case

A 61-year-old man presented with a right thyroid solitary thyroid nodule which was present for the last 6 years but had recently increased in size. On examination, he had a 7 × 6 cm swelling in the right thyroid lobe without any palpable LAP. FNAC was suspicious of MTC but his serum calcitonin turned out to be normal (5 pg/ml). He underwent TT+ CCLND. HPE revealed papillary carcinoma thyroid, pT2N0 (right lobe, multifocal, 4 cm, No ETE, 0/12). Post-Operative Course showed normal Tg levels—1.01 ng/dl, ATG—<20 IU/ml and WBRAI scan showed uptake in the right thyroid bed remnant for which he received 65 mCi of RAI for ablation. Post therapy scan showed increased tracer uptake in the left thyroid bed & paratracheal region. He was started on Levothyroxine 200 µg OD and was on regular follow-up. One year later he presented with a left neck recurrent LN which on CECT neck was a 3.6 × 2.0 cm enhancing lesion in the left paratracheal region. Guided FNAC was suggestive of metastatic PTC. At that time his Tg levels were 22.8 but his WBRAI was negative and PET scan revealed a left paratracheal uptake. Selective LN dissection was done. Subsequently, his Tg started rising (Fig. 1). At Tg level of 22.8 his WBRAI was negative (Fig. 2). He was kept on follow-up and after 1 year after which his Tg levels were 243 ng/dl with ATG levels—<20 IU/ml. However, his WBRAI scan was negative. 18F-FDG PET showed left supraclavicular mass with multiple mediastinal LN and non-FDG avid multiple pulmonary nodules (Fig. 3).

Amit Agarwal is the lead author of this chapter.

A. Agarwal et al., *Case Studies in Thyroid and Parathyroid Tumors*,
https://doi.org/10.1007/978-981-99-0938-4_81

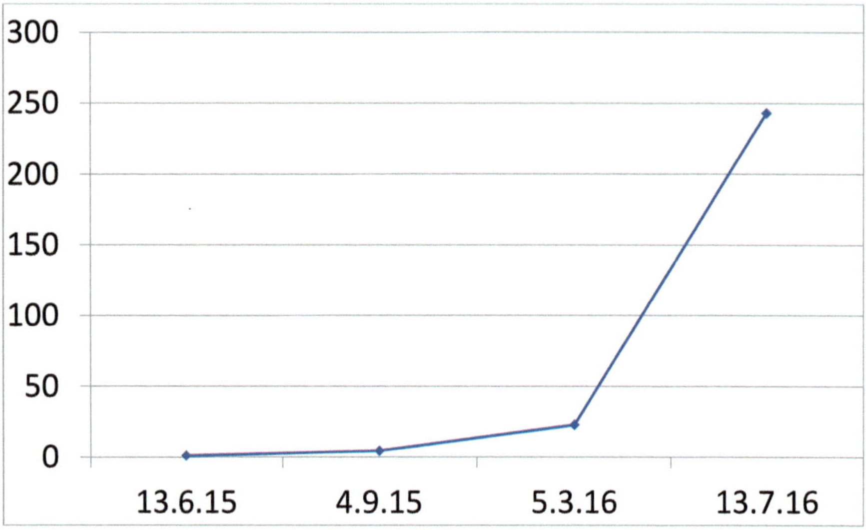

Fig. 1 Rising serum thyroglobulin

Fig. 2 Negative WBRAI with elevated Tg

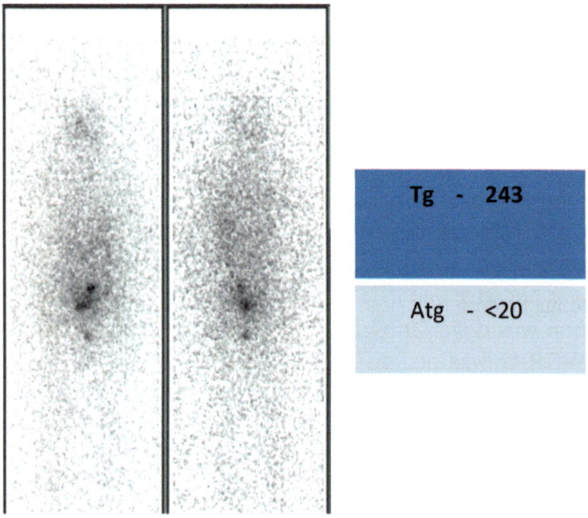

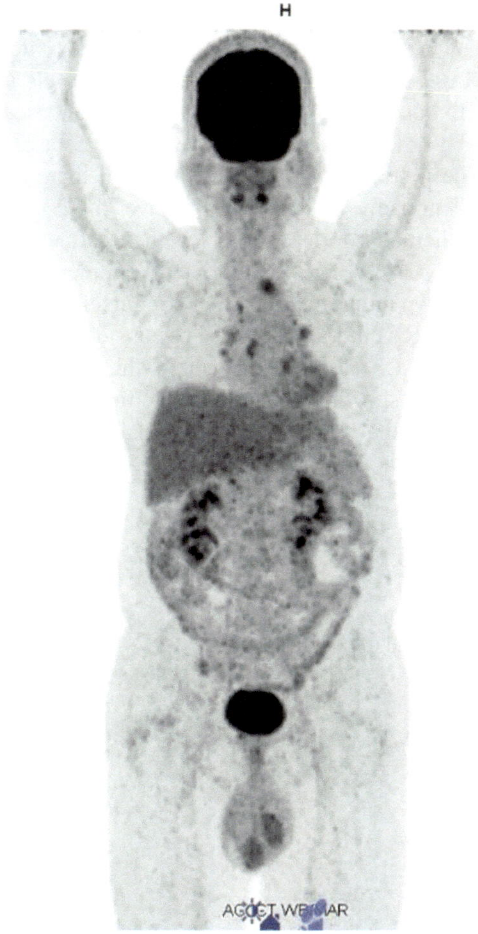

Fig. 3 PET scan showing metastatic disease

Discussion

Sometimes during the course of thyroid cancer management, a situation arises where there is no radiologically or clinically evident disease, but serum thyroglobulin (Tg) levels remain detectable or even significantly elevated. This situation has been referred to as TENIS syndrome (thyroglobulin elevated negative iodine scintigraphy) [1]. This leads to biochemical evidence of persistent or recurrent thyroid cancer as evidenced by the Tg levels but no obvious disease to treat with 131-I. This is one of the most challenging situations because treatment options in such a situation are very limited. One must rule out causes of negative iodine scans such as iodine interference, inferior imaging characteristic features of I^{131} as compared to I^{123} or false-positive elevation of antibody levels (ATG). Sometimes nodal recurrences do not show up on thyroid scan. Once these causes are ruled out a PET scan should be ordered which might reveal metastases. The treatment is usually stepwise. The first approach is to document if there is an operable disease (e.g., neck lymphadenopathy, solitary brain or liver metastases) as the sole site of metastatic disease, then appropriate surgery is the treatment of choice given the fitness of the patient for surgery. The second line of treatment is of empiric radioiodine therapy in scan-negative individuals, though not universally accepted [2] (11 of full). Empiric 100 mCi of RAI therapy needs to be considered when surgery is not feasible, the Tg level is high (the usual consensus is that the value should be at least more than 10 ng/ml), or showing a fast doubling time [3] (3 of basu). In unresectable disease, external radiotherapy is an option in painful bony metastases and brain metastasis (that has lost the ability to concentrate 131I). The fourth option is to start TKI.

References

1. Mallick U, Charalambous H. Current issues in the management of differentiated thyroid cancer. Nucl Med Commun. 2004;25(9):873–81.
2. Ma C, Xie J, Kuang A. Is empiric 131I therapy justified for patients with positive thyroglobulin and negative 131I whole-body scanning results? J Nucl Med. 2005;46(7):1164–70.
3. Mazzaferri EL. Empirically treating high serum thyroglobulin levels. J Nucl Med. 2005;46:1079–86.

Aggressive Sporadic Medullary Thyroid Cancer

Case

A 61-year-old gentleman presented to us with a history of anterior neck swelling for 3 years which was slowly progressive initially but rapidly increased since 3 months. He also gave a history of diarrhea for 6 months with 3–7 episodes/day and secretory in nature. On examination he had 12 × 9.5 cm swelling in Lt lobe of thyroid which was multilobulated, firm, moving with deglutition, trachea deviated towards Rt side, left carotid bruit present, and Pemberton sign was positive. He also had multiple bilateral level II, III, IV deep cervical LN, largest 2 × 1 cm left level III LN. USG neck revealed large soft tissue mass of size 5.3 × 6.4 × 7.5 cm involving Lt lobe, isthmus, and Rt lobe with no e/o retrosternal extension along with b/l cervical L.N.(LT > RT). LEVEL 1B, 2, 3, 4, 5, 6, largest 2.3 cm. Guided FNAC from thyroid mass and left cervical lymph node was positive for medullary carcinoma with nodal metastasis. IDL: showed b/l vocal cords mobile. Investigations were as follows (Table 1):

Amit Agarwal is the lead author of this chapter.

A. Agarwal et al., *Case Studies in Thyroid and Parathyroid Tumors*,
https://doi.org/10.1007/978-981-99-0938-4_82

Table 1 Investigation results of the patient

T4	13.2 pmol/L	12–22
TSH	2.75 mIU/ml	0.4–4
Sr. Calcium—Total	9.1 mg/dl	8.5–10.5
Ionized	1.17 mmol/L	1.13–1.32
iPTH	3.2 pmol/L	1.6–6.9
24 h UMN	186	<600
24 h UNMN	579	<600
S.Calcitonin	>2000	
S.CEA	12.5 μg/dl	<6
MDP bone scan	No evidence of metastases	

CECT Neck and Thorax showed a large well defined, heterogenous mass of 4.7 × 6.2 × 10 cm in Lt lobe and isthmus with mediastinal extension; nodular calcification in mass with multiple enlarged mediastinal nodes abutting major vessels and multiple enlarged left cervical nodes in 2, 3, 4, 5 groups along with narrowing of tracheal lumen and multiple small miliary nodules in b/l lung. He was taken up for surgery and TT + CCLND + LT MRND + RT SLND + MEDIAN STERNOTOMY + SUPERIOR MEDIASTINAL NODE Dissection was done. At operation besides central compartment (level VI) LN, conglomerate mass in superior mediastinum (level VII): largest 5 × 4 cm was found extending retrotracheally and behind Lt brachiocephalic vein. On grossing weight of the specimen was 136 gm. Histopathology confirmed medullary thyroid carcinoma with nodal metastases (34/35). Post-operative calcitonin done after 2 months was still elevated. On follow-up at 1 year his calcitonin was still found to be elevated and hence ^{18}FDG PET-CT Whole Body Imaging was done which revealed Faintly FDG avid sub-centimetric left level II cervical lymph nodes are seen.; mild FDG uptake is noted in ill-defined soft tissue like lesion of size 3.2 × 2.1 cm in left para tracheal region; FDG uptake is noted in sub-centimetric right lower para tracheal, subcarinal, right peribronchial lymph nodes. Non-FDG avid multiple sub-centimetric lung nodules are seen. FDG uptake is noted in lytic lesions of body of C6 (SUVmax 2.2) and D5 vertebrae and sacrum (SUVmax1.5). Annual calcitonin was elevated but Calcitonin doubling time was more than 1 year (Table 2). At 3 years of follow-up his calcitonin values increased substantially along with CEA values and he was referred to Nuclear Medicine for therapy. He underwent Ga-68 DOTANOC Scan which revealed multiple skeletal, bilateral pulmonary, hepatic, cervical, and mediastinal lymph nodes metastasis, with thyroid recurrence. He was given 3 cycles of 200 mCi of Lu-177 DOTANOC each was infused intravenously along with amino acid infusion with well-maintained hydration under supervision at 2 months interval. However, post-therapy scan (after 24 h) did not show any improvement in metastatic lesions and he ultimately succumbed to florid metastatic disease.

Table 2 Serial Calcitonin levels over a period of 3 years

Lab Reports | PACS Reports | Procedure Reports | Old HIS Reports

Endocrine Surgery Lab

Investigation	Value	Unit	Refrence Range	Order No	Received Date	Result Status	Specimen	Test On	Remarks
Serum calcitonin		pg/ml	.6-11.5	ORDER20151456648	01-12-2015 15:29	V	Blood - Plain	Blood - Plain	
Serum CEA	166.0	ug/l	.5-8.8	ORDER2015940892	11-08-2015 13:08	V	Blood - Plain	Blood - Plain	
Serum calcitonin		pg/ml	.6-11.5	ORDER2015940892	11-08-2015 13:08	V	Blood - Plain	Blood - Plain	
Serum CEA	126.0	ug/l	.5-8.8	ORDER2014861620	24-09-2014 16:02	V	Blood - Plain	Blood - Plain	
Serum calcitonin		pg/ml	.6-11.5	ORDER2014861620	24-09-2014 16:02	V	Blood - Plain	Blood - Plain	
Serum calcitonin		pg/ml	1-12	I0813023418	29-08-2013 16:27	V	Blood - Plain	Blood - Plain	
Serum CEA		ug/l	0-6	I0813023418	29-08-2013 16:27	V	Blood - Plain	Blood - Plain	
Serum calcitonin		pg/ml	1-12	I0113016311	10-01-2013 09:51	V	Blood - Plain	Blood - Plain	
Serum CEA	18.6	ug/l	0-6	I0113016311	10-01-2013 09:51	V	Blood - Plain	Blood - Plain	
Serum calcitonin		pg/ml	1-12	I1012080694	22-12-2012 10:47	V	Blood - Plain	Blood - Plain	

Parameter	Value
Serum calcitonin -female	
Serum calcitonin	>20000.0
Serum calcitonin -male	

Prev

Discussion

About 75% of medullary thyroid cancer cases present in sporadic form and 25% in a hereditary pattern. However, even in sporadic MTC, 50% will show somatic RET mutation. MTC demonstrates a more aggressive clinical course, and it is characterized by a poorer prognosis than differentiated thyroid cancers (DTC). Stage III or stage IV MTC is observed in nearly half of the patients at diagnosis. Ten-year survival rates for patients initially stratified according to AJCC/UICC TNM classification as stage I, II, III, or IV are 100, 93, 71, and 21%, respectively [1]. At initial diagnosis, neck disease is usually amenable to surgery but even after R0 resection, recurrences are frequent and are often associated with, or precede, the discovery of distant metastases. Advanced medullary thyroid cancer includes patients with a locally advanced disease not amenable to surgery, those with R1 resection, and those with distant metastases. Clinically detected distant metastases are present at diagnosis of medullary thyroid cancer in 4–17% of patients [2, 3]. Although distant metastases are often not clinically detectable they might be present initially in an even larger proportion of patients with medullary thyroid cancer; this might account for persistent high calcitonin levels after complete surgery. Distant metastases will be detected during follow-up in another 18–38% of patients.

The risk of lateral lymph node metastases in the contralateral neck and the mediastinum increases with the size of the primary tumor, the incidence of a coexistent thyroid tumor, and every additional central lymph node metastasis. Though there is no controversy regarding the need for total thyroidectomy in MTC, due to the high prevalence of central compartment lymph node metastases (50–75%), most surgeons suggest performing central compartment lymph node dissection (CCLND) with total thyroidectomy as initial treatment. Considering that this prevalence is the same whether the primary tumor is less than 1 cm or greater than 4 cm, prophylactic CCLND should be performed independently of the primary tumor size and the presurgical evidence of lymph node involvement. More recent evidences suggest using preoperative calcitonin values to determine the extent of lymph node dissection. It seems that there is virtually no risk of lymph node metastases when preoperative calcitonin level is less than 20 pg/mL (normal reference range <10 pg/ml). In these cases, the prophylactic CCLND might be avoided. On the other hand, calcitonin values higher than 20 pg/mL, 50 pg/mL, 200 pg/mL, and 500 pg/mL seem associated with the presence of lymph node metastases in the ipsilateral central and ipsilateral lateral neck, in the contralateral central neck, in the contralateral lateral neck, and in the upper mediastinum, respectively. Ipsilateral lateral neck dissection should be added if the primary tumor is larger than 1 cm in size or there is evidence of positive nodes in the central neck, although some surgeons advocate bilateral neck dissection for all patients with MTC, since cervical lymph node metastases are frequent and can occur at an early stage. A contralateral lateral neck dissection should be considered in patients with bilateral tumors or extensive lateral adenopathy on the side of the primary tumor. Extensive lymph node dissection will cure approximately 60% of node-negative and 10% of node-positive patients. Subjects who are still having low but detectable calcitonin values (<150) after initial surgery can present distant metastatic disease but in a majority of cases persistent/recurrent disease is confined to neck lymph nodes. These patients can be followed every 6 months to 12 months with physical examination, neck US, and measurement of serum basal calcitonin and CEA. Detectable serum calcitonin levels are compatible with long-term survival during which calcitonin may remain stable over time or slowly increase. In cases of postoperative basal calcitonin values higher than 150 pg/mL or in those in which calcitonin increases substantially over time, patients should be evaluated with imaging studies. In particular, patients with calcitonin higher than 5000 pg/mL present distant metastatic disease in more than 50%, and sites of metastases can be detected in almost all cases in which calcitonin is higher than 20,000 pg/mL. The most sensitive imaging studies to detect MTC in different sites PET with different tracers (fluorodeoxyglucose F 18 [18FDG], dihydroxyphenylalanine F 18 [18F-DOPA], dotatate gallium Ga 68 [68Ga-DOTATATE]) may be useful. To avoid repeated and unnecessary imaging studies in patients who are usually long survivors, after initial staging, except in rare cases, CT scans should be performed no more than annually and according to the serum calcitonin trend of increase. Both serum calcitonin and CEA levels doubling times (DTs) are good predictors of survival, in particular the former and can also predict disease progression [4].

Lymph node metastases have been found in small (5 mm) MTCs. Patients with clinically evident disease are best treated with a minimum of a total thyroidectomy and bilateral central neck dissection.

Lymph node metastases have been proven to be the main prognostic factor in MTC. As survival is significantly better for patients after systematic versus selective lymphadenectomy, using the technique of a compartment-oriented microdissection of cervicomediastinal lymph nodes, node dissection represents the preferred surgical treatment as well as the optimum technique in primary as well as secondary node-positive MTC. Moley and DeBenedetti [5] recommend a routine central and bilateral neck dissection in all patients with palpable MTC. In their study, lymph node metastases were found in 81% of all central neck dissection specimens. In 81% of the ipsilateral neck dissection specimens and in 44% of the contralateral neck dissection specimens, pathological lymph nodes were found. Scollo et al. [6] also recommend a central and bilateral neck dissection for all patients with MTC with proven lymph node metastases on one side.

Assessing progressive disease Serial (at least four) measurements of CTN and CEA allow the determination of their doubling time (DT), the interval of time in which the level has increased twofold. Among MTC patients, DTs may vary widely from a few months to several years, but DT remains rather unchanged in a given patient during his lifetime. Because in a given patient, the serum CTN level is closely related to the tumor volume, the DT is a strong predictor of tumor progression and survival [7]. In some patients, the serum CEA increases progressively, whereas the CTN does not or even decreases and this suggests cellular dedifferentiation. Therefore, both CTN and CEA DTs should be taken into account for prognosis and also to determine the frequency at which imaging is performed.

Treatment of Metastatic Disease Surgical treatment of distant metastatic lesions is not indicated unless the lesions have the potential to compromise vital structures and/or be life-threatening. Liver metastases, particularly if solitary may be amenable to surgical treatment in some cases. Multiple liver lesions can be treated by radiofrequency ablation, thermablation chemoembolization, cryo embolization, and transarterial radioembolization. External beam radiotherapy (EBRT) can be reserved for treatment of lung metastases that are symptomatic (cough, dyspnea, difficulty in swallowing). However, because of the high risk of radiation fibrosis and respiratory failure, it is used very rarely. Skeletal metastases are treated by local RT for painful bone metastases, by 3-weekly intravenous infusion of zoledronic acid or a monthly subcutaneous administration of denosumab or by local treatment approaches to prevent/delay fractures such as radiofrequency ablation, vertebroplasty, or kyphoplasty. Brain metastases may also be treated with EBRT or stereotaxic radiosurgery to prolong survival and improve quality of life. Classical doxorubin-based cytotoxic chemotherapy for advanced metastatic MTC has shown limited response rates (15–20%). Treatment with several radiolabeled molecules has been widely explored. A promising approach documenting complete remission or partial remission seems to come from the treatment of MTC patients with radio-labeled (yttrium 90 or lutetium 177) peptides targeting somatostatin receptors. MTCs are known to express SSTR 2 that facilitates imaging with 99mTc-labeled and especially 68Galabeled analogues. Hence, tracer concentration at disease sites confirms SSTR expression making it amenable to therapy with similar peptides bound to therapeutic radioisotopes like 177Lu or 90Y. Most studies have used four cycles of 200 mCi 177Lu-DOTATATE with 6–10-week intervals between cycles. Many responders reported improvement in quality of life and cancer-related pain and there were few grade III or IV hematological or renal toxicities.

Since 2005, a new interest for targeted therapy in MTC has been growing. The rationale for this interest was represented by the presence of RET mutation in 50% of advanced sporadic MTC cases. In addition to RET, other important targets (i.e., vascular endothelial growth factor receptor [VEGFR], epidermal growth factor receptor [EGFR], hepatocyte growth factor receptor [MET]) and RAS were demonstrated to be overexpressed in this tumor and represented the molecular basis of treating this disease with tyrosine kinase inhibitors (TKIs).

According to the current ATA guidelines, a postoperative MTC risk stratification and long-term follow-up are mainly based on histopathological data, including tumor stage, the presence of lymph node and/or distant metastases (TNM classification), and serum concentration of two biomarkers: calcitonin (Ctn) and carcinoembryonic antigen (CEA). However, even if histopathological or clinical features allow to predict a long-term prognosis, they are not sufficient to select the patients showing aggressive MTC courses requiring immediate treatment or those, who are refractory to different therapeutic methods. Hence, there is a role of RET mutation in predicting aggressive MTC. Patients without somatic RET mutation demonstrated significantly longer survival than those harboring RET mutation in tumor cells. Moreover, the detection of RET M918T cfDNA allowed predicting a worse outcome better than Ct doubling time. Further, the RET mutation M918T predicts a better response for treatment with cabozantinib, a multikinase inhibitor. Although the evaluation of the MTC somatic mutation profile so far is not recommended in daily clinical practice, it is worth considering in patients with advanced disease before qualification for systemic treatment. It seems of particular importance in the coming era of new, very promising selective RET-inhibitors LOXO 292 (selpercatinib) and BLU 667 (pralsetinib).

References

1. Wells SA, Asa SL, Dralle H, Elisei R, Evans DB, Gagel RF, Lee N, Machens A, Moley JF, Pacini F, et al. Revised American Thyroid Association guidelines for the management of medullary thyroid carcinoma. Thyroid 2015;25:567–610.
2. Mehrotra PK, Mishra A, Mishra SK, Agarwal G, Agarwal A, Verma AK. Medullary thyroid cancer: clinico-pathological profi le and outcome in a tertiary care center in North India. World J Surg 2011;35:1273–80.
3. Pelizzo MR, Boschin IM, Bernante P, et al. Natural history, diagnosis, treatment and outcome of medullary thyroid cancer: 37 years experience on 157 patients. Eur J Surg Oncol 2007;33:493–7.
4. Tamatakos M, Paraskeva P, Katsaronis P, Tasiopoulou G, Kontzoglou K: Surgical approach to the management of medullary thyroid cancer: when is lymph node dissection needed? Oncology 2013;84:350–5.
5. Moley JF, DeBenedetti MK. Patterns of nodal metastases in palpable medullary thyroid carcinoma: recommendations for extent of node dissection. Ann Surg. 1999;229(6):880–7; discussion 887–8.
6. Scollo C, Baudin E, Travagli JP, Caillou B, Bellon N, Leboulleux S, Schlumberger M. Rationale for central and bilateral lymph node dissection in sporadic and hereditary medullary thyroid cancer. J Clin Endocrinol Metab. 2003;88(5):2070–5.
7. Soussan M, Nataf V, Kerrou K, Grahek D, Pascal O, Talbot J-N, et al. Added value of early 18F-FDOPA PET/CT acquisition time in medullary thyroid cancer. Nucl Med Commun 2012;33:775–9.

Poorly Differentiated Thyroid Cancer

Case

A 47-year-old woman presented to us with a history of anterior neck swelling for 4 years which was gradually progressive, painless, and without compressive symptoms. On examination she had a 4 × 5 cm swelling present in the isthmus of thyroid, all margins palpable, without retrosternal extension and without deep cervical LN enlargement. FNAC was suggestive of FLUS. She was taken up for total thyroidectomy and at operation no extra-thyroidal extension was present. Histopathology was reported as poorly differentiated carcinoma (insular variety) and mutation analysis revealed that she was BRAF negative, PIK3 negative, RET negative but NRAS positive. Post-operatively she had elevated thyroglobulin (339.8 ng/ml) and WBRAI revealed uptake in the thyroid bed and she was treated with 125 mci of I-131 orally under supervision. Subsequent scans showed no evidence of uptake or metastasis and she did well without evidence of disease at 6 years of follow-up.

Discussion

As compared to differentiated thyroid cancer (DTC), poorly differentiated thyroid cancer (PDTC) exhibits significant aggressive features like larger tumor size, higher incidence of extrathyroidal extension (ETE), lymph node metastasis, and distant metastasis. Furthermore, unlike DTC, PDTC tends to present with locally invasive extrathyroidal disease, particularly the aerodisgestive tract in more than half of the patients [1, 2]. PDTC metastasizes to regional lymph nodes in up to 50–85% of cases [3], in comparison to 40–75% lymph node metastasis in DTC [4]. Similarly, distant metastases are much more frequent in PDTC, occurring in up to 85% of cases [4] when compared to 10–33% of cases in DTC [5]. It has been suggested that

Amit Agarwal is the lead author of this chapter.

A. Agarwal et al., *Case Studies in Thyroid and Parathyroid Tumors*,
https://doi.org/10.1007/978-981-99-0938-4_83

PDTC is a heterogeneous group of tumors and it will be worthwhile to identify more favorable PDTC tumors. Although the morphologic criteria for PD tumors are well-defined in the "Turin criteria" [6], it is still not clear as to how much of a PD area besides a well-differentiated component is required to allow such a diagnosis and whether it is of any prognostic significance. In the study by Dettmer et al. [7] the authors concluded that the presence of even 10% PD area in a tumor that otherwise fulfills Turin Criteria would justify a diagnosis of PDTC and that the presence of even minor amount of PD area in the PDTC is an adverse prognostic marker. However, in another study by Gnemmi et al. [8] they reported no significant relation between percentage of PD area and Cause-Specific Survival. Pathological factors that impact prognosis are presence of atypical mitosis, necrosis, capsular and vascular invasion. Unlike DTC, treatment of PDTC has not been standardized due to the rarity of the disease and heterogeneity of inclusion criteria. Therapeutic decisions on PDTC have thus been mainly extrapolated from the treatment experience on DTC. It is accepted that in general terms a more aggressive approach is needed to treat these tumors as compared with standard low-risk thyroid carcinomas. Total thyroidectomy with or without LN clearance of central/lateral neck should be attempted and is feasible in cases where there is no extra-thyroidal extension. However, unlike DTC, because of frequent extrathyroidal extension in PDTC, thyroidectomy is never easy in these cases and it may be difficult to achieve a R0 resection. Secondly, lot of these cases would have undergone 1 or 2 surgeries (usually less than total thyroidectomy) before presenting with recurrence (either in thyroid bed or lateral neck) making completion thyroidectomy very difficult. Also, radioiodine refractoriness is observed in a high proportion of patients (50%). Presence of TERT mutations correlates with RAI refractoriness. The study by Landa et al. [9] using the MSK-IMPACT NGS platform has showed molecular level evidence for the intermediate position of PDTC. BRAFV600E and RAS mutations remain the mutually exclusive main driver mutations in PDTC, occurring in 33% and 45% of PDTCs, respectively. The higher frequency of RAS family mutations compared with BRAF mutations suggests that more PDTCs may be related to FTC or follicular variant of PTC than classical type PTC. Interestingly, in PDTC, the BRAF/RAS signatures are closely correlated with the histologic phenotypes and dictate distinct metastatic patterns—those with RAS-mutated PDTC tend to metastasize to distant sites while BRAF-mutated PDTC tend to spread to LN only [10]. In various studies, PDTC was the most common cause for disease-specific death (DSS) in fatal non-anaplastic follicular cell-derived thyroid carcinomas [11]. PDTC shows a more aggressive course compared to DTC regardless of focal or diffuse presence of PDTC, with a higher propensity for local recurrence. Indeed, PDTC holds an intermediate position on a progression scale from DTC to ATC in terms of 5-year overall survival (OS), DSS, and disease-free survival (DFS). PDTC is not invariably lethal as ATC and has a 62–85% 5-year OS [1] and a 66% 5-year DSS. Recent reports show that satisfactory 5-year locoregional control can be achieved in PDTC patients (5-year locoregional control in 81% of cases) [1], if all gross disease is cleared at initial surgery. This improvement in locoregional control in patients with PDTC may reflect more comprehensive initial surgery and successful gross disease clearance achieving a R0 resection. However, distant disease represents the major cause of death in PDTC, accounting for up to 85% of disease-related deaths. PDTC tumors have aggressive presentation (increased age, large size, more ETC, rapid growth). Aggressive surgical resection in the form of extended/radical thyroidectomy may result in better loco-regional control and improve survival. RAS is the commonest mutation detected in our series. It will be worthwhile to identify adverse prognostic factors like presence of atypical mitosis in an attempt to identify less favorable PDTC tumors.

References

1. Ibrahimpasic T, Ghossein R, Carlson DL, Nixon I, Palmer FL, Shaha AR, Patel SG, Tuttle RM, Shah JP, Ganly I. Outcomes in patients with poorly differentiated thyroid carcinoma. J Clin Endocrinol Metab. 2014;99:1245–52.
2. National Cancer Institute. Surveillance, epidemiology, and end results (SEER) program. SEER stat fact sheets: thyroid cancer. Available at: https://seer.cancer.gov/statfacts/html/thyro.html. Accessed 31 July 2018.
3. Chao TC, Lin JD, Chen MF. Insular carcinoma: infrequent subtype of thyroid cancer with aggressive clinical course. World J Surg. 2004;28:393–6. 37.
4. Shaha AR. Management of the neck in thyroid cancer. Otolaryngol Clin N Am. 1998;31:823–31.
5. Shaha AR, Ferlito A, Rinaldo A. Distant metastases from thyroid and parathyroid cancer. ORL J Otorhinolaryngol Relat Spec. 2001;63:243–9.
6. Volante M, Collini P, Nikiforov YE, Sakamoto A, Kakudo K, Katoh R, Lloyd RV, LiVolsi VA, Papotti M, Sobrinho-Simoes M, Bussolati G, Rosai J. Poorly differentiated thyroid carcinoma: the Turin proposal for the use of uniform diagnostic criteria and an algorithmic diagnostic approach. Am J Surg Pathol. 2007;31:1256–64.
7. Dettmer M, Schmitt A, Steinert H, Haldemann A, Meili A, Moch H, Komminoth P, Perren A. Poorly differentiated thyroid carcinomas: how much poorly differentiated is needed? Am J Surg Pathol. 2011;35:1866–72.
8. Gnemmi V, Renaud F, Do Cao C, Salleron J, Lion G, Wemeau JL, et al. Poorly differentiated thyroid carcinomas: application of the Turin proposal provides prognostic results similar to those from the assessment of high-grade features. Histopathology. 2014;64:263–73.
9. Landa I, Ibrahimpasic T, Boucai L, Sinha R, Knauf JA, Shah RH, Dogan S, Ricarte-Filho JC, Krishnamoorthy GP, Xu B, Schultz N, Berger MF, Sander C, Taylor BS, Ghossein R, Ganly I, Fagin JA. Genomic and transcriptomic hallmarks of poorly differentiated and anaplastic thyroid cancers. J Clin Invest. 2016;126:1052–66.
10. Volante M, Rapa I, Gandhi M, Bussolati G, Giachino D, Papotti M, Yuri E. Nikiforov RAS mutations are the predominant molecular alteration in poorly differentiated thyroid carcinomas and bear prognostic impact. J Clin Endocrinol Metab. 2009;94:4735–41.
11. Xu B, Ibrahimpasic T, Wang L, Sabra MM, Migliacci JC, Tuttle RM, Ganly I, Ghossein R. Clinicopathologic features of fatal non-anaplastic follicular cell-derived thyroid carcinomas. Thyroid. 2016;26(11):1588–97.

Assessing Operability in Anaplastic Thyroid Cancer

Case

A 58-year-old female complained of swelling over front of the neck for 30 years (Fig. 1) with rapid increase in size for the last 3 months. It was not associated with weight loss, proximal muscle weakness, palpitations, and hyper defecation. There were no features of any local compression. On examination about 8x8 cm hard fixed thyroid swelling extending from ant border of rt. SCM to and border of left SCM but lower border was reachable. Trachea was not palpable. Bilateral carotids were palpable and there were multiple right level 3 and 4 cervical LN. CECT neck showed large heterogenous thyroid swelling with thyroid cartilage and cricoid cartilage invasion but with maintained fat planes with trachea and CCA with suspicion of lung metastases (Fig. 2). Tru-cut biopsy was suggestive of poorly differentiated/anaplastic/mesenchymal tumor. Operative findings included strap muscles invasion by tumor in center, but grossly free superiorly and inferiorly. Both lobes and isthmus enlarged with part of left lobe and isthmus infiltrating into cricoid, thyroid cartilage, and cricothyroid muscles. Strap muscles were resected with tumor. B/L RLN identified and saved. All parathyroids except right superior were identified and saved. After mobilizing the lateral part of both lobes, tumor could not be dissected free from thyroid and cricoid cartilage and hence part of the tumor left (R2 resection done). Tumor remnant marked all around and in center with radio-opaque Liga clips (Fig. 3). Histopathology was suggestive of anaplastic/mesenchymal tumor. However, on immunohistochemistry the tumor cells show diffuse positivity for CK-7 and Vimentin and focal positivity for S-100.SMA, Desmin, TTF-1; calcitonin is negative in tumor cells. Immunohistochemistry favors diagnosis of Anaplastic carcinoma of thyroid. She was given 5 fractions of EBRT but she succumbed to advance disease within 6 months.

Amit Agarwal is the lead author of this chapter.

A. Agarwal et al., *Case Studies in Thyroid and Parathyroid Tumors*,
https://doi.org/10.1007/978-981-99-0938-4_84

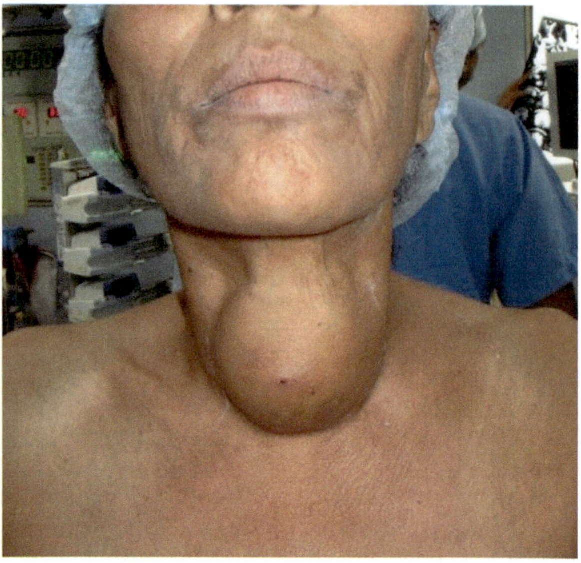

Fig. 1 Clinical pic of the patient with large thyroid mass

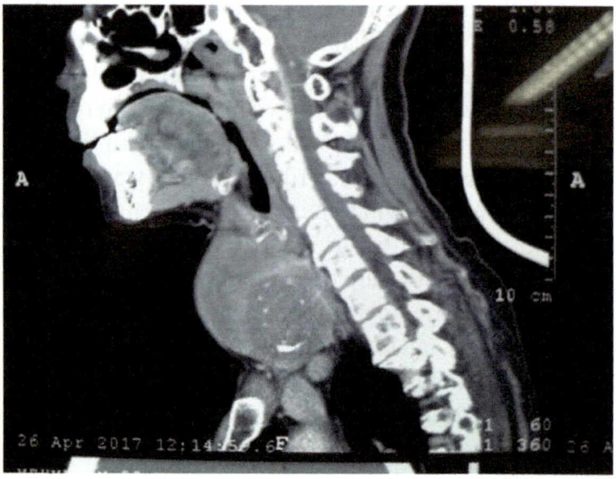

Fig. 2 CECT showing invasion of thyroid cartilage

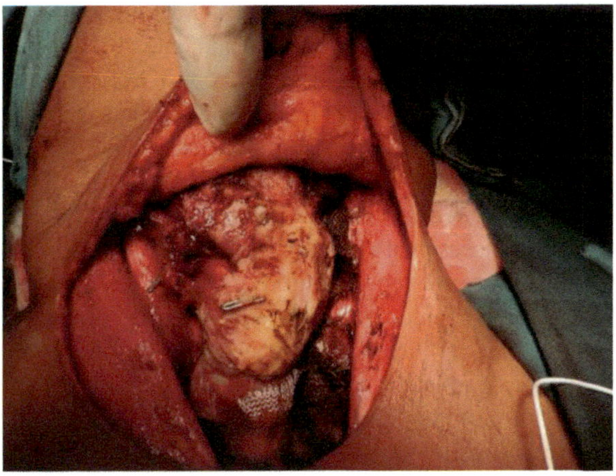

Fig. 3 Intra-operative view showing tumor tissue left behind on thyroid and cricoid cartilage

Discussion

Anaplastic thyroid cancer (ATC) represents one of the most lethal solid organ malignancies, with an overall median survival of 5 months and 1-year survival rate of 20% [1]. Given the poor prognosis, the American Joint Committee on Cancer (AJCC) staging system considers all patients diagnosed with ATC to have stage IV disease [2]. Subcategorization into stages IVA, IVB, and IVC is based on whether the cancer is confined to the thyroid gland, has extrathyroidal extension, or has metastasized to distant sites, respectively. A combined treatment approach of surgery, radiotherapy, and chemotherapy and recently off-label use of TKI may result in improved outcomes for patients with stage IVA and IVB disease [3].

The role of surgery in the treatment of ATC has been controversial. Most clinicians offer surgical resection to ATC patients only if risks and morbidity remain minimal [4]; other investigators have reported prolonged survival in a few selected patients who underwent extensive radical surgery, leading them to recommend en bloc resection of any infiltrated neck structure [5, 6]. Most studies that discuss surgery refer to thyroidectomy only for intrathyroidal ATC and report that extrathyroidal extension represents unresectable disease [7]. Another study [8] presents favorable experience with complete surgical resection of patients with ATC who have extrathyroidal extension but no evidence of metastatic disease. According to this author the patients who are candidates for surgical resection are those without any evidence of distant metastases by preoperative CT or PET scans and whose local disease does not extend lateral to and encase the carotid arteries. In such patients, authors advocate complete excision of the local disease en bloc, including any necessary laryngectomy, tracheal resection, or esophagectomy. Authors arguments in favor of such extensive resections include prolongation of long-term survival in a disease with median survival of only a few months and availability of good options for voice rehabilitation of tracheal esophageal prosthesis or using an electrolarynx to overcome the morbidity of such procedure. The authors recommended that for those patients with superior mediastinal lymphadenopathy that cannot be safely or completely removed through a transcervical approach, a median sternotomy can provide good visualization and access to thoroughly remove all disease and thus concluded that having superior mediastinal spread of disease is not a contraindication to surgical resection and that such patients may also attain long-term survival. Studies have shown that the addition of EBRT to surgery for stage IVB patients showed much greater survival benefit than for stage IVA patients [9].

References

1. Neff RL, Farrar WB, Kloos RT. Anaplastic thyroid cancer. Endocrinol Metab Clin N Am. 2008;37:525–38.
2. American Joint Committee on Cancer staging system. 2014. http://www.cancer.org/cancer/thyroidcancer/detailedguide/thyroid-cancer-staging.
3. Haymart MR, Banerjee M, Yin H, Worden F, Griggs JJ. Marginal treatment benefit in anaplastic thyroid cancer. Cancer. 2013;119:3133–9.
4. Akaishi J, Sugino K, Kitagawa W, et al. Prognostic factors and treatment outcomes of 100 cases of anaplastic thyroid carcinoma. Thyroid. 2011;21:1183–9.
5. Smallridge RC, Ain KB, Asa SL, et al. American Thyroid Association guidelines for management of patients with anaplastic thyroid cancer. Thyroid. 2012;22:1104–39.
6. Sugitani I, Hasegawa Y, Sugasawa M, et al. Super-radical surgery for anaplastic thyroid carcinoma: a large cohort study using the Anaplastic Thyroid Carcinoma Research Consortium of Japan database. Head Neck. 2014;36:328–33.
7. Cobin RH, Gharib H, Bergman DA, et al. AACE/AAES medical/surgical guidelines for clinical practice: management of thyroid carcinoma. Endocr Pract. 2001;7:202–20.
8. Brown RF, Ducic Y. Aggressive surgical resection of anaplastic thyroid carcinoma may provide long-term survival in selected patients. Otolaryngol Head Neck Surg. 2013;148:564–71.
9. Chen J, Tward JD, Shrieve DC, et al. Surgery and radiotherapy improves survival in patients with anaplastic thyroid carcinoma. Am J Clin Oncol. 2008;31:460–4.

Intracranial Metastasis from Follicular Thyroid Carcinoma

Case

A 64-year-old female was referred to our General Surgery clinic with a posterior scalp lump. She had presented to her GP, with a lump in her occipital area of about 3 cm in diameter, which was gradually increasing in size. Due to the unclear etiology, a CT scan was performed (Fig. 1a). This scan showed a large soft tissue mass lesion eroding through the left occipital bone. As it was suspected that this lesion was a metastasis, a CT scan of the chest and abdomen was subsequently performed (Fig. 1b). This showed bilateral thyroid nodules with a dominant solid-cystic nodule occupying most of the left lobe causing mild mass effect and narrowing of the trachea.

The patient was then referred to our Endocrine Surgery clinic. Here, her enlarged thyroid was noticed. A bed-side US scan demonstrated a 4 cm hypo-echoic mixed solid/cystic nodule, which was very vascular. Cytology of this nodule came back as insufficient sample with presence of blood only. Her thyroid profile was within the normal range, her thyroglobulin was >5000 μg/L [3.5–77]. Based on these findings, the most probable diagnosis was thought to be a metastatic follicular thyroid carcinoma (FTC), and the patient was planned for a total thyroidectomy (Fig. 2). The histology report confirmed the presence of a 4.7 cm FTC with signs of lymphovascular invasion.

The patient was subsequently referred to the Neurosurgery Department, for resection of her metastatic lesion. She underwent a left occipital craniotomy and

Rajeev Parameswaran is the lead author of this chapter.

A. Agarwal et al., *Case Studies in Thyroid and Parathyroid Tumors*,
https://doi.org/10.1007/978-981-99-0938-4_85

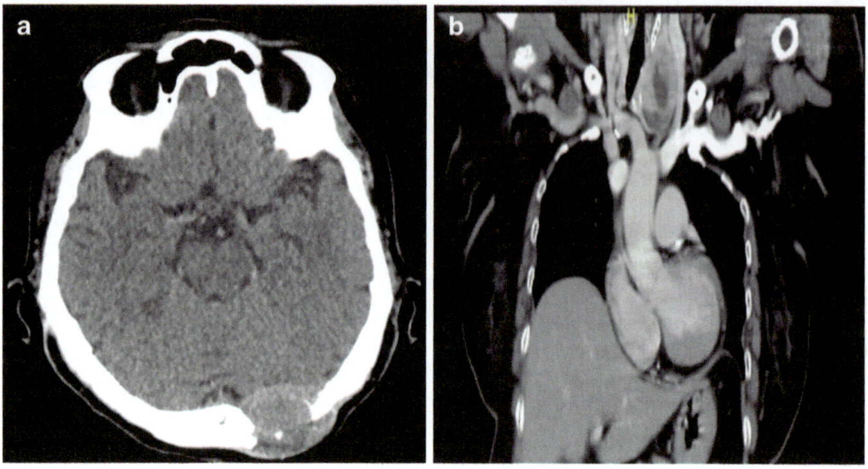

Fig. 1 (**a**, **b**) CT showing the presence of parieto-occipital lesions eroding through the vault and a large heterogeneous lesion in the thyroid

Fig. 2 Excised total thyroidectomy specimen showing the large vascular tumor

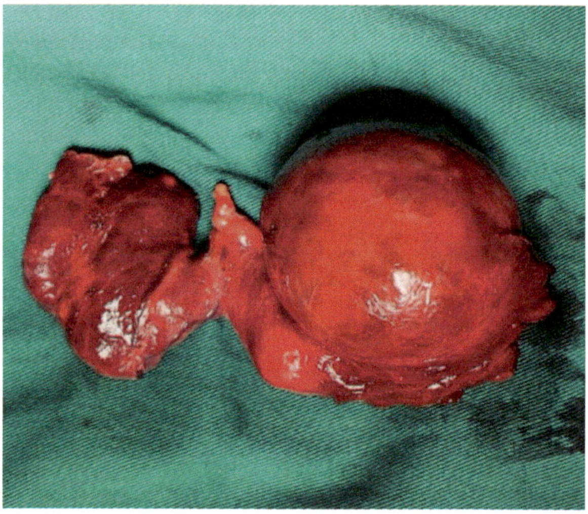

resection of tumor. Peri-operatively, there was a hemorrhagic, highly vascular tumor with indistinct planes, which had eroded through the bone. On histology, this was confirmed to be metastatic carcinoma, consistent with thyroid origin. After recovery from this procedure, she underwent adjuvant radioiodine treatment (200 mCi). Unfortunately, her I131 whole body scan showed both an iodine-avid lytic lesion involving the body of vertebra T9, worrisome for an osseous metastatic deposit, as well as increased radiotracer uptake at the left occipital region, possibly indication residual tumor (Fig. 3). She is currently on a suppressive dose of 175 mcg of levo-thyroxine, awaiting further work-up, and possibly treatment of her lesions.

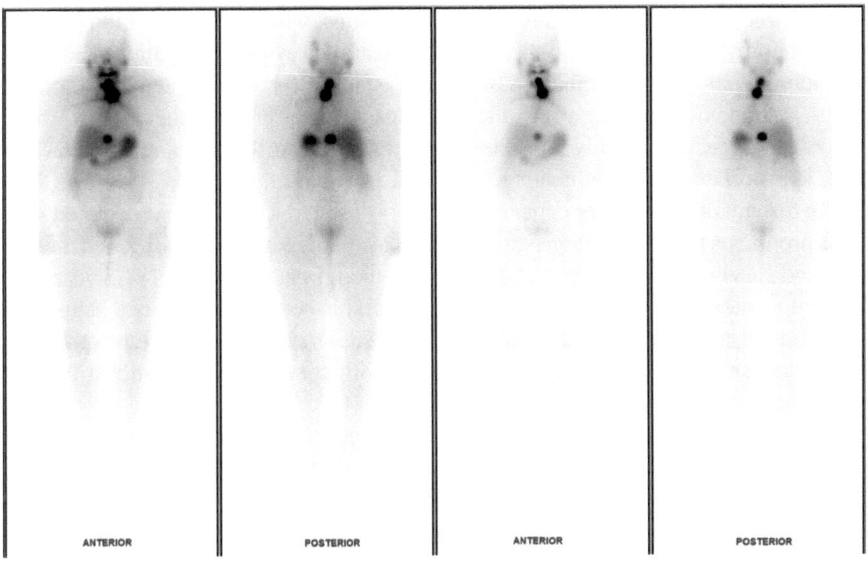

Fig. 3 Whole body scan showing osseous uptake in T9 vertebra along with uptake in the central neck and occiput

Discussion

Follicular thyroid cancer (FTC) is less common than papillary thyroid cancer, and it makes up about 12% all thyroid cancers. FTC metastasizes via hematogenous route, and distant metastasis is not unusual. The most common sites of metastasis are bone and lung, while spread to the liver, bladder, and skin has also been reported [1]. Pooling all differentiated thyroid cancers (DTC), reported incidence of metastasis to the brain is about 1% [2]. Overall, these lesions are located more frequently in the hemispheres, and only very rarely in other regions [3].

Most cranial metastases from FTC are asymptomatic, but there are several cases of patients presenting with symptoms such as headache, visual disturbances, or ocular muscle weakness [3]. Furthermore, due to the high vascularity of metastatic lesions from FTC due to an increase in vascular endothelial growth factor (VEGF) or VEGF receptor expression, these lesions could be perceived as pulsatile [4]. Importantly, cerebral metastasis can also cause acute intra-cranial hemorrhage. It therefore also advised that patients with known thyroid cancer, who present with intra-cranial hemorrhage should be considered as having metastatic disease [5].

The ATA guidelines on differentiated thyroid cancer propose surgical resection or stereotactic radiosurgery for brain metastases from DTC [6]. Generally, surgical resection of all surgically accessible lesions seems to provide the best outcomes, especially for those patients with solitary or oligometastatic metastasis, and for those in whom the lesions are causing significant mass effect. Stereotactic radiosurgery can be considered for those who are too high risk for surgery or if surgery is not possible. For those patients with multiple lesions, whole brain radiation external beam therapy could potentially be used [5]. Treatment with radioiodine can also be considered, although several cases of adverse events after admission of radioiodine, such as sudden hemorrhage into the brain lesion and cerebral edema, have been reported, suggesting to only consider this therapy after resection, and if the lesions have appropriate uptake, which is relatively infrequent [2, 6].

As for any other primary cancer, brain metastases from FTC are associated with poor prognosis [7]. While large series are not available, due to its rarity, the median reported survival from the time of diagnosis is thought to be around 1–1.5 years [2]. Several clinical features, such as age ≤60 years, a better performance status, ≤3 intra-cranial lesions), PS (≤2), number of BM sites), and the absence of other distant metastasis, have shown to be associated with survival [8], but robust data on outcomes for patients with brain metastasis from FTC remain scarce.

There are some features that one may see in metastatic follicular thyroid carcinomas. Metastasis can occur at various time intervals following thyroid cancer surgery and patients with short-term relapse may have a favorable prognosis. Symptoms related to metastasis resolve after therapy and improve the quality of life. Most importantly, longer the interval between primary cancer presentation and onset of cranial or cerebral metastasis, better the survival [9, 10].

References

1. Farina E, Monari F, Tallini G, Repaci A, Mazzarotto R, Giunchi F, et al. Unusual thyroid carcinoma metastases: a case series and literature review. Endocr Pathol. 2016;27(1):55–64.
2. Gomes-Lima CJ, Wu D, Rao SN, Punukollu S, Hritani R, Zeymo A, et al. Brain metastases from differentiated thyroid carcinoma: prevalence, current therapies, and outcomes. J Endocr Soc. 2019;3(2):359–71.
3. Vrachimis A, Schmid KW, Jürgens H, Schober O, Weckesser M, Riemann B. Cerebral metastases from thyroid carcinoma: complete remission following radioiodine treatment. Dtsch Arztebl Int. 2013;110(50):861–6.
4. Bhansali A, Shanmugasundar G, Walia R, Dutta P, Rajwanshi A, Gupta N. Follicular thyroid carcinoma with pulsatile osseous metastases. BMJ Case Rep. 2012;2012:bcr0920103354.
5. McWilliams RR, Giannini C, Hay ID, Atkinson JL, Stafford SL, Buckner JC. Management of brain metastases from thyroid carcinoma: a study of 16 pathologically confirmed cases over 25 years. Cancer. 2003;98(2):356–62.
6. Haugen BR, Alexander EK, Bible KC, Doherty GM, Mandel SJ, Nikiforov YE, et al. 2015 American Thyroid Association Management guidelines for adult patients with thyroid nodules and differentiated thyroid cancer: the American Thyroid Association guidelines task force on thyroid nodules and differentiated thyroid cancer. Thyroid. 2016;26(1):1–133.
7. Wu MH, Lee YY, Lu YL, Lin SF. Risk factors and prognosis for metastatic follicular thyroid cancer. Front Endocrinol (Lausanne). 2022;13:791826.
8. Choi J, Kim JW, Keum YS, Lee IJ. The largest known survival analysis of patients with brain metastasis from thyroid cancer based on prognostic groups. PLoS One. 2016;11(4):e0154739.
9. Fujita T, Ogasawara Y, Doihara H. Solitary cranial metastasis of thyroid carcinoma 13 years after primary surgery: report of a case. Surgery Today (Tokyo, Japan). 2009;39(1):44–7.
10. Parameswaran R, Shulin HJ, Min En N, Tan WB, Yuan NK. Patterns of metastasis in follicular thyroid carcinoma and the difference between early and delayed presentation. Ann R Coll Surg Engl. 2017;99(2):151–4.

Persistent Hypercalcitoninemia

Case

A 45-year-old male presented to the hospital in 2017 with a left thyroid nodule of about 2.5 cm. He had no family history of thyroid disease and endocrinopathies. Thyroid function tests were normal. US scan of the thyroid showed a solid 2.6 cm nodule at the upper pole with mild hypervascularity. Fine needle cytology showed atypia for which the patient underwent a diagnostic hemithyroidectomy. Definitive histology showed medullary thyroid carcinoma. He underwent a completion thyroidectomy which showed no further disease. His postoperative course was uneventful, and his calcitonin at 1 month follow up was 7.6 pg/mL (normal <5 pg/mL). He continued to be well no evidence of any recurrence in the thyroid bed or nodes. His serial calcitonin levels showed a rising trend as shown in Fig. 1.

Rajeev Parameswaran is the lead author of this chapter.

A. Agarwal et al., *Case Studies in Thyroid and Parathyroid Tumors*,
https://doi.org/10.1007/978-981-99-0938-4_86

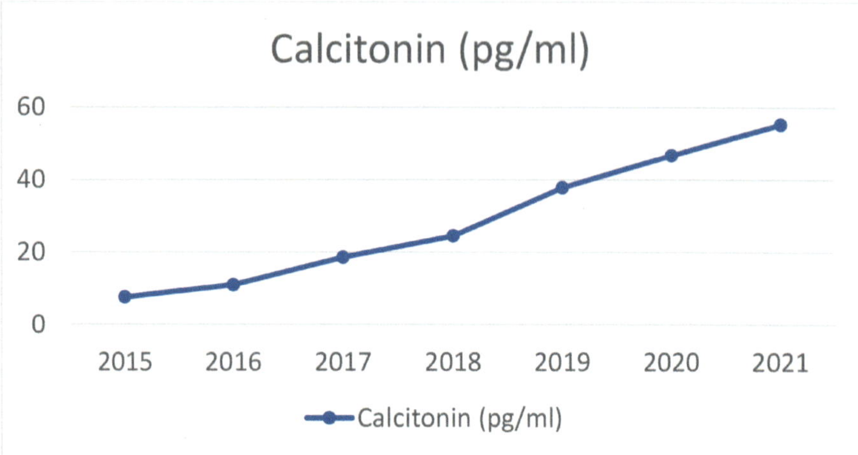

Fig. 1 Showing rising trend in serial calcitonin estimation

Discussion

Medullary thyroid carcinoma (MTC) has a more aggressive behavior than other differentiated thyroid neoplasms, and the presence of residual or recurrent disease after initial surgery is not an unusual finding [1]. MTC is derived from the C cells (calcitonin-producing cells) of the thyroid gland, and about three-quarters is sporadic while one-quarter is associated with the hereditary multiple endocrine neoplasia (MEN) type 2 syndromes. Following total thyroidectomy, it is important to establish cure, by measuring the calcitonin levels, which should be undetectable following complete removal of all thyroid tissue [2, 3]. Calcitonin is a 32–amino acid monomeric peptide which results from cleavage and post-translational processing of procalcitonin, which in turn is a precursor peptide derived from preprocalcitonin [4]. For both patients with sporadic as well as hereditary MTC, determination of serum calcitonin levels is the cornerstone of assessing biochemical remission [5]. The ATA guidelines advise measuring of calcitonin at 3 months postoperatively, and if undetectable or within the normal range, repeat measuring every 6 months for 1 year, and then yearly thereafter [1]. The normalization of calcitonin levels following thyroidectomy is generally associated with a more favorable outcome, [6] although there is some conflicting data on when this normalization should have occurred [7]. Although the ATA guidelines do not differentiate between sporadic and hereditary forms of MTC, others have shown better outcomes (i.e., normal postoperative calcitonin levels and biochemical remission) for patients with CDKN1B mutations and/or polymorphism versus those with sporadic MTCs negative for RET-mutation [8].

Generally, for those patients in whom there is a newly or persistently elevated serum calcitonin following surgery, but this is less than 150 pg/mL, a physical examination and ultrasound scan (US) of the neck are indicated [1], as it has been shown that for a rise in calcitonin until this level, the persistent or recurrent disease is virtually always confined to the neck [9]. If no substrate to cause the elevated levels of calcitonin can be detected, re-measurement of calcitonin (and carcinoembryonic antigen (CEA)) combined with physical examination and US should be conducted every 6 months [1]. For those patients in whom the serum calcitonin levels are beyond 150 pg/mL, more rigorous imaging protocols should be undertaken, as there is an increased chance of the presence of distant disease. This group of patients should thus undergo not only a neck US, but also a chest computed tomography scan (CT), a contrast-enhanced magnetic resonance imaging (MRI) or three-phase contrast-enhanced CT of the liver, and bone scintigraphy and MRI of the pelvis and axial skeleton [1, 10, 11]. Moreover, for those patients with a raised calcitonin above 150 pg/mL but in whom imaging modalities are unable to identify a site of disease recurrence, the use of 18-F-fluorodihydroxyphenylalanine (^{18}F-DOPA) and 18-F-fluorodeoxyglucose (^{18}F-FDG) positron emission tomography/computed tomography (PET/CT) should be considered [12].

The implications of the numeric levels of calcitonin following thyroidectomy have recently been further recognized, [5, 9, 13] and generally it is considered that calcitonin levels of more than 40 pg/mL for those patients who are post-thyroidectomy could already be a sign of nodal metastases. For those patients who already underwent a complete nodal clearance, recurrent nodal disease should be suspected among those in whom levels reach more than 10 pg/mL. Furthermore, among patients following thyroidectomy, distant metastasis was found in half of those in whom serum calcitonin levels exceeded 5000 pg/mL, and were virtually always present when calcitonin was higher than 20,000 pg/mL [5].

However, it is important to realize that calcitonin could be increased for other reasons, not related to MTC [4]. While calcitonin has a high sensitivity for the detection of MTC, it also has a relatively low specificity [14]. It has been shown that calcitonin can be increased in association with several benign conditions, such as chronic renal failure, hyperparathyroidism, autoimmune thyroiditis, as well as with certain other malignancies, such as small cell and large cell lung cancers, prostate cancer, and several neuroendocrine tumors [1]. Thus, when the calcitonin levels are disproportionate to the expected clinical findings, other causes should be evaluated. However, only moderately raised levels of calcitonin are generally seen associated with non-MTC causes, as calcitonin levels >100 pg/mL have a risk of 90–100% for MTC [14].

All patients with persistent or recurrent MTC following thyroidectomy, which is found to be confined to the neck, are considered candidates for repeat neck operations. For this group of patients without signs of distant metastases, the ATA guidelines advise a complete, compartmental dissection of the image-positive or biopsy-positive disease, i.e., a lymph node dissection of the central or lateral neck compartments [1]. There does not seem to be a role for surgical treatment of MTC beyond local disease, while currently available chemotherapy and/or radioiodine therapy regimens have dismal outcomes. Therefore, developing novel treatments aiming at molecular targets must be pursued.

Although compartment-oriented lymph node dissection is the only option for cure, biochemical remission might not be obtained in the majority of these patients who present with serum calcitonin levels above 10 pg/mL [15]. Generally, reoperation is considered indicated if calcitonin levels are elevated in a patients with sporadic MTC who underwent less than a total thyroidectomy or if there is proven locoregional recurrence or lymph node metastases. Additionally, for those patients with hereditary MTC, the presence of any thyroid remnant – even without elevated calcitonin levels – is considered an indication for repeat surgery. Importantly, it has been shown that patients undergoing repeat surgery for recurrent or persistent MTC have more unfavorable disease associated with diminished long-term outcomes [16]. In view of patients' quality of life, the degree of surgery necessary to obtain biochemical cure and tumor control should thus be weighed against the increased risks of post-operative complications associated with repeat surgery, specifically recurrent laryngeal nerve palsy and long-term hypoparathyroidism [16, 17].

References

1. Wells SA, Asa SL, Dralle H, Elisei R, Evans DB, Gagel RF, et al. Revised American thyroid association guidelines for the management of medullary thyroid carcinoma. Thyroid. 2015;25(6):567–610.
2. Engelbach M, Görges R, Forst T, Pfützner A, Dawood R, Heerdt S, et al. Improved diagnostic methods in the follow-up of medullary thyroid carcinoma by highly specific calcitonin measurements. J Clin Endocrinol Metab. 2000;85(5):1890–4.
3. Dottorini ME, Assi A, Sironi M, Sangalli G, Spreafico G, Colombo L. Multivariate analysis of patients with medullary thyroid carcinoma. Prognostic significance and impact on treatment of clinical and pathologic variables. Cancer. 1996;77(8):1556–65.
4. Becker KL, Nylén ES, White JC, Müller B, Snider RH. Clinical review 167: Procalcitonin and the calcitonin gene family of peptides in inflammation, infection, and sepsis: a journey from calcitonin back to its precursors. J Clin Endocrinol Metab. 2004;89(4):1512–25.
5. Machens A, Schneyer U, Holzhausen H-Jr, Dralle H. Prospects of remission in medullary thyroid carcinoma according to basal calcitonin level. J Clin Endocrinol Metabol. 2005;90(4):2029–34.
6. Modigliani E, Cohen R, Campos JM, Conte-Devolx B, Maes B, Boneu A, et al. Prognostic factors for survival and for biochemical cure in medullary thyroid carcinoma: results in 899 patients. The GETC Study Group. Groupe d'étude des tumeurs à calcitonine. Clin Endocrinol (Oxf). 1998;48(3):265–73.
7. Ismailov SI, Piulatova NR. Postoperative calcitonin study in medullary thyroid carcinoma. Endocr Relat Cancer. 2004;11(2):357–63.
8. Accardo G, Conzo G, Esposito D, Gambardella C, Mazzella M, Castaldo F, et al. Genetics of medullary thyroid cancer: an overview. Int J Surg. 2017;41(Suppl 1):S2–6.
9. Pellegriti G, Leboulleux S, Baudin E, Bellon N, Scollo C, Travagli JP, et al. Long-term outcome of medullary thyroid carcinoma in patients with normal postoperative medical imaging. Br J Cancer. 2003;88(10):1537–42.
10. Giraudet AL, Vanel D, Leboulleux S, Aupérin A, Dromain C, Chami L, et al. Imaging medullary thyroid carcinoma with persistent elevated calcitonin levels. J Clin Endocrinol Metab. 2007;92(11):4185–90.
11. Delorme S, Raue F. Medullary thyroid carcinoma: imaging. Recent Results Cancer Res. 2015;204:91–116.

12. Romero-Lluch AR, Cuenca-Cuenca JI, Guerrero-Vázquez R, Martínez-Ortega AJ, Tirado-Hospital JL, Borrego-Dorado I, et al. Diagnostic utility of PET/CT with. Eur J Nucl Med Mol Imaging. 2017;44(12):2004–13.
13. Machens A, Lorenz K, Dralle H. Prediction of biochemical cure in patients with medullary thyroid cancer. Br J Surg. 2020;107(6):695–704.
14. Toledo SP, Lourenço DM, Santos MA, Tavares MR, Toledo RA, Correia-Deur JE. Hypercalcitoninemia is not pathognomonic of medullary thyroid carcinoma. Clinics (Sao Paulo). 2009;64(7):699–706.
15. Rowland KJ, Jin LX, Moley JF. Biochemical cure after reoperations for medullary thyroid carcinoma: a meta-analysis. Ann Surg Oncol. 2015;22(1):96–102.
16. Machens A, Dralle H. Benefit-risk balance of reoperation for persistent medullary thyroid cancer. Ann Surg. 2013;257(4):751–7.
17. Jin S, Sugitani I. Narrative review of management of thyroid surgery complications. Gland Surg. 2021;10(3):1135–46.

Lymphoma of the Thyroid

Case
A 68-year-old male presented with a rapidly enlarging neck mass with pressure symptoms that included dysphonia, dysphagia, and Horner's syndrome (as shown in Fig. 1a). Clinical examination revealed a large thyroid mass with no associated lymphadenopathy. Serum biochemistry revealed subclinical hypothyroidism (TSH-15 mIU/L) and normal thyroid autoantibodies. Fine needle cytology showed the presence of mononuclear and atypical cells. Ultrasound and CT neck showed a large thyroid mass as shown in Fig. 1b. Core biopsy performed showed the presence of DLBCL and Ann Arbor Stage was IIE. He was commenced on (R–CHOP; rituximab, cyclophosphamide, doxorubicin, vincristine, and prednisolone) regime followed by adjuvant EBRT. His thyroid mass subsided following combined chemoradiotherapy. The patient continues to be disease free with no palpable neck mass and no signs of HS at 1 year.

Rajeev Parameswaran is the lead author of this chapter.

A. Agarwal et al., *Case Studies in Thyroid and Parathyroid Tumors*,
https://doi.org/10.1007/978-981-99-0938-4_87

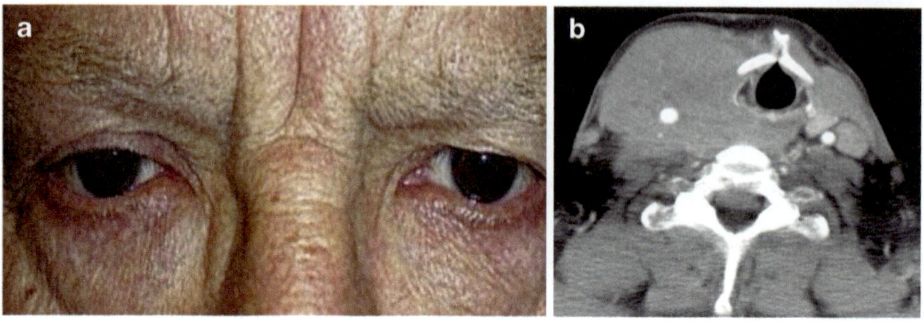

Fig. 1 (**a**, **b**) Patient with Horner's syndrome and CT showing the presence of the large thyroid mass

Discussion

Primary thyroid lymphomas (PTL) are rare malignancies seen in the thyroid gland, accounting for about 2% of all extranodal lymphomas and about 5% of all thyroid neoplasms. These neoplasms usually arise on a background of longstanding Hashimoto's thyroiditis (HT) [1], with a risk being about 40–80 times higher than general population [2, 3]. The transformation from thyroiditis to lymphoma only occurs in a very small proportion of patients [2], probably due to chronic antigenic stimulation of lymphocytes [4]. It is believed that primary thyroid lymphomas arise from mucosa-associated lymphoma tissue (MALT) [5] and hence the initial description of these lesions as MALT lymphomas [6]. However, these lesions are now included under the entity "marginal zone B-cell lymphoma of MALT-type" (MZBL) as proposed by the WHO Classification for Neoplastic Diseases of the Lymphoid Tissues [7] and Revised European-American Classification of Lymphoid Neoplasms (REAL) [8]. Currently, primary thyroid lymphomas are classified into 2 broad categories: extranodal marginal zone B-cell lymphoma (EMZBCL) and diffuse large B-cell lymphoma (DLBCL).

Diffuse B cell lymphoma accounts for over 50% of cases of PTL, followed by EMZBCL lymphomas in nearly quarter of case, followed by rarer types such as follicular lymphoma, Hodgkin's lymphoma, T-cell type, etc. [9, 10]. DLBCL behaves in a more aggressive manner in comparison to the indolent behavior of EMZBCL or follicular types. Most commonly patients present with an enlarging neck mass of a short duration and patients experience a range of compressive symptoms such as dysphagia, dyspnea, or hoarseness [11, 12]. Other presentations include Horner's syndrome [13], pain over the thyroid gland [10, 14], and B-symptoms such as fever, night sweats [14]. Clinical examination usually reveals a hard thyroid mass and about a third of patients may have a history of hypothyroidism secondary to Hashimoto's thyroiditis [10, 11].

Investigations include ultrasound scan of the thyroid, fine needle aspiration cytology, core biopsy or excision biopsy, and staging CT scan. Ultrasound scan may show features based on the nature of presentation such as nodular or diffuse

Table 1 Ann Arbor staging of lymphoma

Stage	Location of disease
I E	No disease seen
II E	Regional lymph nodes
III E	Disease on both sides of the diaphragm
IV E	Systemic disease

enlargement [15]. Though fine needle cytology can help diagnose lymphoma in about 80–100% of cases, problem is that of high rate of false negatives [16], especially in a background of lymphocytic infiltration commonly associated with HT. When FNA is performed without immunotyping or immunohistochemistry, the diagnosis can be difficult, especially MZBL [11, 17]. The alternative therefore would be to perform a core biopsy or open biopsy, especially to distinguish thyroiditis from low-grade marginal zone lymphoma and diagnose aggressive variants. Open biopsies especially are useful in examining tissue for detailed histology, immunostaining, and evaluating any genetic rearrangements [16]. Stage of disease is evaluated with a CT scan of the head, neck, chest, abdomen, and pelvis and staging done using the Ann Arbor staging [18] (Table 1).

The treatment of PTL is primarily radiotherapy (RT) or combined multimodal therapy (CMT) with no or limited role for surgery [19]. RT is more effective for MZBL than DLBCL especially in localized disease using doses ranging from 30–50 Gy [20, 21]. Reported 5-year cause-specific survival rates are around 80 to 100% for MZBL compared to 55% to DLBCL [22, 23]. In patients with aggressive or disseminated disease usually associated with DLBCL disease, CMT is usually required [24, 25]. The common agents used for multimodal therapy are cyclophosphamide, vincristine & prednisolone (CVP), cyclophosphamide, doxorubicin, vincristine, and prednisolone (CHOP) and more recently include rituximab, an anti-CD20 monoclonal antibody (R-CHOP) [17, 25, 26]. CMT was associated with improved survival rates and decreased relapse rates [27, 28]. Factors associated with poor prognosis include increasing age and stage, DLBCL type, large size, rapid progression, mediastinal disease, and presence of B-symptoms [9, 16, 29].

References

1. Pedersen RK, Pedersen NT. Primary non-Hodgkin's lymphoma of the thyroid gland: a population based study. Histopathology. 1996;28(1):25–32.
2. Holm LE, Blomgren H, Löwhagen T. Cancer risks in patients with chronic lymphocytic thyroiditis. N Engl J Med. 1985;312(10):601–4.
3. Abbasgholizadeh P, Naseri A, Nasiri E, Sadra V. Is Hashimoto thyroiditis associated with increasing risk of thyroid malignancies? A systematic review and meta-analysis. Thyroid Res. 2021;14(1):26.
4. Kossev P, Livolsi V. Lymphoid lesions of the thyroid: review in light of the revised European-American lymphoma classification and upcoming World Health Organization classification. Thyroid. 1999;9(12):1273–80.

5. Isaacson P, Wright DH. Malignant lymphoma of mucosa-associated lymphoid tissue. A distinctive type of B-cell lymphoma. Cancer. 1983;52(8):1410–6.
6. Isaacson PG. Lymphoma of the thyroid gland. Curr Top Pathol. 1997;91:1–14.
7. Swerdlow SH, Campo E, Harris NL, Jaffe ES, Pileri SA, Stein H, et al. WHO classification of tumours of haematopoietic and lymphoid tissues. Lyon: International Agency for Research on Cancer; 2008.
8. Sander CA, Flaig MJ, Kaudewitz P, Jaffe ES. The revised European-American classification of lymphoid neoplasms (REAL): a preferred approach for the classification of cutaneous lymphomas. Am J Dermatopathol. 1999;21(3):274–8.
9. Graff-Baker A, Roman SA, Thomas DC, Udelsman R, Sosa JA. Prognosis of primary thyroid lymphoma: demographic, clinical, and pathologic predictors of survival in 1,408 cases. Surgery. 2009;146(6):1105–15.
10. Watanabe N, Noh JY, Narimatsu H, Takeuchi K, Yamaguchi T, Kameyama K, et al. Clinicopathological features of 171 cases of primary thyroid lymphoma: a long-term study involving 24553 patients with Hashimoto's disease. Br J Haematol. 2011;153(2):236–43.
11. Sarinah B, Hisham A-N. Primary lymphoma of the Thyroid: diagnostic and therapeutic considerations. Asian J Surg. 2010;33(1):20–4.
12. Sitges-Serra A. The rapidly growing thyroid mass. Br J Surg. 2006;93(6):647–9.
13. Donaldson JF, Rodriguez-Gomez IA, Parameswaran R. Rapidly enlarging neck masses of the thyroid with Horner's syndrome: a concise clinical review. Surgeon. 2014;13(2):110–5.
14. Alzouebi M, Goepel JR, Horsman JM, Hancock BW. Primary thyroid lymphoma: the 40 year experience of a UK lymphoma treatment centre. Int J Oncol. 2012;40(6):2075–80.
15. Ota H, Ito Y, Matsuzuka F, Kuma S, Fukata S, Morita S, et al. Usefulness of ultrasonography for diagnosis of malignant lymphoma of the thyroid. Thyroid. 2006;16(10):983–7.
16. Stein SA, Wartofsky L. Primary Thyroid lymphoma: a clinical review. J Clin Endocrinol Metab. 2013;98(8):3131–8.
17. Matsuzuka F, Miyauchi A, Katayama S, Narabayashi I, Ikeda H, Kuma K, et al. Clinical aspects of primary thyroid lymphoma: diagnosis and treatment based on our experience of 119 cases. Thyroid. 1993;3(2):93–9.
18. Carbone PP, Kaplan HS, Musshoff K, Smithers DW, Tubiana M. Report of the committee on Hodgkin's disease staging classification. Cancer Res. 1971;31(11):1860–1.
19. Klyachkin ML, Schwartz RW, Cibull M, Munn RK, Regine WF, Kenady DE, et al. Thyroid lymphoma: is there a role for surgery? Am Surg. 1998;64(3):234–8.
20. Harrington KJ, Michalaki VJ, Vini L, Nutting CM, Syrigos KN, A'Hern R, et al. Management of non-Hodgkin's lymphoma of the thyroid: the Royal Marsden Hospital experience. Br J Radiol. 2005;78(929):405–10.
21. Blair TJ, Evans RG, Buskirk SJ, Banks PM, Earle JD. Radiotherapeutic management of primary thyroid lymphoma. Int J Radiat Oncol Biol Phys. 1985;11(2):365–70.
22. Laing RW, Hoskin P, Hudson BV, Hudson GV, Harmer C, Bennett MH, et al. The significance of MALT histology in thyroid lymphoma: a review of patients from the BNLI and Royal Marsden Hospital. Clin Oncol (R Coll Radiol). 1994;6(5):300–4.
23. Tsang RW, Gospodarowicz MK, Pintilie M, Wells W, Hodgson DC, Sun A, et al. Localized mucosa-associated lymphoid tissue lymphoma treated with radiation therapy has excellent clinical outcome. J Clin Oncol. 2003;21(22):4157–64.
24. Vigliotti A, Kong JS, Fuller LM, Velasquez WS. Thyroid lymphomas stages IE and IIE: comparative results for radiotherapy only, combination chemotherapy only, and multimodality treatment. Int J Radiat Oncol Biol Phys. 1986;12(10):1807–12.
25. Miller TP, Dahlberg S, Cassady JR, Adelstein DJ, Spier CM, Grogan TM, et al. Chemotherapy alone compared with chemotherapy plus radiotherapy for localized intermediate- and high-grade non-Hodgkin's lymphoma. N Engl J Med. 1998;339(1):21–6.
26. Portlock CS, Rosenberg SA. Combination chemotherapy with cyclophosphamide, vincristine, and prednisone in advanced non-Hodgkin's lymphomas. Cancer. 1976;37(3):1275–82.

27. Doria R, Jekel JF, Cooper DL. Thyroid lymphoma. The case for combined modality therapy. Cancer. 1994;73(1):200–6.
28. Ha CS, Shadle KM, Medeiros LJ, Wilder RB, Hess MA, Cabanillas F, et al. Localized non-Hodgkin lymphoma involving the thyroid gland. Cancer. 2001;91(4):629–35.
29. Onal C, Li YX, Miller RC, Poortmans P, Constantinou N, Weber DC, et al. Treatment results and prognostic factors in primary thyroid lymphoma patients: a rare cancer network study. Ann Oncol. 2011;22(1):156–64.

Micro Papillary Thyroid Cancer

Case

A 49-year-old male was referred to the endocrine surgery with an enlarged thyroid gland and neck nodes (Fig. 1a, b). He was found to be euthyroid as his thyroid profile was within the normal range (free T4: 11.9 pmol/L [8.0–16.0]; TSH: 1.00 mIU/L [0.45–4.50]). Ultrasound showed a small subcentrimetric (8 mm) and underwent a thyroid ultrasound-guided biopsy of the nodule and lymph nodes, which showed the presence of papillary thyroid carcinoma.

The patient was counseled for surgical treatment, in the form of a total thyroidectomy and right lateral neck dissection. His surgery was uneventful. Histology

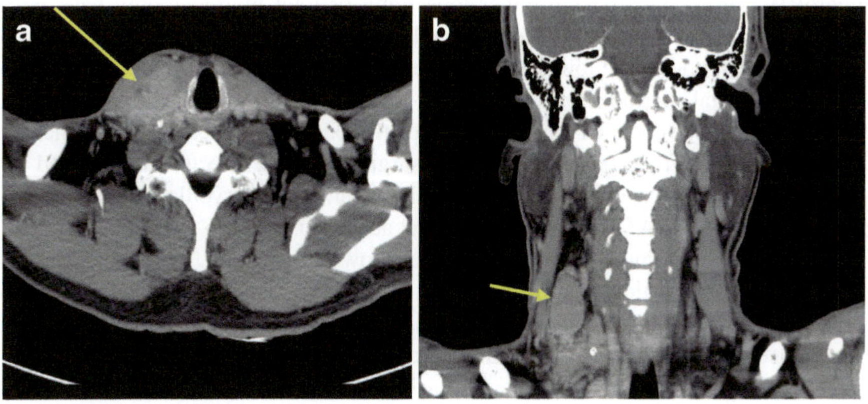

Fig. 1 CECT showing subcentrimetric nodule in thyroid along with large lateral LN. (**a**) CECT Neck showing enlarged thyroid gland with a nodule (yellow arrow). (**b**) CECT Neck of same patient showing enlarged Right level 4 lymph node (yellow arrow)

Rajeev Parameswaran is the lead author of this chapter.

A. Agarwal et al., *Case Studies in Thyroid and Parathyroid Tumors*,
https://doi.org/10.1007/978-981-99-0938-4_88

report showed papillary micro-carcinoma, size 0.7 cm, involving the right lobe with five of 15 lymph nodes with metastatic carcinoma (5/15) and the largest focus of cancer about 5 cm in size.

During his post-operative clinic visit, he was doing well and had no issues regarding scar or voice. His adjusted calcium measured 2.32 mmol/L, with a PTH of 5.4 pmol/L. He was kept on a suppressive dose of levothyroxine, and as his microPTC was considered of the ATA intermediate risk category, he remains under follow-up from our endocrinology team with serial blood tests (including thyroglobulin) and US.

Discussion

Papillary thyroid microcarcinoma (microPTC) is defined as a PTC with a maximum diameter of 10 mm, [1] and it generally has an excellent prognosis. Overall, following surgery for microPTC, disease-specific mortality rates are reportedly <1%, with low loco-regional (i.e., 2–6%) and distant recurrence rates (i.e., 1–2%) [2, 3].

The incidence of microPTC has increased significantly during the last decades, and it is currently estimated that almost 40% of all thyroid cancers are microPTC [4]. Most microPTCs are detected incidentally, either on imaging, or following surgery for benign conditions [5, 6]. The optimal management for microPTCs remains controversial, which has led to a heterogenous treatment paradigm.

Surgical treatment, by removal of (part of) the thyroid gland, has been the traditional cornerstone for the treatment of patients with PTC, and thus also for those with microPTC, protocols advising either lobectomy or total thyroidectomy have been described [7, 8]. Although there are currently no robust studies comparing these two surgical interventions, the low mortality rate for microPTC would suggest the performance of a total thyroidectomy to be over-treatment in the vast majority of cases. Other arguments to consider when deciding on the extent of surgical treatment include the risk of thyroid recurrence, monitoring, surgical adverse effects, and the need for thyroid hormone replacement therapy [9]. Moreover, active surveillance is also a recognized option. The ATA guidelines state that active surveillance 'can be considered' as an alternative to immediate surgery in very-low-risk patients [2]. This strategy is based on the observation that most low-risk microPTCs remain small; and that even among those patients who did undergo surgery none showed any life-threatening recurrence or distant metastasis, and none died of their thyroid carcinoma [7]. This strategy does come with the additional task of minimizing patients' psychological stress when they are diagnosed with microPTC, which is not removed, but which does require active surveillance by undergoing annual US. This could also in part be why the ATA guidelines would not even recommend a biopsy for lesions ≤10 mm without sonographic or clinical signs of potentially high-risk behavior (e.g., extrathyroidal extension on US or voice change) [2]. As alternative treatment strategies, some authors have explored other options, such as US-guided percutaneous ethanol ablation (UPEA) or percutaneous laser ablation (PLA), but larger outcome data on these treatment options is necessary before general recommendations could be made [9].

Regarding the absence of the necessity of adjuvant radioiodine (RAI) for this group of patients (tumor maximum diameter of ≤10 mm confined to the thyroid), there does seem to be consensus [10]. While the need for TSH suppression remains more undecided [11], the ATA guidelines advise against TSH suppression and propose the serum TSH to be kept within the low-normal range (i.e., 0.5–2 mIU/L), for the subgroup with a low risk of recurrence, and without previous RAI [2].

While microPTCs usually have an indolent course, there is a small proportion exhibiting aggressive behavior, associated with disease recurrence. Several high-risk features include extra-thyroidal extension, presence of lymph node metastasis, proximity to either trachea or to recurrent laryngeal nerves, or high-grade features on cytology [12]. Additionally, the is uncertainty regarding a possible different prognosis for preoperatively versus incidentally diagnosed microPTCs [13]. Specifically, there is some suggestion of differences in baseline characteristics, behavior, and outcomes between these two groups, as a meta-analysis comparing outcomes of incidental versus non-incidental microPTC, reported the former to have much lower recurrence rates [14]. Non-incidental microPTC can either be found on imaging, or can be in the form of a palpable thyroid nodule or even lymph node metastasis. Overall, among patients with microPTC, lymph node (LN) metastasis is seen in 2–45% [15–18]. While it seems that patients with a non-incidental microPTC tend to undergo more aggressive treatment (e.g., more extended resection, adjuvant RAI, and TSH suppression), they seem to remain at a higher risk of disease recurrence [14]. Although exact reasons for this remain unclear, this finding does show the clinical importance of microPTCs.

Although various factors remain unknown, patients who present with a microPTC (either prior to or after surgery) should be offered an individualized treatment plan based on the biology of their tumor, and equally on the patient's context and values. In this setting, shared decision-making is imperative [9]. Moreover, it has recently been shown that specific molecular profiles could be utilized as markers for the prediction of more aggressive biological behavior of microPTC, such as the co-existence of BRAF with other oncogenic mutations (e.g., PIK3CA, AKT1), TERT-promoter, or TP53 mutations [2]. And future studies into establishing the impact of molecular profiling and genetic alterations on the clinical management of patients with microPTCs are to be expected.

References

1. DeLellis RA. Pathology and genetics of tumours of endocrine organs. Lyon: IARC; 2004.
2. Haugen BR, Alexander EK, Bible KC, Doherty GM, Mandel SJ, Nikiforov YE, et al. 2015 American Thyroid Association management guidelines for adult patients with thyroid nodules and differentiated thyroid cancer: the American Thyroid Association guidelines task force on thyroid nodules and differentiated thyroid cancer. Thyroid. 2016;26(1):1–133.
3. Cecoli F, Ceresola EM, Altrinetti V, Cabria M, Cappagli M, Montepagani A, et al. Therapeutic strategies and clinical outcome in papillary thyroid microcarcinoma: a multicenter observational study. Eur Thyroid J. 2016;5(3):180–6.
4. Lim H, Devesa SS, Sosa JA, Check D, Kitahara CM. Trends in thyroid cancer incidence and mortality in the United States, 1974-2013. JAMA. 2017;317(13):1338–48.

5. Miccoli P, Minuto M, Galleri D, Dagostino J, Basolo F, Antonangeli L, et al. Incidental thyroid carcinoma in a large series of consecutive patients operated on for benign thyroid disease. ANZ J Surg. 2006;76(3):123–6.
6. Ito Y, Higashiyama T, Takamura Y, Miya A, Kobayashi K, Matsuzuka F, et al. Prognosis of patients with benign thyroid diseases accompanied by incidental papillary carcinoma undetectable on preoperative imaging tests. World J Surg. 2007;31(8):1672–6.
7. Miyauchi A, Ito Y, Oda H. Insights into the Management of Papillary microcarcinoma of the thyroid. Thyroid. 2018;28(1):23–31.
8. Liu Z, Huang T. Papillary thyroid microcarcinoma: an over-treated malignancy? World J Surg. 2016;40(3):764–5.
9. Brito JP, Hay ID. Management of papillary thyroid microcarcinoma. Endocrinol Metab Clin N Am. 2019;48(1):199–213.
10. Lamartina L, Durante C, Filetti S, Cooper DS. Low-risk differentiated thyroid cancer and radioiodine remnant ablation: a systematic review of the literature. J Clin Endocrinol Metab. 2015;100(5):1748–61.
11. Sugitani I, Fujimoto Y, Yamada K. Association between serum thyrotropin concentration and growth of asymptomatic papillary thyroid microcarcinoma. World J Surg. 2014;38(3):673–8.
12. Walgama E, Sacks WL, Ho AS. Papillary thyroid microcarcinoma: optimal management versus overtreatment. Curr Opin Oncol. 2020;32(1):1–6.
13. Haymart MR, Cayo M, Chen H. Papillary thyroid microcarcinomas: big decisions for a small tumor. Ann Surg Oncol. 2009;16(11):3132–9.
14. Mehanna H, Al-Maqbili T, Carter B, Martin E, Campain N, Watkinson J, et al. Differences in the recurrence and mortality outcomes rates of incidental and nonincidental papillary thyroid microcarcinoma: a systematic review and meta-analysis of 21 329 person-years of follow-up. J Clin Endocrinol Metab. 2014;99(8):2834–43.
15. Noguchi S, Yamashita H, Murakami N, Nakayama I, Toda M, Kawamoto H. Small carcinomas of the thyroid: a long-term follow-up of 867 patients. Arch Surg. 1996;131(2):187–91.
16. Pelizzo MR, Boschin IM, Toniato A, Pagetta C, Piotto A, Bernante P, et al. Natural history, diagnosis, treatment and outcome of papillary thyroid microcarcinoma (PTMC): a mono-institutional 12-year experience. Nucl Med Commun. 2004;25(6):547–52.
17. Kwak JY, Kim EK, Kim MJ, Son EJ, Chung WY, Park CS, et al. Papillary microcarcinoma of the thyroid: predicting factors of lateral neck node metastasis. Ann Surg Oncol. 2009;16(5):1348–55.
18. Ito Y, Tomoda C, Uruno T, Takamura Y, Miya A, Kobayashi K, et al. Papillary microcarcinoma of the thyroid: how should it be treated? World J Surg. 2004;28(11):1115–21.

Part VIII

Case Snippets

Retrosternal Dermoid

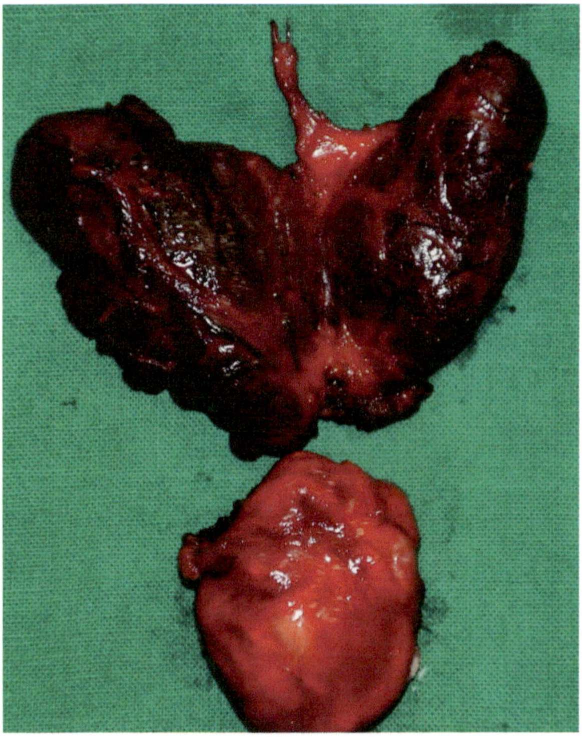

Retrosternal dermoid

Ranil Fernando is the lead author of this chapter.

A. Agarwal et al., *Case Studies in Thyroid and Parathyroid Tumors*,
https://doi.org/10.1007/978-981-99-0938-4_89

Case

A 60-year-old female presented with multinodular (MNG) goiter of 10 years duration with compressive symptom. She was assessed to have a euthyroid Grade 2 MNG.

At surgery a MNG and a retrosternal dermoid cyst (confirmed histologically) was found and removed. The dermoid cyst may have contributed to the compressive features. This is again an uncommon cause of compression.

Ancient Treatment Practices for Goiter

Case

Two cases of multinodular goiters are presented here to demonstrate the ancient practices of managing goiter. The first case was a 62-year-old lady who presented with a large multinodular goiter of 40 years duration, showing tattoo marks on the goiter which were made to beautify the goiter as an ancient practice to remove stigma from the goiter (Fig. 1). The second case was a 40-year-old male who also presented with a multinodular goiter of 20 years duration showing scalding marks on the skin of the goiter (Fig. 2). On questioning it was revealed that the marks were made with hot iron instrument to burn the skin and to drain the blood to decrease the size of goiter. These two cases demonstrate that in far flung interior areas of the country, ancient practices of managing goiter were still prevalent.

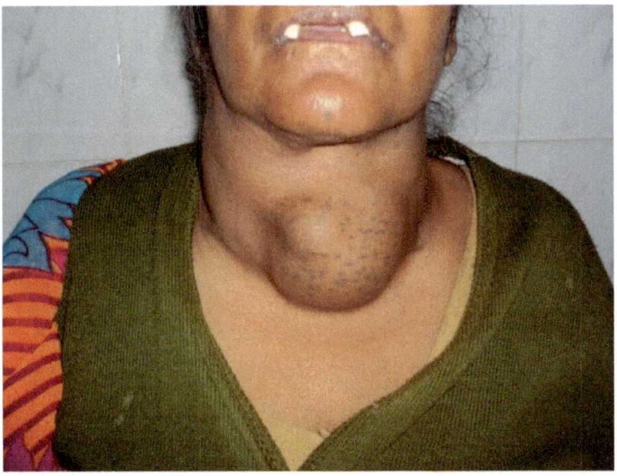

Fig. 1 Permanent tattooing of the goiter

Amit Agarwal is the lead author of this chapter.

A. Agarwal et al., *Case Studies in Thyroid and Parathyroid Tumors*,
https://doi.org/10.1007/978-981-99-0938-4_90

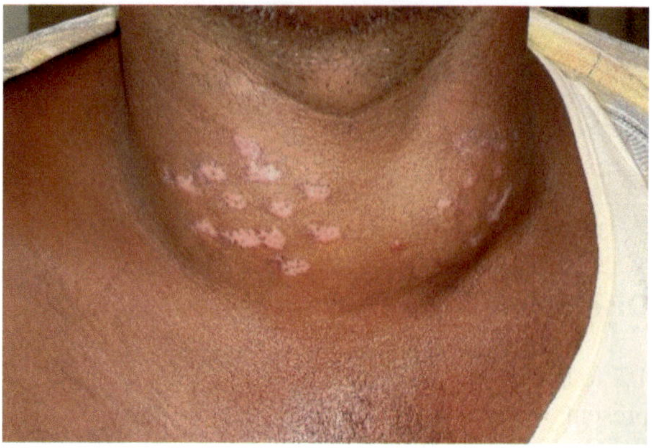

Fig. 2 Scalding marks on the skin over the goiter

GPSR Compliance

The European Union's (EU) General Product Safety Regulation (GPSR) is a set of rules that requires consumer products to be safe and our obligations to ensure this.

If you have any concerns about our products, you can contact us on ProductSafety@springernature.com

In case Publisher is established outside the EU, the EU authorized representative is:

Springer Nature Customer Service Center GmbH
Europaplatz 3
69115 Heidelberg, Germany

Batch number: 10166008

Printed by Printforce, the Netherlands